Massage Therapy Career Guide
For Hands-On Success
Second Edition

Massage Therapy Career Guide

For Hands-On Success

Second Edition

by Steve Capellini

THOMSON ™

DELMAR LEARNING

Australia Canada Mexico Singapore Spain United Kingdom United States

THOMSON

DELMAR LEARNING ™

Massage Therapy Career Guide for Hands-On Success, Second Edition
by Steve Capellini

Vice President, Health Care Business Unit:
William Brottmiller

Editorial Director:
Matthew Kane

Acquisitions Editor:
Kalen Conerly

Product Manager:
Juliet Steiner

Editorial Assistant:
Molly Belmont

Marketing Director:
Jennifer McAvey

Marketing Coordinator:
Christopher Manion

Production Director:
Carolyn Miller

Production Manager:
Barbara A. Bullock

Production Editor:
John Mickelbank

Library of Congress Cataloging-in-Publication Data

Capellini, Steve.
  Massage therapy career guide for hands-on success / by Steve Capellini.—2nd ed.
    p. cm.
  Includes index.
  ISBN 1-4180-1051-0 /
     978-1-4180-1051-5
  1. Massage therapy—Vocational guidance. 2. Massage therapy—Practice. I. Title.
  RM722.C37 2006
  615.8'22023—dc22
                              2005033977

NOTICE TO THE READER

Dedication

For my wife, Atchana, who has helped turn my dreams into reality.

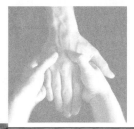

Contents

Acknowledgments / **xi**
About the Author / **xiii**

Introduction / 1

A Meaningful Career Choice / **1**
My Transition from Amateur to Professional / **3**
What You Will Learn / **5**
Using This Book—Now and Later / **8**

Chapter One

Massage Therapy: A Career Without Limits / 9

The Development of Massage in the United States / **10**
Current Growth Rate in the Field / **12**
The Aging Baby Boom Generation Creates a Demand for Massage / **13**
The Mainstreaming of "Alternative" Therapies / **15**
Dozens of Directions for Postgraduate Study / **17**
A Wealth of Opportunities / **17**

Chapter Two

Is There a Healer Hidden Inside You? / 19

The Psychology of Touch / **21**
The Spirituality of Touch / **24**
Realistic Expectations / **26**
Overcoming Sexual Issues / **35**

Chapter Three

Choosing a Massage School: Making the Best Decision / 41

Massage-School Hunting / 42

Developing Your Skills: Massage Schools and Training Programs / 43

Setting Educational Goals / 48

The Learning Trap Versus the Earning Trap / 51

Faculty Versus Facility / 52

Standards / 53

The Importance of Finding a Mentor / 58

Chapter Four

Discovering Your Ideal Work Space / 63

Status: Independent Contractor or Employee? / 63

A Special Focus on the Spa Industry / 76

Job Interviews and Test Massages / 92

Working with Massage Therapists: A Manager's Guide / 94

When Clients Originally Made in your Business are Co-Opted
   by Your Therapists / 97

Chapter Five

Massage Clients: Finding Them and Treating the Whole Person / 99

Clients—Where to Find Them / 100

Getting Referrals and Introductions / 105

Advertising / 106

Consultations and Evaluations: What You Can Realistically Hope
   to Accomplish and What Cases You Should Refer Out / 107

Special Cases / 107

Establishing Boundaries / 122

Clients Who Become Friends / 124

Chapter Six

Touch and the Law / 127

The Parameters of the Profession: What You Legally Can and Cannot
   Do As a Massage Therapist / 128

Licensing / 134

Zoning / 145

Establishment License / 145

Liability Insurance / 146

Safety Concerns / 147

Third-Party Billing / 147

Taxes / 150

Chapter Seven

Creating the Perfect Space: How to Set Up and Maintain the Optimal Environment for Your Massage Therapy Practice / 157

Creaing Your Space: Points to Keep in Mind / 157

Setting Up a Professional Space / 163

Elements Common to All Massage Environments / 177

Computerizing Your Massage Business / 195

Chapter Eight

Day-to-Day Realities: Dealing with the Details of a Thriving Massage Practice / 201

A Nightmare Day in the Life of a Massage Therapist / 202

Scheduling and Managing Your Time Effectively / 204

Record Keeping: Client Records and Financial Records / 211

Fees: Setting Them, Bartering, Keeping the Books / 215

Keeping Yourself in Shape Mentally and Physically: Combating the Burnout Syndrome / 228

Rewards: Vacation Time and Therapy for the Therapist / 232

Rewards: From Financial Planning to Financial Freedom / 233

A "Dream" Day in the Life of a Massage Therapist / 239

Chapter 9

Creating a Professional Image / 243

Image Enhancers / 244

Advertising Options / 258

Marketing / 259

Business Plans / 264

Chapter 10

The Path Ahead: How to Advance Your Career in Massage / 267

Resources / 268

Beyond the Basics: Advanced Trainings / 281

Specialized Massage Pursuits / 288
Moving into Other Professions / 299
Expanding Your Reach / 301
Conclusion / 323

Appendix A: Resources / 325
General Resources / 325
Books / 327
Business Tools / 330
Magazines / 330
Associations / 330
Schools / 331
Massage Equipment Manufacturers / 331

Appendix B: Advanced Trainings Chart / 333

Index / 337

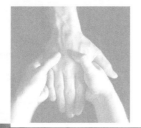

Acknowledgments

I am grateful to Umpun, Rangsan, Tasana, Lek, and Pat Chuaindhara (and Rolando), my extended Thai family who helped support me (and feed me!) during the writing of this book. Thanks to my parents for paying $500 for my first massage class over 20 years ago; it paid off. My "California family" also gave their support. Thanks to Rob, Suzzane, Chris, Ari and Nicole. Thanks to Nancy Downey, Suzanne Nelson, Kalen Conerly, Juliet Steiner, and the other folks at Thomson Delmar Learning who provided a thorough and friendly editing experience. Rebecca Kollaras deserves special credit for helping immeasurably to get my career in gear; thanks so much.

Perhaps to an even greater extent than most other fields, massage is a business of networking and interconnectedness. People literally reach out and touch each other, helping each other to grow in many different ways.

I owe a large debt of gratitude to a long list of massage people who have helped me throughout my career and especially during the writing of this book: Ed Wilson, who let me know about this project in the first place, and his bride, Iris, for being both friends and inspirations; Carole Spellman, for her friendship and belief in the dream; Tara Grodjesk, for the high quality and integrity of everything she does; Phyllis Sandler, for being the greatest massage client ever and continually inspiring me to grow; Dan and Telka Ulrich, for the great experience at their school and for their friendship and continued inspiration; Don Payne, for his supportive and honest ways—I learned some massage business lessons with your help, Don; Nancy Dail and her family, for heartwarming experiences at a great school in a beautiful setting; Julia Cowan, for her help and connections and eloquence; Dave Kennedy, for his insights and for understanding what I've been trying to get across all along; the professionals at the AMTA; all the helpful folks at the ABMP, who went out of their way to get me information, especially Kris Centeno; and Will Green and Pricilla at the IMA.

A special thanks to all the people who agreed to be interviewed for profiles: Valerie Sasso, Noel Martin, Bob Bottorf, Doug Rasmusson and his wife Kim, Zach Thomas, Kara Mathenia, Charlotte Applegate, Brian Glotsbach, John Fanuzzi, Elaine Stillerman, Vivian Madison-Mahoney, Ellen Porr, Ernesto Fernandez for his mentoring expertise, and especially Mirka Knaster for her knowledge and wisdom and the many other contacts she suggested. The publisher would like to thank the following professionals for their expertise in reviewing this manuscript: Ginny Burge, Houston, Texas; Nancy Dail, Waldoboro, Maine; James Mally, MD, Roseville, California; Kathy Ozzard, Miami, Florida; and Ed Wilson, Miami, Florida.

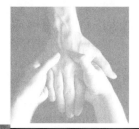

About the Author

Steve Capellini has dedicated the past 20 years to spreading the word about massage and how *you* can make massage therapy an enjoyable, profitable part of your life. He is a spa specialist and has helped hundreds of therapists and business owners achieve profitability and fulfillment in this quickly growing industry. Steve Capellini has been a licensed massage therapists since 1983, and for his first job he worked for $8.00 an hour doing 13 half-hour massages a day, so he feels confident about having started lower on the totem pole than most therapists. In addition to thousands of hours of hands-on therapy, he also has had years of teaching experience, plus a James Michener fellowship for writers; he hopes this combination has created a book that you will find eminently usable and perhaps even fun to read. He wishes you the best in your career and encourages you to get in touch with him via e-mail if you have any questions. See his Web site, *http://www.royaltreatment.com*, for contact information.

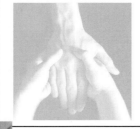

Introduction

For those of you just beginning your exploration of the field of massage therapy, I'd like to extend a warm welcome. Soon you will discover the many resources you have available to learn more about the profession: the hundreds of helpful and knowledgeable people, the expanding number of massage schools and learning centers around the country, all the tools of the trade and where to find them, plus much more. This book can serve as a guide while you become familiar with new territory, new concepts, and new possibilities. It is filled with practical advice and how-to information that will get you up and running in your successful new business.

However, the most important information I hope to share in the following pages has much more to do with you than it does with any business form, insurance bylaw, or tax code.

A MEANINGFUL CAREER CHOICE

Massage therapy, more than any other profession available as a career choice today, will bring you back into direct and meaningful contact with your fellow human beings. Whether we acknowledge it or not, we seek out ways to contribute to society, to give back to the family of mankind that supports us and that we are an integral part of. Yet, at the same time, we are forced by economic realities to engage in many occupations that don't give us the sense of giving and joy that come from working wholeheartedly at a contributive, ethical livelihood. We feel stuck, chained to a system that offers no escape from the daily treadmill.

Choosing massage therapy as a career is a way to escape from that disappointing cycle, to add more enjoyment and satisfaction to your work life, and to make a very good living at it in the bargain.

An Alternative to the Technological Lifestyle

Most physicians begin their careers in medical school with the noble goal of relieving the suffering of other people; but by the time they graduate and enter the modern world of high-tech medicine, many find that something is missing. Even though they are highly trained and excellent at what they do, they've lost touch with the people they want to heal. A barrier of machinery and technology often comes between them and their patients.

I am not proposing a back-to-nature plan that would do away with the advances of science. In fact, my own father's life was saved by sophisticated medical intervention, and I fully support the use of the ingenious tools that save lives and increase the quality of life for so many people. Yet, at the same time, something has been lost. John Naisbitt writes about this in his book, *Megatrends:*

> The more high technology around us, the more the need for human touch. The more high tech in our society, the more we will want to create high-touch environments, with soft edges balancing the hard edges of technology . . .[1] Our response to the high tech all around us was the evolution of a highly personal value system to compensate for the impersonal nature of technology. The result was the new self-help or personal growth movement, which eventually became the human potential movement.[2]

Massage therapy and other body-oriented techniques are not new, but they are even more important to us now than they were in years past. The more technology pulls us away from each other, the more we feel a need to get back in contact. As we fly apart from each other on jet planes and bullet trains and fast cars, we feel a little tug within that calls us back to each other, back to our own bodies, and back to the quiet stillness and healing energy of our planet that is always there.

---

1. John Naisbitt, *Megatrends* (New York: Warner Books, 1982), 45.

2. Ibid., 36.

How often do you spend an hour in a tranquil, softly lit room with a person, speaking quietly about things that matter, or simply not speaking at all, while working diligently to restore suppleness and health to that person's body, mind, and spirit? This scenario makes up the bulk of a working massage therapist's day. The quality of human interaction in this field is unsurpassed by any other profession.

The profession of massage therapy has become a way of life and a livelihood for thousands of people in this country. It is in a period of explosive growth right now—and for very good reasons: It is a way to serve; it is a way to communicate; it is a way to transform your good intentions into concrete benefits for your fellow human beings; and it is a way to train your sense of touch, refining it and turning it into an instrument for healing, compassion, and love.

Throughout this book, I am going to be introducing you to some very interesting people who have chosen massage therapy as a profession and who have then gone on to create stimulating careers. Their real-life stories are called Profiles, and they will serve as inspiration and guidance for you as you take the first steps in the same direction.

MY TRANSITION FROM AMATEUR TO PROFESSIONAL

Let me begin by introducing myself. After graduating from college, I was living in Venice Beach, California, spending my days roller-skating down the boardwalk and searching for ways to make ends meet while still enjoying the bohemian lifestyle the neighborhood was famous for. I was friends with actors, musicians, street people, writers, and health food fanatics, and I was working in a juice bar for $4 an hour.

My roommate was a young filmmaker named David who was also a licensed massage therapist. I went to the screenings of his movies, and we traded massages occasionally, just for fun. I had never been trained in massage, but it felt natural to me, and David suggested that I check out a local massage school in Santa Monica and get my license, too, because that might be a good way to make some money while doing what I enjoyed.

I went to the massage school, but in my heart I felt that massage was something I could never charge people money for. It was too personal and I enjoyed doing it too much. It was more an act of friendship, support, and shared pleasure than a business transaction; and I assumed that my course work and licensing were all formalities, that I would continue as I had before when I graduated—giving free massages for fun to people I liked.

Then I lost my job at the juice bar and graduated from massage school at the same time. David told me he knew a man who wanted a professional massage. David was too busy making a movie to do the massage himself. Was I interested?

At first it was a dilemma. Would I willingly give up the image of massage I had as an intimate gift, turning it into a commodity to be traded for the almighty dollar? On the other hand, I literally did not have enough money in my wallet to buy a sandwich for lunch the next day.

I called the man. His house was beautiful, perched on a mountainside above the waves in Pacific Palisades. I walked in there with my friend David's battered homemade massage table, set it up in this man's den, and proceeded to give him the same kind of caring, nurturing, soul-communicative massage I'd shared with friends for years, all the while trying to push the idea of a money exchange out of my mind.

At the end of the massage, the man was extremely grateful and reported feeling better than he had for a long time. Then, reaching into his wallet, he extracted two $20 bills and handed them to me, smiling. "Thank you so much," he said, looking me straight in the eye.

That was a magical moment for me. Something clicked in my mind, and suddenly I knew that it wasn't "wrong" to be paid for doing something I loved that also made other people feel great! In fact, the entire concept of having to suffer and work for somebody else and perform some unwanted task just to get money seemed like a very bad idea. Who had thought up that idea in the first place? Why had so many people bought into it, including me?

I saw a new light shining at the far end of the tunnel of pennilessness I'd been living in since leaving my parents' home. As I left my first client's house, carrying David's table to my beat-up old Toyota, I considered the numbers: Forty dollars for a one-hour massage was worth 10 hours of work in the juice bar. If I could get just two paying clients like that five days a week, that would be like working a 100-hour week just for doing 10 massages! The light at the end of the tunnel exploded with a flash, and I saw a sign.

Yes, a dollar sign. I had been converted. It was OK to make some money now that I knew I could do something I loved, not hurt anybody, and probably even make lots of other people feel much better.

It's been a long road since then, filled with hundreds of challenges and rewards I never could have imagined back in Venice Beach, and I haven't regretted a minute of it. Of course, there have been many ups and downs. The straight road to riches and fulfillment has been strewn with unexpected obstacles, and that is precisely why I am writing this book—to help you avoid some of the worst potholes and hazards.

WHAT YOU WILL LEARN

In **chapter 1,** we'll explore the development of massage therapy in this country and how the profession has grown. We'll see why now is the perfect time to become involved in the expanding market as traditional health care is gradually forced to broaden its scope, allowing more "alternative" therapies like massage to become accepted parts of our system. Baby boomers are reaching their 50s and 60s now, and alternatives for maintaining youth and health are tops on their list of ways to spend their vast discretionary income. Massage therapy is a broad field that offers multiple ways to capitalize on these demographic trends. Opportunities for continued education and expanding salability are limitless, as well.

In **chapter 2,** you'll find out if massage therapy is the optimum profession for you. Some people enter the field for the wrong reasons, and they find their enthusiasm quickly runs out. Take the test in this chapter and discover whether you have any of the 10 traits of a "born therapist." Learn about the psychology of touch and how to deal with people on such an intimate basis when they are frequently at their most vulnerable. Often massage sessions can become spiritual experiences, and we'll meet a minister/massage therapist who has worked to help people discover the spiritual aspects of massage. Then I will give you some realistic facts and figures about what you can expect your first year in practice and in subsequent years as your practice develops. As your career develops, sexuality may well be an issue that must be confronted, acknowledged, and examined honestly to move past it and assume your role as a true healer, and this is discussed in this chapter.

Once you've decided that massage is the path to follow, there are many schools and institutions to help you. **Chapter 3** will reveal how to scout out the best ones in your area and across the country. Finally, to help you on your way, you'll be given some advice about forming relationships with mentors and guides.

Chapter 4 focuses on what you can do once you've taken the plunge and made massage therapy a part of your life. You'll learn about all the job options that are open to you as you search for entry-level positions, and I'll offer guidance to help send you in the direction that's right for you.

Chapter 5 is my opportunity to introduce you to that special class of people you will be spending most of your time with—the massage client. Very specific needs and concerns arise when someone becomes a massage client. Often, the relationship between client and therapist becomes extremely close. I'll show you how to move people swiftly from being strangers to being loyal customers by using tools such as evaluation charts and referral systems. I'll also give you some tips for dealing with problem clients and establishing clearly defined boundaries even while allowing opportunities for friendship to flourish.

In **chapter 6,** "Touch and the Law," we'll get down to some basics about what you will have to know to operate your business up to the highest standards. I will fill you in about zoning, licensing, taxes, insurance, third-party billing, safety issues, and more.

Chapter 7 is filled with information to help you create the most conducive environment for your new business. Massage therapy is a profession unlike any other, and you'll require some very specific design savvy when you are creating your space. This chapter will give you everything you need to know from choosing the right location to picking the right colors. You'll also learn how to sort through a panoply of equipment choices that can be somewhat confusing at first. Massage tables, chairs, linens, oils, creams, mats, tools and more will all be explained; and I'll get you in touch with some of the best distributors and manufacturers in the country.

Once you've settled into your new work space and your new lifestyle, you'll be faced with the challenge of optimally organizing your schedule. **Chapter 8** will address the issues of scheduling your time, staying in good enough condition to keep up with a demanding practice, and battling a common complaint of many massage therapists—the burnout syndrome. I'll teach you 14 key techniques to help you create yourself and your practice anew year after year to stay fresh and continue to offer clients the very best you have. In this chapter you'll find two day-in-the-life scenarios of a typical busy therapist. One will be a dream day, when everything is going right; I'm including it so you will know how wonderful this life can truly be. The other will be a nightmare, when everything that can go wrong for a therapist does and there seems to be no escape. You will most likely never experience all of these potential difficulties at once, but I am including them here so you can be prepared. In the last section of this chapter I'll talk about money: how you can determine your fees, how to set up the successful bartering systems that so many therapists use, and how to keep track of your income and expenses. Of course, one of the ultimate goals you'll have as a successful therapist is a new degree of personal and financial freedom. I'll discuss how to achieve this state most effectively and then offer some ideas about enjoying it once you get there.

In **chapter 9,** I'll teach you how to create a professional image for yourself as a massage therapist. You'll learn how to develop an inexpensive promotional package that will set you apart as a therapist and business person. Marketing and advertising will play a part in this discussion. I'll also talk about business plans for therapists and the associates who plan on going into business with them such as salon owners, doctors, and chiropractors.

In **chapter 10,** the last chapter, I am going to talk about the vision you have of yourself as a successful, evolving practitioner of the multifaceted art form and healing science of massage therapy. I'll explain many of the paths you can choose to further your knowledge, perhaps learning one of the advanced techniques in the field such as Watsu™ (water shiatsu), or the massaging of prize racehorses, or working hands-on with AIDS patients. I am going to give you the information you need to keep up with your dynamic new career through the professional journals, professional organizations, trade magazines, and a plethora of excellent books targeted to practitioners. Then, at the end of the book, I'll offer some advice about creating a name for yourself in the massage business and perhaps moving to the next level, which includes writing your own articles or books, teaching your own workshops, and branching out into the lucrative consulting opportunities available with corporations, medical facilities, salons, and spas.

This book can also be used in conjunction with Thompson Delmar Learning's core massage textbook, *Theory and Practice of Therapeutic Massage 4th edition,* by Mark Beck. Many of the chapters included here fit well into Chapter 19, "Business Practices". Earlier topics fit into the beginning chapters of Beck's book, "Historical Overview of Massage" and "Requirements for the Practice of Therapeutic Massage."

USING THIS BOOK—NOW AND LATER

The best way to use this book is to read quickly through each of the chapters, getting an idea of where the information you need most is located. Slow down and absorb those sections that seem most relevant to you at this stage of your life. Pay special attention to the *profiles* in each chapter, reading them closely, because they will provide the real-life inspiration you need to turn ideas into accomplished goals. Later you can jump around from chapter to chapter, extracting the data most relevant to your situation and absorbing the material about each subject as it arises in your career development.

You'll be able to use this book as a reference while your practice grows and while you gradually become more accustomed to thinking of yourself as a massage therapist. Over the years, if you stick with it, some of your clients may become friends—even very good friends. Your fellow therapists will definitely become friends, you will network and grow, and new doors will begin to open. Your world will gradually begin to spin more and more around an axis of massage, and your life will evolve into something you cannot fully imagine right now. It will be a good path to follow.

I know. It has happened to me.

Massage Therapy: A Career Without Limits

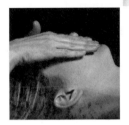

What do you think of when you see or hear the word *massage*? An hour of blissful relaxation at an exotic luxury spa? Thirty minutes of back-and-neck tension relief at a local salon or day spa? Perhaps the sober examination room of a doctor's office, where a skilled neuromuscular therapist eases nerve pain using maneuvers prescribed by the physician? The end of a 10K run, and hundreds of athletes waiting their turn on one of the many massage tables lined up near the finish line? Or the safe, nurturing environment of a private massage therapist's studio?

These scenarios and many more pop into the heads of people everywhere when they hear the word *massage.* Just a few years ago, most people would have considered massage something foreign, outside the scope of their lives. Now, a growing number of people look upon massage therapy as not only an acceptable part of their lifestyles but as a necessity. In 2003 more than one in five adults received a massage (twenty-one percent), which constitutes a 13-point jump from 1997, when the first edition of this book was published. Twenty-eight percent of adults said they expected to receive a massage in the next 12 months. Clearly, this is a profession that is expanding rapidly.[1]

Where do you fit into this newly emerging picture in the field of massage therapy? Are you considering a career as a therapist? Do you have aspirations of opening a spa facility? Do you simply want to help others feel better and relieve pain and stress in whatever way you can? Whatever your circumstances, you'll benefit by knowing a little about the history of massage therapy and how it developed to its present state of popularity.

THE DEVELOPMENT OF MASSAGE IN THE UNITED STATES

Massage has been around for a long time. Before it was ever classified as a distinct therapy, people the world over were using their instincts and "rubbing away the hurt" when a family or tribe member was injured. Shamans and medicine men included the use of touch in their healing rituals. With the development of organized religion, the practice of "laying on of hands" became popular. Many biblical references were made to "anointing with oil" and other forms of compassionate touch. We'll talk more about this in "The Spirituality of Touch" in chapter 2.

The Greeks are credited with making touch an official part of modern medicine. Hippocrates, often called the father of modern medicine, recommended massage as an important part of a health and healing regimen in his treatise *On Articulations.* The early Egyptians used massage also; many of their hieroglyphs depict foot massage in the royal temples. And throughout the Roman Empire, massage was used extensively for the restoration of wounded soldiers and the health of the population in general. The Romans' famous baths became the centerpieces of their daily lives.

The practice of massage in the East has an even more ancient and diversified tradition that includes acupressure, shiatsu, ayurveda, Jin Shin Jyutsu, and many others, some of them thousands of years older than our oldest methods. For more information about these and other therapies, refer to *Discovering the Body's Wisdom* by Mirka Knaster and her profile in chapter 10.

---

1. "2003 Massage Therapy Consumer Survey Fact Sheet" (Evanston, IL: American Massage Therapy Association).

In the Western world, after the end of the Roman Empire, massage became taboo for many centuries. This was probably due to the influence of the church, which considered touch to be the path toward sin. For a long time, the human body was terra incognita, and nobody was allowed sufficient knowledge of it. For example, the artist Michelangelo was denied access to cadavers to study anatomy and had to sneak into a Florentine morgue at midnight to perform his own clandestine autopsies.

Massage gradually came back into favor in the late 1800s, when it was used again for medical purposes. However, the rise of technology in the late 19th and early 20th centuries soon led us to forsake touch as something "old-fashioned." Before this unfortunate decline, medical practitioners of all sorts included some form of massage in their healing repertoire. Even Sigmund Freud used touch in the early days of his development of psychotherapy, employing a type of hand massage to help his patients relax and get their minds into a receptive state.

As technology took over in the field of medicine, massage was given a "second place" behind mechanical and surgical techniques. The hands-on aspect of healing was still recognized, but it no longer played a dominant role. Even so, pioneers like Per Henrik Ling in Sweden developed protocols and techniques that are still being used today. Modern "Swedish" massage is so named because of Ling's work in the field.

In the late 1800s and into the first part of the 1900s, massage was practiced mostly in health clubs, spas, and sports and country clubs. These were the days of good, old-fashioned rubdowns, during which businessmen would carry on conversations with each other while being massaged on adjoining tables. Also, physicians prescribed "health-club rubs" for women who had nervous conditions. By the First World War, massage in the medical setting had developed into what is now known as physical therapy.

In the middle part of the 20th century, massage suffered a time of lowered prestige due to the proliferation of "massage parlors," which were simply fronts for prostitution activities. These places still exist in some states, but during the 1960s and 1970s a renaissance of massage occurred and a much wider appreciation for its therapeutic benefits began to emerge. Much of the renewed interest in massage in this country started in California, particularly at Esalen Institute in Big Sur, where traditional Swedish massage techniques were blended with modern body awareness to form a new, "open" way of applying healing touch.

The last quarter of the 20th century saw a tremendous growth in the massage industry, with new styles emerging and ancient Eastern systems coming into renewed popularity as well.

CURRENT GROWTH RATE IN THE FIELD

Some massage therapists I have talked with have complained about saturation in the massage market in certain parts of the country. They say that there are too many massage therapists and not enough customers. They are afraid that all the new people choosing to go to massage school will take away customers from an already dwindling supply.

In my opinion, these people are practicing a self-defeating philosophy known as scarcity mentality, and they are literally talking themselves out of success. We have only begun to tap the most superficial layers of a customer base that potentially includes almost half of the people in this country. Those therapists who spend time worrying about shrinking supplies of customers would benefit by instead spending an equal amount of time instructing the public about the benefits of massage, thus constantly increasing their marketplace.

In terms of massage therapy, what this country needs more than anything else is education. The more people hear about massage, the more they'll know how to incorporate it into their lives. Fortunately, this is exactly what is happening. For example, logging on to America Online, I found a special section featuring massage workshops displayed on the welcome menu—and this was seen by millions of other people. Books and videos on massage instruction can be found in every bookstore in every city and in the backs of many magazines. (See "Suggested Reading" in appendix A.)

In 2004 the American Massage Therapy Association (AMTA) had 46,000 members, and the Associated Bodywork and Massage Professionals (ABMP) had 52,000 members. In 1980 the ABMP didn't even exist, and the AMTA had only 1,400 members. There is no way to tell exactly how many people are practicing massage therapy in this country, because many states still do not require licensing and many practitioners have not joined any organizations; but the ABMP estimates that the figure is over 165,000 and growing. At a minimum, an additional 45,000 students are graduated from over 800 U.S. massage schools every year. The new National Certification Exam was first administered in 1992; since then, over 60,000 therapists from everywhere in the country have taken it and become certified. Massage promises to continue as one of the fastest-growing segments of the job market.

If these figures depress you and make you think that you have found massage too late, banish that thought. This is a profession that is here to stay, and those individuals who are willing to put forth enough positive energy and effort are bound to succeed. Sometimes a beginning therapist, flushed with enthusiasm and fresh ideas for a new practice, will end up more successful than an established therapist who isn't pursuing new goals or advanced education. Don't worry about the profession itself starting to slow down. Enough indicators in our society point to a continuation of this field's growth, as highlighted in the following section.

We haven't even begun to reach our full potential market for massage. By some estimates, only 25 percent of U.S. adults have ever received a professional massage. My personal feeling is that we should strive to have at least as many massage therapists as bartenders and as many massage clinics as bars. When people go to a bar and order a drink, they are looking for relaxation and camaraderie. Massage therapy offers that and much more. It certainly feels as good or better than a cocktail makes you feel. It's not *that* expensive, costing the equivalent of 5 to 10 cocktails, depending on where you go. Plus, it has the added attraction of being good for you instead of depleting your body's health and vitality. I'm not proposing that we abolish bars; what I'm saying is that massage can be brought to an extremely wide level of acceptance if we approach it in the right way and educate the public about its benefits. That education is already happening, and it will continue.

THE AGING BABY BOOM GENERATION CREATES A DEMAND FOR MASSAGE

A number of factors combined to turn the past decade into a time of tremendous growth for massage. By far the most dramatic shift that has taken place is the aging of the baby boom generation. The largest segment of the U.S. population is now approaching and passing the 50-year mark, and people in this group are searching for ways to stay in shape and retain their youthful looks for as long as possible. Simultaneously, they are finding themselves with more disposable income than people of other generations. If massage therapists can successfully market their skills to this group, there is no limit to the success they might find.

According to baby boom expert Hershel Chicowitz, four million baby boomers turned 50 in 2004. That is a lot of people who will be potentially seeking your services. We are talking about some profound demographic forces that will be shaping our society as we collectively age. This shift is already becoming apparent, as attested to by the dramatic rise in popularity of spas (see more about spas in chapter 4). Read what Chicowitz has to say:

> We are amused when people write and ask what effect the boomers are having on the economy. Folks, in 2003, the economy IS the boomers! We represent the vast majority of the workforce. There are 76 million of us: we ARE the economy. That is not bragging; that is just a statistical reality. The huge growth in the economy in the [19]90s was due in no small part to 76 million of us working up to our peak earning and spending years.[2]

This point is important: the baby boom generation is not only the largest in this country; it is the wealthiest. When you realize that your potential customer base includes millions and millions of people who can *all afford your services,* you will develop the perspective of a glass half full instead of one half empty. One surefire way to hamper your own potential for success is to assume that only a limited number of people are out there, assiduously counting their pennies and shying away from anything they perceive as a luxury—such as massage.

As an exercise, try repeating the following words to yourself and see if you can really believe them:

> The market for massage therapy in this country is *huge.* More people every day are discovering that massage is not a luxury but a necessity—and one that they can definitely afford. I can create a great lifestyle for myself doing massage therapy while at the same time helping the people I touch.

Do you find yourself doubting the reality of these statements? Don't worry; many people feel the same way. At the end of this book, I'll have you try this exercise again. You may be surprised at how different you feel.

---

2. Hershel Chicowitz, "The Birth of the Boomers," Baby Boomer Headquarters, http://www.bbhq.com/bomrstat.htm (accessed 2004).

THE MAINSTREAMING OF "ALTERNATIVE" THERAPIES

One other large shift in our society bears mentioning in regard to its effect on massage therapy. You are probably aware that physicians have been facing new challenges recently because of the proliferation of managed health-care systems. HMOs and similar organizations have made it more difficult for many doctors to earn the living they've been accustomed to. Because of this, doctors are beginning to take alternative therapies, including massage, more seriously. In fact, we are seeing the words "alternative therapy" deleted in this context and the phrase "complementary and alternative medicine (CAM)" used in its place. No longer a second-class adjunct, massage is being recognized as a distinct field within the health-care spectrum and a complement to much of what doctors do in their everyday practice. See Figure 1-1 to get an idea of just how popular these "alternative" therapies have become.

Massage, spa treatments, and elective aesthetic procedures like laser resurfacing and body contouring are all being performed in doctors' offices today. Many physicians have taken this idea one step farther and opened

Figure 1-1 | Complementary and alternative medicine (CAM) use in 2002 (including massage, chiropractic, homeopathy, dietary supplements, ayurveda, traditional Chinese medicine, and more). (Reprinted with permission from the National Center for Complementary and Alternative Medicine, August 8, 2005, http://nccam.nih.gov/news/camstats.htm.)

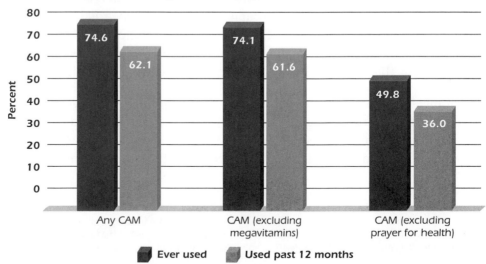

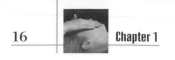

Figure 1-2 | Conditions for which complementary and alternative medicine was used in 2002 (these figures exclude the use of megavitamin therapy and prayer). (Reprinted with permission from the National Center for Complementary and Alternative Medicine, August 8, 2005, http://nccam.nih.gov/news/camsurvey__fs1.htm.)

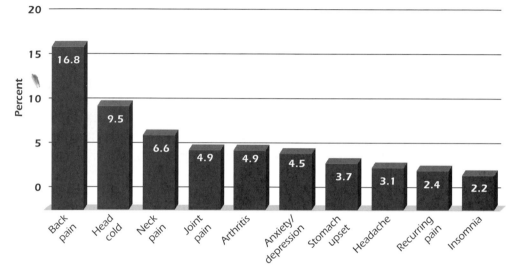

their own medical day spas. The reasons for this are threefold: first, most of these procedures are not covered by insurance, so patients have to pay directly, increasing a doctor's income; second, the effectiveness of alternative therapies is finally being recognized and taken seriously by a large number of physicians; and third, the public in general is becoming more convinced that alternative therapies work—and they are demanding them. As you can see in Figure 1-2, the condition for which people most frequently seek out alternative therapies is back pain; neck pain is number three. Both of these conditions are often improved with massage therapy.

The simple fact is: Mainstream doctors will have to broaden their scope or their patients will go elsewhere. According to a nationwide government study, 36 percent of U.S. adults aged 18 and over use some form of complementary and alternative medicine.[3] Physicians are watching their business head out

3. National Health Review Survey, conducted by the National Center for Complementary and Alternative Medicine (NCCAM) and the National Center for Health Statistics (NCHS, part of the Centers for Disease Control and Prevention), May 2004, http://nccam.nih.gov/news/camsurvey.htm.

the door, and they are starting to do something about it. This is good news for a public that deserves choices in their health care. It's also good news for the massage therapists who are ready to work with these doctors. Therapists working in conjunction with knowledgeable doctors can help to make a difference in the lives of thousands of patients.

DOZENS OF DIRECTIONS FOR POSTGRADUATE STUDY

Massage therapists are reacting to these trends by increasing their level of skill and offering more advanced forms of therapy. It is rare to find a therapist who has been practicing for a few years who hasn't mastered at least one advanced alternative to the basic massage routine, and many are going much further. Thousands of therapists use massage as a stepping stone toward training in chiropractic, naturopathic medicine, herbology, and even acupuncture. Once you've decided upon a career in massage, the learning is never finished.

A WEALTH OF OPPORTUNITIES

Massage therapy is here to stay, and the time is right to join the thousands of other people who have set out upon this path toward helping others while creating for themselves a successful, independent lifestyle. Opportunities are everywhere:

- ❋ More doctors and chiropractors are realizing it makes sense to employ massage therapists.

- ❋ To stay competitive, every new quality resort hotel that opens now comes equipped with a spa. Qualified staff is needed to work these properties.

- ❋ Through education, the public is quickly becoming aware of the importance of massage.

- ❋ According to the *Wall Street Journal*, home-based businesses are being recognized as more stable than large companies. Massage therapists who become their own bosses and work out of their own homes or small offices are positioning themselves to make large profits in America's changing work environment.

Today it's possible not only to survive as a massage therapist but also to thrive, using your skills, intuition, and creativity to forge a career unique to you. Once you get started, you may surprise yourself with the variety and depth of experiences you'll have, the new relationships you'll form, and the directions this lifestyle will take you.

2 | Is There a Healer Hidden Inside You?

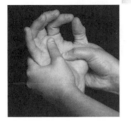

Many people find their way to the career of massage therapy because it is a viable, promising business opportunity. It is especially attractive to those who consider themselves "free spirits" who plan on moving around quite a bit, taking their skills with them wherever they go. Many artists, writers, musicians, housewives, aerobics instructors, manicurists, stylists, nutritionists, psychologists, and others find massage to be the perfect complement to their lifestyle. Some people do quite well as therapists working only part-time while they concentrate attention on some other area of their life. However, those who go the furthest and have the most impact in the world are therapists who are dedicated and who have come to the profession out of a desire to help others feel better. Many among these have had their own healing experiences with massage, which is how they decided to get into the field. I know several people who had car accidents or illnesses and were subsequently helped by massage. They usually decided right there on the therapy table that this was something they wanted to do—something important, something meaningful, something that helps. People choose massage when they have one of those what's-really-important-in-life kinds of moments. If you look within yourself and focus on what you know to be true on the deepest level, you'll see that health, wholeness, and vitality top the list. Does part of you want the opportunity to spend more time offering that to others? Do you want to develop your innate abilities to help others feel better? Do you want to delve into the mysteries of the human body/mind and find ways to help harmonize its inner workings?

If you've had inklings lately that would lead you toward becoming a therapist but you aren't really sure if this is the right direction, you will probably benefit from taking the following test. In it, you'll find out if you have any of the telltale traits of a "born therapist." Go easy on yourself. This test isn't the final word on who should become a massage therapist and who should not, but it will at least give you some important issues to think about during the decision process.

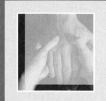

THE TEN TRAITS OF A BORN THERAPIST

1. Do people swoon and tell you that you have "great hands" when you simply place them on their neck and shoulders and squeeze a little? Yes ☐ No ☐

2. Do you feel sympathetic pain someplace in your own body when other people tell you about their own pain? Yes ☐ No ☐

3. Do you feel very comfortable with your own and others' bodies? Are you free from excess inhibition and body-image hang-ups? Yes ☐ No ☐

4. Do you have or are you willing to develop the ability and desire to work several hours a day at a very physical endeavor requiring significant stamina? Yes ☐ No ☐

5. Is it easy for you to remain silent for an entire hour (or several hours in a row) without indulging in conversation if a client doesn't wish it? Yes ☐ No ☐

6. Have people ever told you that your presence makes them feel peaceful or calm? Yes ☐ No ☐

7. Do you take your own health seriously by exercising, watching what you eat, and following the principles of moderation? Yes ☐ No ☐

(continues)

8. Does the idea of changing your lifestyle and livelihood seem exciting rather than horrible? Yes ☐ No ☐

9. Is the human body a source of wonder and intrigue for you, making you want to learn more about how it works through intensive study? Yes ☐ No ☐

10. Are you willing to invest a significant amount of time and money for schooling, supplies, association memberships, and equipment? Yes ☐ No ☐

If you answered Yes to _____ questions, then . . .

9–10　Head to the nearest massage school to enroll.

6–8　Begin serious investigation about the possibilities; send away for more information from massage schools.

3–5　Seek out established therapists in your area who may be able to give you some advice, inspiration, and insight about daily life in the massage field.

0–2　Consider more deeply what your needs and motivations are for looking into massage as a career.

THE PSYCHOLOGY OF TOUCH

It takes a special kind of person to be able to go up to a stranger and say, "Take your clothes off and lie down. Relax, everything's going to be OK."

People have to be able to trust you. And for that to happen, you have to trust yourself. You have to know yourself quite well. Handling live human bodies is not like handling produce at the supermarket or data on a computer. You've got a whole complex, fragile, consciousness-infused being there beneath your hands when you work on people. They know right away what you're up to when you lay your hands on them.

This fact was pointed out in an unlikely place. Ken Blanchard's classic best-selling book on business and management, *The One Minute Manager,* had these words of wisdom about touch:

> Touch is a very powerful message. Touch is very honest. People know immediately when you touch them whether you care about them, or whether you are just trying to find a new way to manipulate them. **When you touch, don't take.** Touch people . . . only when you are **giving** them something—reassurance, support, encouragement, whatever.[1]

When you touch someone during massage, at times you may awaken feelings within them that have to be dealt with very professionally. Not everyone is capable of dealing with these stirred-up feelings. In many societies and religions, there existed—and still exists today—strong taboos against close physical contact. Through the prohibition of touch, religious and societal leaders have attempted to maintain control over people. They know that touch is the instigator of private, primitive experiences, bringing people a sense of safety and security or deep relaxation or healing or sexual arousal or emotional release.

Experiencing these sensations and knowing that they are OK gives people a sense of autonomy and freedom from repression that is *not* OK with certain kinds of authority. In much of our early training, we are taught to believe that we should not feel certain feelings and that if we do feel them, there is something wrong with us. Therefore, we are taught from a young age to repress anything that is unseemly in our parents' eyes or our churches' eyes or society's eyes. Those feelings, however, remain.

Often in a massage therapy session, especially a good one, some of these repressed feelings may be reexperienced because they are being released from their storage places in the body. These types of memories are called somatic, or body-based, memories. To become an effective massage therapist, you'll have to learn how to communicate with people on a meaningful level about their bodies and their feelings. To do that, you'll have to be mature and responsible. This is something to keep in mind when you are thinking about becoming a therapist or already training to be one.

You may downplay the significance of the nonphysical aspect of touch and claim you are going to use only straightforward, mechanical, no-nonsense, muscle-focused therapy. That is probably not the best approach. Touch is always about people, about their hearts and minds, and sometimes even about their souls.

---

1. Kenneth, Blanchard, Ph.D., *The One Minute Manager*, p. 95, William Morrow & Company, 1981.

PROFILE: Zach Thomas
Spirituality, and Massage

After graduating from college as a premed student at Duke University, Zach Thomas decided that his true calling was in the seminary. He became a parish minister for seven years but continued to feel a strong pull toward medicine. Eventually he began working as a chaplain, first in a rehabilitation hospital, then in a long-term nursing home, and finally in an acute-care hospital, for a total of 13 years. "When the opportunity to work as a chaplain presented itself, I was truly thankful for the chance to utilize my interest in the medical fields and my spiritual training," he recalls. He accomplished some dynamic work in his field and became the founding president of Hospice at Charlotte in North Carolina.

Zach was happily working as a chaplain, running marathons, and raising a family when, during a trip to Switzerland, he received a professional massage that ended up radically changing his life. "I was turned around, struck, impacted, opened up—still can't find the right verb—by that massage," remembers Zach. "For several months after returning home I was really confused. I could neither avoid the profound meaning of the bodywork experience, nor could I see any practical way of combining chaplaincy work and bodywork. The profound meaning of professional touch had two dimensions. The

immediate connection for me was with the image of Jesus' healing touch, which appears on practically every page of the gospel. In the seminary, the healing reality of Jesus' life never was fully appreciated."

Zach kept his massage work quiet for several years, honing his skills by working on friends and others by word of mouth two days a week. Eventually, he earned his massage license.

The biggest problem he encountered was the church's attitude toward touch and healing. The mainline church played down the role of hands-on healing in Jesus' life, even when faced with plenty of biblical references. Fundamentalists (such as some televangelists and traveling charismatic preachers), on the other hand, took "healing" to an extreme. The result was that the mainline church perpetuated a mind-body split by teaching a "no-touch" approach to pastoral care.

Today, however, things are changing. The mind-body duality is slowly beginning to dissolve. The church is rediscovering the "laying on of hands," and medical practitioners are beginning to appreciate healing touch, prayer, and meditation. Within this new atmosphere, Zach was able to form a group of colleagues within the church who had a similar interest in massage and healing touch. Nuns, priests, pastoral counselors, and others joined

(continues)

Zach Thomas (continued)

him in forming an alliance called the Resource Group on Human Touch, and in the late 1980s, the National Association of Bodyworkers in Religious Service (NABRS) was formed. Zach served as president for eight years.

Now Zach teaches workshops for churches and religious professionals about the whole project of reclaiming a healing ministry and a more healthy personal and spiritual approach to touch. "Obviously, for a male to find a mode of touch free of sexual content or intent is a huge breakthrough. The issues of intent, boundaries, and ethics have never been stressed enough. As a result, many would-be bodyworkers enter the field fairly naively."

Zach stresses the importance of proper preparation for all massage students. "Begin working on your professional scope of practice early," he counsels. "Have a goodly number of other professionals; MDs, RNs, DDSs, PTs, et cetera, to whom you can refer. And above all, don't assume you are also a psychologist as well as a bodyworker. Also, go to a counselor or spiritual director to attend to your own inner sense of boundaries and self-esteem. The major pitfall by far for new

therapists is the ego. It inevitably assumes it can address far more than the therapist is capable of or trained for. How little is the window of our opportunity to serve is not the wisdom of the novice."

In recent years Zach has traveled to Thailand to learn the ancient healing massage techniques taught there. In fact, he wrote down the comments contained in this profile while sitting beneath a mango tree in the northern Thai city of Chiang Mai. He has also written an interesting, informative book, *Healing Touch: The Church's Forgotten Language.* In the book's epilogue, he talks about bridging the gap between the East and the West, between the mind and the body, through the use of simple healing touch. It is certainly a worthwhile, and exciting, journey to be on.

Healing Touch can be ordered from the Presbyterian Publishing Corporation at (800) 227-2872 or at http://www.wjkbooks.com.

You can contact the National Association of Bodyworkers in Religious Service (NABRS) at 5 Big Stone Court, Baltimore, MD 21228-1018; (410) 455-0277; nabrs@aol.com.

THE SPIRITUALITY OF TOUCH

Many people begin to practice massage therapy because they find it is a way for them to communicate in a direct, spiritual way with other people, with themselves, and with their God.

How is this possible? you ask. What does massage have to do with God?

In my opinion, massage can be considered a spiritual experience because it involves communication. The root of the word communication is the Latin *communicare*, from *communis*, meaning "common." When we communicate with another person through the medium of massage (Figure 2-1), we are letting ourselves be equal to them; the same as them; with common feelings, aspirations, fears, repressions, ecstasies, and ideas.

On one level, massage actually has little to do with muscles and joints and hands and backs. It has to do with the person inside the body giving the massage and the person inside the body getting the massage. The real massage is the transmission of a message from the giver to the receiver and back again; and that message is likely to contain elements of gratitude, understanding, compassion, and shared awareness.

Massage can be that kind of communion. For many of the most wonderful massage therapists in the world, communion is the focus of their work. Massage therapy can be a form of worship, one in which no feelings or

Figure 2-1 | **Massage is a form of communication. (Reproduced with permission of Xanterra Parks & Resorts.)**

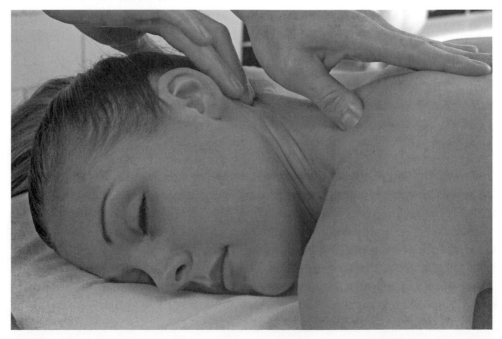

experiences are repressed; in which a healing communion with other human beings, one at a time, is the only required practice; and which accepts every color, race, and social background with open arms.

This may sound like a grandiose vision when what we're essentially describing is a back rub. Right? Believe me, I wouldn't be talking this way if it weren't for the hundreds of examples I've seen of people who have turned massage into just this kind of communion. In fact, a growing number of massage practitioners used to be or still are members of the clergy. Zach Thomas of North Carolina, for example, helped found the NABRS (National Association of Bodyworkers in Religious Service). I'll let his story speak for itself.

REALISTIC EXPECTATIONS

With all this talk about psychology and spirituality, you may be wondering what exactly is going to happen to you if you decide to become a massage therapist. Will your friends still recognize you? Will you wear only white clothes, pray with people over the massage table, and sport a turban wrapped around your head?

No need to worry. Besides the potentially "esoteric" aspects of the massage business, it is also filled with some reassuringly normal and down-to-earth matters. What can you realistically expect from your new lifestyle if you decide to become a massage therapist? The answer to that question changes depending on who's asking it. However, many therapists find that several new experiences are shared by a majority of their colleagues. Certain rites of passage must be faced. Certain self-concepts must be redefined. Certain new habits must be cultivated, others left behind.

Although everyone's situation will be unique, it may be helpful for you to hear some of the things other people have gone through during their gradual metamorphoses into massage therapists. The challenges and opportunities change as time goes on. I'm going to give you an idea of what you can expect at four different stages of your new career.

Stage One: The Neophyte

You've just graduated from massage school. Your skills have been sharpened through hundreds of hours of practice. You have stars in your eyes as you contemplate the myriad new adventures and opportunities that await you. You have already gotten started, yet at the same time you are feeling like you can't wait to get started. It's a paradoxical time of rapid growth that almost always seems too slow.

During this period, normally throughout your entire first year as a therapist, you can:

✳ Expect to struggle at first. It's never as easy as it sounds on paper. If you're like most new therapists, you've taken the average fee for a massage in your area, multiplied it by eight hours in the workday, and come up with some staggering numbers for your soaring new income. If you charge $50 for a massage right out of the gate, you'll expect to be making $400 a day—and that's an expectation that can cause you some personal pain. Tone down those expectations, and you'll have an easier first year. Instead of multiplication, try some division, and you'll probably end up much happier.

current minimal monthly
living expenses

$\div$ $=$ number of massages to aim
                                                                    for per month

the fee you receive per
massage

✳ Expect to try a couple different approaches before settling on one that works for you. Many new therapists think that they can see a seamless career path already custom designed to take them into the future, and this may indeed happen to you, but the majority of people entering the profession find that they continue along a steep learning curve for their first year and their projected trajectories change one or more times, sometimes dramatically.

✳ Expect to run into some less-than-desirable clients. Not everyone comes to massage out of purely therapeutic motives. You may have to overcome some sexual issues at the beginning of your career (see "Overcoming Sexual Issues" later in this chapter). It will take a while for you to develop your own way of spotting potential problems before they happen and dealing with these situations if they occur. Besides customers soliciting sexual favors, you may run into several other annoyances that include (1) people with poor personal hygiene, (2) clients who nag and complain and whom you can never please, (3) people who are chronically late and don't respect you professionally, and (4) people who undervalue your skills and think of massage as merely a "rubdown." You will find that all of these problems gradually dissipate if you are persistent and learn from each experience.

✳ Expect to be misunderstood by an employer. Maybe it's your boss at the new day spa. Maybe it's the chiropractor at the clinic where you work. Employers in general may not completely understand you or appreciate your art, especially when you first start as a therapist. It will take some time for you to prove to others, and to yourself, just how necessary and beneficial your services are to other people.

✳ Expect to experience a minor identity crisis. What do your friends think of your becoming a massage therapist? How about your family? When I asked for money to help put me through massage school, my parents assumed I was going through just another "phase" and that sooner or later I'd get a "real" job. My new massage friends knew what I was up to (and I had the added benefit of living in California at the time, where it seems everybody understands massage therapists), but old friends thought I had lost a few marbles. How about you? How will your current colleagues or co-workers or buddies view you if you start touching others therapeutically for a living? You'll have to deal with the social context of your new identity. This is especially evident when you're lugging around your big massage table to people's apartments, through lobbies, up elevators, with all the world seeing what you do. It can be exciting, but it can also take some adjusting to.

✳ Expect to wonder if you have made the right decision. When you become a massage therapist, everything is suddenly different. Most of it is wonderful, but you may find yourself alone one night, with barely enough money to buy food for your cat (which happened to me more than once during my early years), waiting for the phone to ring, or settling for a temporary low-paying position in another field just to make some money. You know you're heading the right direction in your life, but in the meantime you are suffering a little, and you wonder: "Is this really for me?" I've found that the only way to get through those times is to get through them. On the other side of those trials, you'll find out whether you're really a massage therapist or not. The way to tell is if you're still doing massage. Usually at least once during your first year, there comes a moment when you must demonstrate to the Higher Power

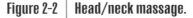

that you have faith and will continue in spite of any obstacle or setback or problem. Remember: At the end of this trial lies the goal you dreamed of before starting—a career and a way of life dedicated to helping others and at the same time achieving personal financial freedom and respect for yourself. It's worth it.

Stage Two: Becoming Established

You are actually making your living with your new skills, and you are even starting to get ahead. Paying the rent is probably not as much of a problem, and people are treating you with a little more respect (because you're feeling more self-respect from within). You have shifted from wondering what it would be like to be a massage therapist to knowing what it's like (Figure 2-2). You've gotten used to the physical work involved, and your body feels stronger. After working on dozens, even hundreds, of people, you begin to know intuitively what people need when they walk through the door. You've made it through the tests of faith that distinguished you from the other would-be therapists who have now moved on to some other pursuit. For many therapists, this is the true honeymoon stage of their career, sweeter and easier than it was right at the beginning.

Figure 2-2 | Head/neck massage.

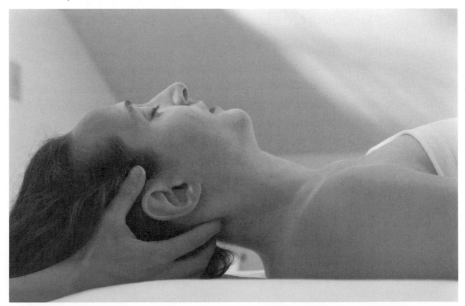

During this period, which begins somewhere near the end of your first year as a therapist and continues into your second or third year, you can:

❋ Expect to earn more money. The financial dreams spawned by your early calculations begin to take form. You may find yourself demanding a higher percentage of the gross massage income from the establishment where you work, and you'll probably have a few more private clients to work with. This will bring your monetary reality more into line with your monetary expectations. It is not, however, the final step on your road to riches. You will incrementally increase your income over time. This first step along that road may not even be the biggest jump in income for you, but it will probably feel the best.

❋ Expect to find your own "rhythm." Some therapists are built to work long, hard hours, performing eight or nine back-to-back massages all day long without wilting or complaining. Others find that one or two appointments in the morning and one or two in the afternoon are plenty, and they can't offer their best work if they are forced to work too many hours. Everyone is different, and by the time you reach this stage in your career, you will have settled on a method that allows you to work to your maximum without overextending yourself. The important thing to remember is that you are OK just the way you are. If a colleague seems fine performing twice as many massages as you, don't fall prey to self-judgment. There really does seem to be a magical number of treatments per day for each therapist beyond which they should not go.

❋ Expect to start taking vacations. Massage is demanding work, and therapists quickly find that they need breaks to stay refreshed and do their best work. Usually those breaks are a little more frequent and more extended than the vacations of many other people, due to a combination of factors—not the least of which is the independent, adventurous nature of most therapists. I know of several who work very hard from September through May and then take off for three months each year. Often, these "vacations" include some kind of massage work, as well. In my second year as a therapist I had the opportunity to visit Europe for several months, living on $10 a day, and through a friend I found a job doing massage for a film crew that was making a documentary about the life of Ernest Hemingway. With the money I made on that job, I was able to stay in Europe for half a year.

✳ Expect to start thinking about the future. Even if you're still quite young, you'll soon realize that you have limits. Your hands and the rest of your body won't last forever under the constant stress of performing massages all day long. Accordingly, start to plan ahead and wonder what other avenues you'll be able to branch out into—usually within the same line of work but sometimes in others, perhaps related. Many therapists become spa managers or open their own spas, for example. Others open massage schools or get jobs teaching at one. That way they continue to work in a field they know intimately, yet they are not engaged in the physical work all day every day.

✳ Expect to start feeling some peace of mind. You've done it. You've made the change and have become something you truly wanted to be, perhaps for the first time in your life. You are helping people and helping yourself and working hard; a long road stretches ahead with a lot of potential enjoyment along the way. You may find moments at this stage when your career choice seems eminently right to you, and that knowledge will offer you a contentment that you may not have had before. You may, like so many therapists do, begin to explore forms of meditation, yoga, and Eastern mysticism. A new internal space opens inside you once you've committed yourself to an external form of service in this world.

✳ Expect to keep on struggling nonetheless. There will always be issues and challenges to face. Days will still come when you're grasping for the right path to take through particularly thorny problems. But you'll have a certain strength inside you now, born of the confidence that has been gathered with experience.

Stage Three: The "Mid-Career Crisis"

You are an established, well-known therapist in your circle. People refer clients to you. You refer clients to other professionals. You've joined one or more of the professional organizations available, and you've made many treks to annual massage conventions around the country and perhaps around the world. You've traveled to study massage techniques in other cultures, and you've given literally thousands of treatments. Three years passed after receiving your license, then four, then five. Now it's been almost 10 years. Perhaps you've bought a house with the money you've earned as a therapist.

Or you met your spouse who started as a colleague in the massage field. Things have changed for you, and all because of massage. Somewhere around this time, in the 7- to 12-year range, you may go through a professional midlife crisis. This is when some people switch out of the massage field altogether, becoming a salesperson or an investment banker. This may never happen to you, but it is a common enough occurrence that I wanted to mention it here. At this stage of flux in your career you can:

✳ Expect to know what you are doing but experience resistance to doing more. There may come a point when you feel stuck. Often this type of dissatisfaction can be positive because it impels you to act and take the next step in your career. That point is usually when a therapist will decide that extensive further education is a necessity, for example.

✳ Expect to be quite attached to your lifestyle. Even if you are seriously thinking about changing careers, the life of a therapist has become second nature to you and the thought of giving it up is mostly unpleasant. You treasure the meaningful interaction you have with your clients, and you treasure your independence.

✳ Expect to feel some aches and pains. Most therapists, no matter how careful they are, end up at some point with joint stiffness, a sore back, or tired arms or legs, a result of the physical nature of the work. When it happens to you, you may feel like throwing in the towel before your body suffers any damage. Usually, though, these problems can be greatly improved with some increased awareness of body mechanics; smarter working habits; the addition of other therapies to your repertoire; and a few good applications of ice, mud, paraffin, or other products (see chapter 8 for details).

✳ Expect to get involved with certain business deals. Whether it's negotiations to buy your own massage studio property or hiring therapists to work for you or seeking a rung on the many multilevel marketing opportunities available today, you may be looking around for something to supplement your income. Massage may always be your first love, but you've realized by now that there will always be a limit to trading your hours for a specified amount of money. You'll be looking for ways to grow exponentially in the financial sense. And if you're like most motivated therapists, you'll find it.

Stage Four: Long-Term Success

You've made it through, somewhere past the 10-year mark, and you're still a therapist. In a way, now you will always be a therapist, because you've done it for so long that you and others consider you a therapist no matter what. Even if you do something else now for a while, you'll be a therapist who is temporarily doing something else. Your life will be forever colored by the experiences and realizations you've had through your work in massage. Once you reach this stage, which will last the rest of your life, you can:

✳ Expect to start teaching others, either officially in a massage school or in workshops or unofficially as a mentor and guide to newer therapists. This comes naturally to most people. Without even trying, you will find yourself encouraging and offering advice to others. People will come to you automatically when they see and sense that you've gone through the other stages that they are now on the brink of entering. (See "The Importance of Finding a Mentor" in chapter 3.)

✳ Expect to spread the news somehow. Many therapists end up promoting themselves and their work in ways they never would have conceived of in the beginning of their careers. People who had never written even a letter will write whole articles and essays on massage and health. People who were afraid to speak in front of 10 people will get up in front of hundreds to express the things they've learned through helping others. You have become known, and you stand for something in other people's minds. If you've followed your original intentions, you stand for health and healing and relaxation and wholeness. People may expect you to act a certain way, to eat a certain way, or to dress a certain way when they meet you because they've formed an opinion about you before getting to know you. You will have learned to live with being "known" in this way.

✳ Expect to charge more for your treatments—and be worth it. There's no use in underpricing your services. By this time, you've gained enough knowledge and experience and created a good enough reputation to demand the higher fees that once seemed out of reach to you. You can do this easily now because you have paid your dues.

✳ Expect to create something new. Most therapists find that the long years of work and service have been leading up to something uniquely their own, some special offering that nobody else can give. Perhaps it's a seminar they've envisioned or a new form of therapy or an excellent new technique to add to the canon of massage maneuvers. Or maybe they've found a way to reach out more, give more, offer higher value, touch people who never have been touched therapeutically before in their lives. It may be big or small, but it will always be something creative. Massage therapy seems to bring out the artist in people eventually.

- Expect to be relishing new challenges. Something will always come up in life—maybe a disaster or maybe a great opportunity or maybe both. Whatever life brings your way, you will now react to it through the use of your skills as a therapist. When Hurricane Andrew devastated much of South Florida, for example, I joined dozens of other therapists and we headed down to the epicenter of the damage to offer free massage to soldiers, Red Cross volunteers, police officers, and 911 operators. For days we braved the heat and the privations with everyone else and did what we could to help. Right after the Oklahoma bombing, some therapist friends headed in their camper trailer straight to Oklahoma City to perform similar services (see the profile of Bob Bottorf in chapter 5). The same thing happened after 9/11 in New York City, and after hurricane Katrina on the Gulf Coast. The Red Cross is getting used to the sight of massage chairs being set up on the scene at most disasters. People in those situations are in dire need of reassuring human touch.
- Expect to be witnessing your life as it turns into an adventure. You will continue to travel and meet new people and branch out in directions you never thought of before. If you keep following your heart and using your hands to heal, you will probably not experience boredom very often.

A Positive Attitude

Your single greatest asset, especially as a beginning massage practitioner, is your positive attitude. In fact, if you don't nurture a positive attitude about this line of work, one of two things are going to happen: Either you're going to find yourself *not* working as a therapist eventually or you're going to find yourself working in a dead-end position somewhere, scratching your head and wondering why clients aren't flocking to you automatically and why your dreams haven't come true.

It is especially important for you to cultivate and display this positive attitude during your first year as a therapist. As an example, one young therapist I know found a position in a physician's office for a base salary of about $15 per hour. The doctor was not particularly interested in helping her develop her career. He just needed someone to operate a new body-contouring massage machine that was going to make his practice a lot of money. The therapist had three choices: decline the position in the first place, accept the position and work there grudgingly while seeking other employment, or accept the position and give it all she had, knowing that her *attitude* was going to be the ultimate arbiter of her success or failure.

If you choose the third path, you'll never know what glorious surprises may be waiting for you. Opportunities abound for those who concentrate on their *inner attitude* first and then worry about the exterior trappings of success.

That young therapist in the doctor's office? She achieved such spectacular results using the massage device that the manufacturer of the machine hired her to be a consultant and trainer. She ended up with a high-paying job, opportunities for travel, media exposure, and lots of invaluable experience. The job she found did not exist before she came to work for the company. It was created just for her to take advantage of her enthusiasm and skill. This is the way it can work for any therapist who is willing to put forth sufficient effort, both outer *and* inner, in pursuit of his or her goals.

OVERCOMING SEXUAL ISSUES

One unavoidable reality of the massage profession is its association with sex in the minds of many people. There is a good chance, especially if you are a woman, that you will be propositioned by a man for sex at least once during your career; and the sad fact is that many therapists experience this *many* times over.

In a number of states, massage is still associated with massage parlors, and it's easier to find sexually oriented massage than it is to find good therapeutic practitioners. Countless men have had sexual experiences during a massage. If one of these men winds up on your table, the fact that you are saying that you don't give "that kind of massage" could very likely just be taken as a challenge, and the man will end up even more stimulated because of that challenge. This has happened to many female therapists and even a few male therapists.

More than most people realize, this is not so much an issue of sexuality as it is one of power and money and control. An older man with money to spare has a certain edge over a young woman who is struggling to pay her bills. It can be difficult to factor out these realities from the equation of a massage, but it *can* be done. The secret to doing it can be summed up in one word: *intention.*

A therapist's intention is the foundation of the ethical practice of massage. The basic truth is that, short of a forced encounter or rape, the therapist holds the ultimate control. He or she can put a halt to the massage at any moment and ask the client to leave. Sometimes this is exactly what has to happen. If a client is behaving badly or making inappropriate suggestions, the massage should be stopped immediately. If half or more of the massage has already been completed, then the client should be charged full price. If less than half the massage has been completed, a portion of the fee should still be charged to cover the therapist's time. Of course, sometimes what the therapist wants more than anything is to just get the client *out.* If that is the case, make no mention of the fee. Just get the client to leave as quickly as possible.

At times, you may have clients who seem to be "just kidding around" about sexuality or sexual issues. This can happen regardless of the client's nationality, race, religion, sex, or age. Even if the client is elderly or seems "respectable," he or she may still make one or more of the following comments that should serve as a red flag for you:

- ✳ "From this position, I get a great view of your legs."
- ✳ "I'm just a harmless old guy/gal."
- ✳ "You don't really need to cover me with a towel, do you?"
- ✳ "My inner thighs are really sore. Can you work there?"
- ✳ "Do you give 'full body' massage?"
- ✳ "Do you offer any extras?"
- ✳ "Will this be a 'full' massage?"
- ✳ "How much would you like to get tipped today?"
- ✳ "Do you offer 'relief' or 'release' massage?"

You may wonder at times how far you should go in letting the "guys just be guys." What should you let them get away with and brush off with a grain of salt, and what should you put your foot down about? In general, it is best to cut off all sexual "kidding around" the moment it starts because it almost invariably is an attempt on the client's part to test the waters and see how much he can get away with—always with the intention of going further if allowed.

Make sure to find out exactly how any new client has found out about you and your services. Personal references are best, but even that is no guarantee. One time a client was referred to me by a close friend, but I failed to inquire how this client knew my friend. It turned out that they did not know each other. This man had called my friend about an ad he'd placed in a newspaper advertising health food products. He asked if massage was included, and my friend referred him to me without thinking twice about it. The man called a number for health food products in search of sexual massage services. This is how desperate many people are. Five minutes into the massage, I terminated the session and sent him packing.

Problems with Female Clients

Although men do the lion's share of propositioning in this business, it is by no means their exclusive domain. Women customers do occasionally proposition male therapists, and at times this can be a more confusing situation. In all cases, it is the therapist's responsibility to remain clinical in intention and avoid sexual contact with the client. But, whereas women have learned to repel the blatant advances of men whom they don't know, men have learned that any advance from a woman gives the green light, and their instincts are to go forward. This situation calls for a high level of self-control on the part of the male therapist.

What if—in spite of a therapist's best intentions and a long track record of giving ethical, professional massages—the client on the table turns out to be extraordinarily attractive and suddenly makes it clear, either verbally or nonverbally, that she is open to a sensual encounter? In my opinion, there is nothing morally wrong with a therapist who feels desire in that situation. It is a natural response. There are therapists who have been drawn into sexual situations, and the most serious consequence of their actions has been an internal one: They've had to review their own *intentions* and their level of commitment to the practice of therapeutic massage. However, in other cases the consequences can be very grave, and I would like to caution all therapists and would-be therapists in case they ever find themselves tempted in this way.

The issue of sexuality and massage is a dilemma not so much about moral principles as it is a conflict between two drives within the human psyche and body. One is the drive toward consciousness and compassionate, therapeutic work to aid and uplift others. The other drive is toward erotic pleasure and sexual release. Both have their root in the same, larger driving force within all of us—to connect, to communicate, to have meaningful and/or stimulating experiences with other people. It is a fact that sexual thoughts and feelings can emerge for some people during a therapeutic massage. If such arousal should occur, it should not present a problem as long as the therapist has the right intentions and remembers to exercise proper control of his actions.

Other Challenges for Male Therapists

In general, our society approves of males who are competent, commanding, and somewhat cold. We value a man who is strong and detached, calmly doing the job he is paid for and doing it well. For a man to be a good massage therapist, however, he must display a large degree of warmth and compassion on a daily basis. Although many people, especially women, would claim to appreciate the traits of gentleness, caring, and vulnerability in a man, there is a slight stigma attached to such a "soft" fellow. We want our men to be soft and kind, but we also want them to be strong and effective, perhaps even violent, if we need their protection.

For these reasons, some men find it difficult to move forward successfully in their careers as caring massage therapists. Often they gradually move away from massage into new roles in allied modalities like physical therapy, chiropractic, medical massage, neuromuscular techniques, and so on. This is understandable, yet also saddening. We *need* nurturing men, and massage therapy is a great way for men to cultivate their nurturing qualities. I encourage all males interested in massage therapy to keep a close watch on their own feelings in this regard. Is society subconsciously talking you out of your role as "just a massage therapist"?

In the practical world, it is more difficult for male massage therapists. Fewer jobs are available in spas and resorts. Some employers refuse to hire males because they say their clients prefer women. And even those men who do find jobs in clinics or spas sometimes find themselves sitting on the sidelines while their female counterparts are chosen by more clients. What can we males do?

A CAUTIONARY TALE

I was the supervisor in charge of forty therapists at a large spa. One quiet day, in the middle of the afternoon, two security men approached and told me I had to pull one of the therapists off the floor *immediately*. I protested because he was about to begin a massage, but the security men looked extremely serious, and I went to find the therapist.

He looked surprised when I told him there were security guards waiting to take him away. My heart went out to him. He was one of the most popular therapists on the staff. What could he have possibly done wrong?

Within minutes, he was whisked away out the employee entrance, and nobody saw him at the spa again. It wasn't until a few days later that I found out what had happened. The therapist was being sued by a woman guest who was accusing him of rape. After the alleged incident, she went to a hospital, and evidence was found that proved intercourse had occurred.

The woman claimed that the therapist had "put her in a trance" and taken advantage of her. Whatever happened, she hadn't stopped the therapist during the experience. Only afterward did she decide that what had happened was inappropriate.

What really happened in that room? Was it consensual? Forced? Was she really in a trance? Nobody but the two of them knows for sure. But whatever did happen cost the therapist his job. And his reputation.

Whenever sexual energy is raised during a professional massage therapy session, the best course of action is always to stop the massage or communicate any feelings of discomfort immediately and correct the situation, thus avoiding potentially unfortunate repercussions.

The truth is, in many cases it's a little more challenging for men to get their massage careers off the ground because of these issues. This is not a good reason to switch your path, however. With some extra perseverance and a good understanding of the societal pressures at play, you *can* move forward, gaining the confidence of employers and clients alike who will eventually come to see you primarily not as a male but as a person (Figure 2-3). We can become role models for men in many professions who would rather be known for their inner qualities than their outer ones. Successful male massage therapists have had to overcome obstacles uniquely their own, and they should be recognized as having achieved something special for themselves, for everyone they touch, and for society as a whole, which needs more examples of caring, compassionate men in *all* walks of life.

Figure 2-3 | The world needs more compassionate, caring men working at massage.

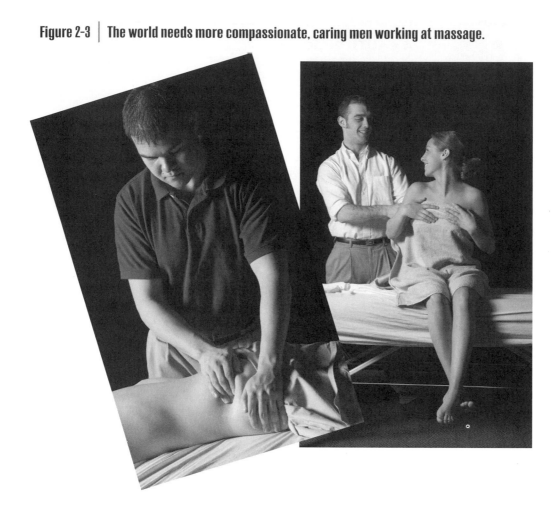

3

Choosing a Massage School: Making the Best Decision

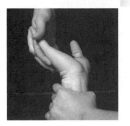

You will probably not face many bigger decisions in your massage career than the decision of where to go to school. You can feel it in your bones, can't you? Somehow, you know you've got to make the perfect match for yourself. With all the choices out there, you are experiencing an emotion that may be approaching anxiety. You are making a decision about how to best train yourself to help other people relax, and yet you yourself are a basket case! This, you may think, is not the way things should be. "Is there something wrong with me?" ask many people in this same situation. "Do I really have what it takes to become a therapist?"

Have no fear. The process of researching, finding, enrolling in, and then beginning your course at the perfect massage school is often a difficult one, but if you trust in your instincts and follow the simple guidelines in this chapter, you will do just fine. Experiencing doubts and fears all along the way, even after you've already begun your program, is completely natural, and you should not let it stop you from moving forward. I recently had lunch with a friend of mine who is going through precisely this situation. She is currently enrolled at a school in Las Vegas. "I can't believe this," she told me. "I moved all the way from New York City, which I love, and now I have to live in the middle of the desert for months, dealing with all these different personalities at the school, and studying harder than I have for years. Do you think I made the right decision?" All I could do is offer her the same advice I am offering you right now: Stick with it. You have followed your heart and finally done something that you've known you want to do for quite some time now. The reality of it may not mesh perfectly with the ideal you had envisioned in your mind, but this does not mean that you are not getting exactly what you need to further your dream.

Of course, there are occasions when students enroll in a massage school that is just not right for them. In this case, it is best to make the conscious decision to change environments. I have another friend who faced exactly this situation. After making a big initial investment, he decided that he needed to change paths anyway and he ended up leaving his original massage school and enrolling in a smaller training program that eventually certified him as an advanced practitioner of "structural integration," a technique similar to Rolfing®. That was right for him. You have to do what is right for you.

MASSAGE-SCHOOL HUNTING

I hope you can use this chapter as a guide to point you in the right directions as you navigate your way through the labyrinth of choices out there in massage education. In a way, at this stage you will be going massage-school hunting in the same way that people go house hunting, and you are going to need the same qualities that prospective first-time home buyers have:

- **Stamina:** That's right. It's not necessarily going to be all peaches and cream as you head out looking for your perfect massage school. You may be one of the lucky ones who has a school right down the street all picked out beforehand, but the majority will have to go through a process that includes a bit of hand wringing and hair pulling before they come to their final decision.

- **Healthy skepticism:** Yes, you should enter any massage school with a slightly critical eye, looking for flaws as well as selling points, just as you would in a house. Those nasty little surprises that come up later in your education were usually there for the observing right from the beginning, but people have a tendency to get starry-eyed and dumb if they fall in love with a school's outward appearance or slick image.

✳ **Knowledge about the marketplace:** How are you going to know which house to buy (or which school to choose) if you are clueless about the marketplace? If you have no idea which schools have a better reputation among potential employers or which schools have graduated the most students who pass their licensing exams, how are you going to make an informed decision? The schools themselves will usually give you this information, but it is coming from a biased source; you have to check it out elsewhere, too.

✳ **An understanding of your own needs:** Although your needs will change over time, it helps to have some long-term goals in mind so you can match the school to your vision.

DEVELOPING YOUR SKILLS: MASSAGE SCHOOLS AND TRAINING PROGRAMS

When you decide to go out massage-school hunting, the most important thing you'll need to do is find the right match for your needs and your personality. The school you choose has to fit like a finely tailored suit. After several years in this profession and experience teaching in several schools, my advice to you is the following: Undertake a thorough study of the owner of each prospective massage school, as well as the people you are going to be spending most of your time with—the instructors and other students. Do this before you lay any of your hard-earned cash on the line. One excellent way to meet the owners and administrators of a school you are interested in is to attend the open houses that many of them offer. Alternately, ask to sit in on a class and observe from the back. You can only use this for an approximation of what your own class will be like, however, because massage classes have a tendency to be dramatically different from each other, even in the same school. Each class quickly develops its own unique "personality." (To learn more about choosing the right school for you, see the sidebar "Massage School: A Transformational Experience" later in this chapter.)

Because there are nearly 800 massage schools to choose from, you may feel a bit overwhelmed at first, but if you follow the subsequent steps, you will quickly zero in on the one that's right for you. When you are ready to start checking out schools, begin by asking massage professionals for their recommendations. Check the yellow pages in your town under Schools and Vocational Institutes. Try studying the list in the back of any issue of *Massage*

Therapy Journal. There you will find the programs of schools that have been accredited by the Commission on Massage Therapy Accreditation (COMTA). To become eligible for accreditation, the programs must offer courses with a minimum of 600 hours of supervised class time, be at least six months in duration, and have been in business for at least two years, graduating two complete classes. The applicant school then completes a process of self-study before a peer team reviews the program with an on-site visit. The commission reviews the on-site report and makes a final decision on the school. Accreditation is a voluntary process.

Throughout the *Massage Therapy Journal, Massage & Bodywork,* and *Massage Magazine,* dozens of massage schools advertise their programs. See appendix A for the magazines' contact numbers. Also, a comprehensive guide, *The Touch Training Directory,* featuring over 800 somatic training institutions, can be viewed for free on the Associated Bodywork & Massage Professionals (ABMP) Web site at http://www.massagetherapy.com/careers/training.php. ABMP also has its own school accrediting agency, the International Massage & Somatic Therapies Accreditation Council (IMSTAC).

Another tactic is to attend one of the professional organization meetings held periodically in different cities on both the national and regional level. A number of the massage school owners and managers participate, often speaking in seminars or on panels. It's an excellent way to get to know them and see how they present themselves and their schools. You can also speak with other attendees and ask their opinion of the schools you have under consideration. Though growing rapidly, the massage community is still relatively tight-knit (Figure 3-1), and the reputation of each school is a matter of communal debate. Most people agree that certain schools are superior, and you should find out which ones they are.

During the several months that you are attending massage school, you'll be worshipping the gods of physiology, anatomy, technique, theory, and practice. Before you decide which altar to devote yourself to, consider the ALTAR factors (**a**ccreditation, **l**ocation, **t**uition, **a**dministration, **r**eputation) to see which school is best for you:

1. **Accreditation:** Not all schools are accredited by COMTA or one of the other accrediting bodies. Becoming accredited is a voluntary procedure, which many excellent schools have not had the time or desire to undergo

Figure 3-1 | Classmates in massage school often become fast friends. (Courtesy of Downeast School of Massage, Waldoboro, Maine.)

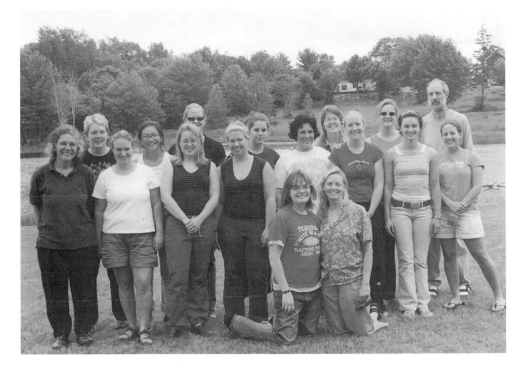

yet. However, most good schools are registered with local business associations such as the Chamber of Commerce or the Association of Vocational and Technical Schools. The key here is to look for how seriously the school takes itself as a business. As time goes on, more and more schools will become licensed, just like the trade schools in other professions. If your state does not yet have licensing for therapists or schools, check to make sure the curriculum will prepare you to pass the National Certification Exam (see chapter 6). You'll be assured of an education that will prepare you for work in the real world. For example, in Maine, to be certified as a therapist, you must either graduate from a COMTA-accredited program or have taken the National Certification Exam. To take the exam, you have to graduate from a state-licensed school—unless, of course, there is no licensing in your state. You can see how tricky this issue gets. Most important for you, before you sign up for school, dig deep and verify the quality and acceptability of the program you're entering.

2. **Location:** The school closest to where you already live will probably be the most convenient. Or, perhaps you are ready for a change and you are looking for the massage school with the most beautiful location available. I have one friend who moved from Florida to Santa Fe, New Mexico, just to attend the school there. In either case, you'll have to judge location along with all the other pros and cons. Do not immediately discount schools that are distant or in exotic locations. The most important thing is to find the match that is most appropriate for you, even if at first the location seems inconvenient. Then, once you have narrowed the field to a few schools where you really want to go, decide based on a full spectrum of factors, including the location of each.

3. **Tuition:** Is the school in your price range? Many offer financial assistance. Be sure to ask the enrollment officer. Sometimes, you get what you pay for in a massage school.

4. **Administration:** Are the people you speak with on the phone and deal with at the school's office courteous, friendly, and enthusiastic? If not, their sour attitude may point to deeper problems at the school that you would eventually uncover if you were to enroll. Also, job-placement assistance is an important factor to consider. Does the administrative staff offer meaningful aid to the students *after* they've graduated and are looking for work?

5. **Reputation:** Ask, ask, ask. Word of mouth is the best advertisement for massage schools, and it is the most certain way for you to come up with some important data regarding the schools you are considering. One school I've worked with is so confident in their reputation that they sponsor periodic "Massage Career Seminars," which they advertise to the general public. They invite outside speakers and even instructors and students from rival schools in the area to give a balanced picture of the local massage school scene. This is the kind of word of mouth that really matters. (See the sidebar, "East West College, Portland, Oregon," later in this chapter.)

A perfect match doesn't come easily. You may find that the teacher that inspires you the most lives in another state. Or, if you know of one school with a great reputation, it may turn out that it is too expensive. You'll have to weigh all these points carefully before making your final decision. Once it's finally made, though, you can relax because one of the most fun, memorable and transformative experiences of your life is about to begin.

Generally speaking, private massage schools founded and run by caring members of the profession offer in-depth, comprehensive, and spirited curricula. Also, more and more vocational institutes are getting on the bandwagon with massage programs and hiring talented individuals to run them; and many of the teachers at these schools are excellent, dedicated people. Private schools sometimes have better facilities and a more upbeat atmosphere—but, on the down side, they are generally more expensive. If price is a definite concern for you and you're determined to study hard and become a great therapist no matter where you get your basic training, just make sure to sit in on a class or two at the school of your choice and ask a few graduates their opinion of the program before you enroll. Also, make sure the school offers an officially recognized program so that you'll be able to use your transcript to obtain a license after graduation if licensing is required in your state.

Since the profession of massage therapy has been growing at such an astonishing rate lately, the number of massage schools has grown tremendously, too. As I've already mentioned, the vast majority of them are run by fine, upstanding people who invest their heart and soul in the business. But some are not. Several entrepreneurs, having spotted a trend and having decided to capitalize upon it, have set up schools with neither heart nor soul. You can tell which ones they are by the "assembly-line" feel you get when you visit them. They may be successful, and many of their students may indeed find paid employment after graduation. But ask yourself if you want to invest some of the most transformative months of your life in such an impersonal atmosphere. Ask yourself again why you've decided to go to massage school. If you really want to grow and become a new person with new skills, you will seek out like-minded, inspiring individuals to help you get there. The world of massage is filled with such people. When you find yourself in a classroom full of them, you'll feel right at home.

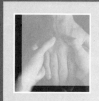

MASSAGE SCHOOL
A TRANSFORMATIONAL EXPERIENCE

A lot of massage schools are run by extremely professional, knowledgeable, giving, caring, fun, creative, adventurous individuals. Massage-school owners are some of the greatest people from many walks of life, people who care about other people and want to build their careers around that fact. In addition, the people who attend massage schools are usually at a very open, experimental, "humanistic" stage of their own lives. They are taking a time out from mainstream lives and typical jobs as bank tellers, law clerks, laborers, and receptionists. They are opening their eyes to new possibilities and new ideas, just like you are. Also, most of them have reached a transformational point in their lives, and enrolling in massage school was a pivotal choice. They are ready to make new friends. Often the bonds formed among class members last throughout a lifetime.

You'll learn more about your classmates than you would in most other school environments. You become vulnerable to each other because you are using your own bodies as the basic learning material of the class. Your tensions, your painful memories, and your injuries are exposed. Usually, any insensitivity is quickly observed and dealt with, which encourages all students to become better communicators.

Many students also have the shared dream of building a successful new business on their own. They will be leaving behind, perhaps for the first time in their lives, the security and routine of a regular salaried position. Or they may be just entering the workforce, still very young and filled with enthusiasm.

You'll learn more from the instructors and owners and other students than just massage techniques. You'll also discover more about what it means to be a human being. You'll discover more about yourself. In fact, the odds are very good that the experience you have in massage school will be one of the most memorable and transformative of your entire life. Once you've made the decision and taken the plunge, go for it all the way. Make lots of new friends, learn everything you can, open yourself to every available opportunity, and *enjoy* the transformation while you are going through it.

SETTING EDUCATIONAL GOALS

You may wonder how it is possible to have goals about your massage education before you've even been exposed to the core concepts of massage. For example, how do you know if you want to be a sports massage therapist if you're not really sure what that entails? Many people experience this same difficulty in deciding their college major. Probably the majority of students begin college without a clear idea of what their major focus of study is going to be. It is through living and growing that they come to know what is right for them, and they often change majors over time. Nobody frowns upon this ongoing decision-making process. Everyone accepts it. Why shouldn't you accept it, too. There is no need to judge yourself at an early stage for not knowing what you will want at a later stage.

In spite of the inevitable uncertainties that you undoubtedly have, however, it is still a very good idea to set some goals for your massage-school education. What should these goals include? What kinds of things should you be asking yourself and hoping for yourself? I'm glad you asked. Following is a list of the goals you would be wise to set for yourself when it comes to education. Of course, these are generic categories. You'll have to fill in the details yourself; and, to stimulate your thinking, I've included a few questions about each topic. Let yourself ponder these ideas and see where they lead you.

- ❋ **Occupation goals:** How do you want to be spending your time after you graduate? Does the school offer placement in a program that is particularly strong in one industry, such as the spa or chiropractic industries? If you can determine where you want to work, it will help you determine where to go to school. (See the next chapter, "Discovering Your Ideal Work Space," for more information on this.)

- ❋ **Revenue goals:** This is discussed at length in chapter 8, "Day-to-Day Realities." At this point, simply jot down some relevant information about yourself and your needs in this area. If money is not a big priority for you, you may do well in a school that focuses on the spiritual and clinical aspects of the work. If you are a born entrepreneur, you'll want a school that emphasizes business mastery, marketing, and success strategies.

- ❋ **Social goals:** After your education is over, how do you want to be perceived? What social status do you wish to attain? Will you be on your way to becoming a physical therapist? A doctor? Will you be content with a job as a therapist for the long haul? How will you wish to think of yourself? Some schools, through their clinical emphases, are better equipped to speed you on your way toward these higher educational pursuits.

✳ Friendship goals: With whom do you want to spend your time over the several months you will spend in massage school and then afterward? Who do you want your peers to be? You will find yourself among a much different peer group if you attend a basic vocational massage school in a big city center than you would if you attended an esoteric massage retreat in the mountains of northern California.

✳ Spiritual goals: As discussed in the previous chapter, many people find a deep spiritual satisfaction in the practice and sharing of massage. If this is highly important to you, you will want to attend a school that has a spiritual focus or at least a culture of openness to spiritual ideas. If daily life there is meditative and dedicated to the raising of consciousness, you may just find a home there.

✳ Aesthetic goals: Face it. Some schools are much more beautiful than others. And some are set in much more beautiful surroundings than others. If the environment is important to you, you may want to choose a school in a rural setting or in an urban area known for its beauty and outdoor draws, such as Santa Fe, New Mexico, or Portland, Oregon, or upstate Maine.

✳ Mysterious goals: All of the goals listed above will impact the final decision of where you end up going to school. Yet there is something else, too, something that is hard to say in words, something that will draw you to a particular place for reasons that you may remain completely unaware of for years but that are nonetheless overwhelmingly compelling. You may call it destiny. You may call it higher purpose. There is something waiting for you out there, and you know it; and, though you do not know at this moment exactly how to access this life-to-be, you feel strongly drawn to the next step. If that next step is attendance at a particular massage school, there is no power in the world that will keep you away from it. There is a quote I love by the poet David Whyte. In his book, *The Heart Aroused* (1996), he says, "The unawakened yet youthful soul within us is so entangled with the world and so physically alert, even in unconscious ways, to the tug of its own future, that it does not need to keep track of every detail in order to find its way in the world." That's right. When it boils right down to it, you are finding your way in the world. Massage school is simply a part of this larger process. Trust.

THE LEARNING TRAP VERSUS THE EARNING TRAP

There are two typical traps that you can fall into as you prepare to enter massage school. I call them the *learning trap* and the *earning trap.*

The thinking of "learning trappers" goes something like this: "I really want to make sure that I am ultra-confident and super well prepared before I get my hands on people who are actually paying me to massage them. It will take a long time, but I'm committed to making it happen and eventually I'll be out there working on people."

The thinking of "earning trappers" is more like this: "I'll whip through this program as fast as possible so I can get out there and start raking it in. Massage school is just a formality, really. I already know how to rub people, right? Let me at 'em."

You can no doubt see the difficulties with either one of these positions. On the one hand, learning trappers keep themselves locked in a cycle of perpetual preparation rather than doing. It is a mistake to get stuck in this permanent-student syndrome, thinking that you will never be good enough to ever begin earning a living at massage until you are the best therapist in the known universe and have written seven books on the topic. Becoming a good therapist is a process—and one that often seems, while you're in it, like a painfully slow and gradual one. You will be plenty prepared to give a safe, effective basic massage after completing your preliminary massage studies. In some areas, this may mean as little as a few hundred hours of education. Be realistic about your abilities, but don't sell yourself short.

On the other hand, don't make the mistake of thinking that you can just get out there with minimal skills and start "raking in the dough." There is too much qualified competition these days. Relying on your good looks, bubbly personality, or raw ambition will only take you so far.

The best path is to prepare yourself psychologically for a well-defined period of intensive immersion in your studies. This is not necessarily a bad thing. Even if you were not the greatest whiz in your past forays into the realm of education, you may surprise yourself at how well you do as a massage student. Being a massage student is different than being almost any other kind of student, as you will be able to engage your body as well as your mind in your education.

Thus, if you were the type who was always better on the playground than in the classroom, you're going to have more to work with in the massage classroom. Also, massage school is probably something that you have chosen to do, so you won't be as likely to have that reluctance factor that degrades so much of our formal education.

Remember, this educational process, like all things in life, is going to end. It is best if you start making plans for that eventuality well in advance. (See the following chapters for a little help in that regard.)

FACULTY VERSUS FACILITY

When you start your training, you will actually be entering two different and distinct massage schools, though they go hand in hand and reflect upon each other in many ways. One is the outer school—the physical facility, the building, the classrooms, the chairs and desks and windows and washrooms and carpet in the hallways. Massage schools inhabit an astonishingly wide array of facilities, each with its own unique charms and its own unique annoying qualities. Some of the massage schools where I have taught over the years include:

- A former boy's Catholic school (complete with itty-bitty urinals that you have to crouch down toward when you use the bathroom)
- A homemade houselike structure on a private lake in Maine
- A floor in a huge, multistory, downtown office building in Manhattan
- Several storefronts in strip malls in suburbs across the nation
- A former warehouse with long, meandering corridors going on forever and truck-loading docks out front
- A suite in a medical arts building
- An old, echoing discount store with classrooms separated by 40-foot-high paper-thin walls

There are doubtless many more examples of singular spaces presently inhabited by massage schools. This outer school will give you a certain feeling every time you step into it, a feeling that you should definitely take into account as you decide where to enroll. However, there is an even more important "school" inhabiting the same space as the physical school, and that is the one contained in the minds of the people who teach there: the faculty.

It is important for you to be able to look beyond the physical structure of the building into the hearts and minds of the people who will be imparting their knowledge to you within its walls. This is the real school.

During the process of deciding where to go to school, too many would-be therapists pay little or no attention to the teachers. I suggest that you, instead, get to know them a little. Have a casual conversation after sitting in on a class as a guest. This was particularly important to me when I first went to The Massage School of Santa Monica. One of the instructors there, Garnett, touched me on the shoulder, uttered a few words, and voilà! Like magic, my scapula released and I was hooked not only on massage but on that particular school.

Allow yourself to be wooed by the faculty as much or more than the facility. This emphasis on faculty can and should be extended to the owner of the school as well. As mentioned in the sidebar "Massage School, a Transformational Experience," school owners tend to be a pretty good lot, with much helpful information to share. I'd have to go one step farther and say that many massage-school owners (at least the ones I've had the pleasure of working) are among the most inspired and inspirational people you will find anywhere. You may even say they are on a mission. Look for one of these on-a-mission types at the helm of the school where you are applying and you stand a good chance of having a great educational experience, even if you have very little interaction with the owner during your tenure at the school.

STANDARDS

When you choose a school, you are also choosing a set of standards that you are going to live by while you're in attendance there. You will be wise to choose standards that will lift you up a little rather than let you down. What I'm saying is that you should not shy away from a school that seems, at first glance, to be a little more difficult or time-consuming or nit-picky than you may want. We all have a natural tendency sometimes to want to just slide along, not overexerting ourselves unless absolutely necessary. Massage school may seem like a perfect opportunity to loaf, frankly. I mean, what could be easier, right? Just sign up, then kick back and get a bunch of massages until graduation when you can bust out and start collecting the dough. A curriculum that includes hundreds of hours of anatomy and physiology, a strict attendance requirement, multiple written exams, and a hundred hours of hands-on clinic work may seem like overkill. After all, it's just massage, right? Think again, my friend.

Massage has become a very competitive field in the past several years, with oodles of people ready to outperform you in any number of areas, such as anatomical knowledge, advanced hands-on skills, and marketing ability. This is not the time to coast.

In my opinion, you want to look for a massage school that offers you at least the following standards:

- Five hundred hours of training (and more is better, though it is not necessarily true that *most* is the *best,* as attested to by the ongoing controversy in British Columbia, Canada, where the 2,000+-hour requirement for a massage certification has led some to claim the need for a shorter program for beginning therapists)

- A heavy focus on basic structure and function of the human body, with a faculty that really cares about your learning experience (which translates to "gives difficult tests and grades strictly")

- A structured learning environment complete with rules and regulations and hierarchies, even if this type of thing normally turns you off (some massage schools can be so informal that a certain lack of respect for the learning process creeps into the whole student body and staff)

- A broadly focused training that includes elements from both Eastern and Western models, even if one of these is not of particular interest to you, because it is important to understand the full array of offerings in bodywork even if you end up specializing in one particular form

- A good amount of community involvement, including work at local athletic events, trips to hospitals and spas, exposure to charity work, on-site professional work, clinical work, and relaxation work

- A high percentage (98 percent or higher) of graduates who pass the state and/or local certification exams

- A high teacher-retention rate, meaning that the faculty is not constantly leaving and looking for new opportunities elsewhere

- A good track record, which does not mean that those schools in operation longer are necessarily better than new schools (but in the case of a new school you should do a little research into the track record of the person who is starting it and the team he or she has gathered)

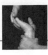
✳ Finally, a high admissions standard (meaning that admissions board members will tell someone who is not good massage therapist material that, in their opinion, the student would not do well there; and, though this may be scary when you face the admissions board, you'll feel better about yourself if you know you're living up to a certain standard right from the start)

Think of massage school as a new beginning and a time to start categorizing yourself as a new kind of individual, a person who holds yourself to the highest standards. The bodywork training institution you end up attending may not be in the Ivy League, but it may just put you in a new league. Take advantage of the opportunity.

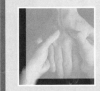

EAST WEST COLLEGE, PORTLAND, OREGON
THE ADVANTAGES OF ATTENDING A LARGER MASSAGE SCHOOL

The East West College in Portland, Oregon, is a large massage school that graduates over 400 students each year. The school had three campuses that were recently combined into one central 53,000-square-foot building, complete with an operating day spa that doubles as a training facility. I have taught several workshops there and knew the school was quite popular, but this really hit home when I was asked to speak at one of its graduations. My own massage-school graduation consisted of 20 or so people in somebody's backyard eating potluck dishes like bright yellow potato salad and shredded carrots with raisins. The East West College graduation where I spoke featured live music in a packed hall at the swank Doubletree Hotel. Energy was high. There were hundreds of shining faces staring up at me in rapt attention.

What could I tell such a crowd? What would help send these graduates on their way toward success in their massage careers? I decided to discuss the obvious differences between my experience and theirs, highlighting the advantages of their graduating from such a well-developed school with a robust program. So, after a thorough description of my own humble beginnings in massage therapy, I spoke of the ways that their big exciting school graduation would act as a launching pad into a big exciting new career. Standing there in front of that packed room, I found myself focusing on what specific things to appreciate about a large massage school. What makes it a good choice for your education? How do you know if a big school

(continues)

with a large student body is right for you? What's the difference between one big school and the next? How do bigger schools compare to smaller schools? I came up with these four points that you may find helpful:

1. Quality of education and interaction
2. Character and personality
3. A meaningful mission
4. Business savvy

Quality of Education and Interaction: There are plenty of good reasons to attend a smaller school: personalized attention, an intimate feeling, camaraderie, more access to faculty, closer affiliation between owners and instructors, and so on. However, if it is run right, a big school offers most, if not all, of these same benefits. Dr. Don Newton, director of education at the East West College, points to the students' pass rate on the NCBTMB national exam, which is 100 percent, while the national average for all massage schools is 75 percent. "Our hands-on bodywork classes are limited to 16 students," states Dr. Newton, "which allows teachers to give personalized attention to each student. Our science lecture classes are a maximum of 28 students, which is significantly smaller than many other large massage institutions."

So, what you're really looking for when you visit a prospective massage school is not so much the size of the building but the size of the individual classes and the feeling that you get while you are in them with other students and a teacher. You should also take a look at the nonclassroom areas that are devoted to students. The cafeteria and lounge areas, for example, are afterthoughts in many schools, even large ones. In some schools, students can wander long hallways, pass through capacious offices, and hear lectures in echoing classrooms; but, when it comes time for lunch, they're packed into a tiny room like sardines in a can.

Character and Personality: Since 1981 the East West College has been owned by David Slawson, and he now co-owns it with his wife Edie Moll. Edie has an interesting perspective on the business because she comes from a nonmassage background. For years she was a high-powered consultant to big companies in the midst of turnarounds and takeovers. To her, we here in the massage business sometimes look like aliens from another world. "The school's character," she says with a smile, "is definitely created by all the characters we have working here. I am amazed at the diversity of people involved in the massage profession. They're not here because they are making a bunch of money but because they feel that what they're doing is making a difference in people's lives and

(continues)

that the school as a whole is adhering to standards of excellence. In that sense, our large school is like a small one in that we allow the personality of each individual to shine through."

Business Savvy: When you attend a massage school, you learn not just from the instructors and not just from books but also from the environment itself. What the school practices, at times, will speak louder than the words it preaches; and just like a parent teaching her children through example, a school will teach you a lot about how to run your massage business by the way it runs its own business. This is a tricky point by which to judge a school because you don't really get a feeling for the school's business savvy until you've been there for quite a while. Students know, though. Make no mistake about that.

"Most schools are started by people with no business background whatsoever," says owner Edie Moll. "Whatever kind of school it is, there has to be a foundation of good business practices for it to sustain itself. . . . The industry is so new and changing that you have to be able to take risks, yet many massage people are risk adverse. Part of our job then is to help these massage students learn through experience what it's like to work within a dynamic, fluid environment. We're changing on a constant basis. For example, we are switching over to online registration because that's what students want. It keeps a big student body happy if you can add personal touches like quick registration and small classes but still offer all the benefits of a big organization, like a well stocked book store, discounts, extensive CE program, class schedule options, diverse faculty, federal financial aid, et cetera."

A Meaningful Mission: For a large school to retain its character and continue to offer the benefits students have come to expect, it must have a valid and meaningful mission statement. In the case of the East West College, it has blended these three components (quality education, character, and business savvy) into a mission that encompasses the entire massage training industry, not just its own institution.

"You have to make your thinking counterintuitive," says Edie Moll. "We try to be more inclusive than exclusive, and one way we do that is through our Massage Career Seminars."

Massage Career Seminars are something I know about personally. Edie has invited me in to speak at several of these events. The attendees are people interested in going to massage school in the Portland area. The interesting thing is that Edie has also invited instructors and students from competing schools to speak, leaving the format unscripted and all topics open for discussion.

(continues)

"That way," says Edie, " we're not just doing a sales job but educating people about what they can expect as they begin their exploration of massage. The whole voyage can be a fun one. Our teachers go out of their way to make the students remember and keep it interesting and interactive. It's all about the student, isn't it? You learn more about yourself than anything else in massage school. You learn about your own body and what you're doing to it and why. You learn about what's going on inside."

And that, in the end, is what matters the most, is it not? Be it large, small, or something in between, as long as the school has "heart" and focuses on what's going on "inside" of its students, then you will be getting the experience you seek from your massage education. As they say, it's all good. One thing, though: when it comes time for a raucous graduation celebration with hundreds of people packed into a swanky downtown hotel, those big schools are sure hard to beat!

THE IMPORTANCE OF FINDING A MENTOR

Massage therapy lends itself well to the traditional practice of mentoring, and this is a subject that is attracting more and more attention in the massage profession. In the same way that young interns learn from experienced physicians as they make their rounds through a hospital ward, you can pick up much valuable information by observing a longtime practitioner and opening a dialogue with him. By doing so, you will learn more than just techniques. As in all systems in which a new member becomes the "apprentice" to an older member, you learn about lifestyle, hardships, rewards, possibilities, and personal growth.

How can you find a mentor? It appears that, to recoin a phrase, "When the massage therapist is ready, the mentor will appear." You may find yourself seeking the counsel of one of the faculty at the massage school you attend. Or an established practitioner in your town may find time to share with you. Perhaps a supervisor at the first establishment where you find work as a therapist will give you some guidance. Or an article you read in a massage journal may inspire you to contact and seek out the author. You will usually feel an attraction or bond to your mentor without knowing why at first. Intuitively, you know that this person can offer you just the right wisdom and advice. Usually the mentor's technique and personality will be similar to your own, and you may think to yourself that you'd like to be in a similar position when you reach a later stage in your own career.

PROFILE: Ernesto J. Fernandez
Massage and Mentoring

Ernesto Fernandez has made a special study of the relationship between massage therapists and their mentors. His book, *The Healer's Journey: Transforming Your Bodywork Career Through Mentoring and Supervision,* is the product of several years of personal experience with mentoring in the massage field as both a giver and a receiver of inspiration and wisdom. He teaches workshops about mentoring for therapists and speaks to groups about the subject at conventions. He has conceived a vision in which a large number of therapists will be able to benefit through the mentoring process and peer group interactions.

"My original vision was to have therapists graduating from massage school get together and form peer groups with working therapists," states Fernandez. "I think there's a need for a network of support, especially for people who are just starting out. What I've discovered in my life, and through interviewing successful therapists, is that the one constant . . . was the amount and degree of support they had received. Bringing in the right advisers, both professionally and personally, helped them build confidence. The confidence was inside of them all along, but the energy and support of a mentor is what helped them to bring it out."

Fernandez stumbled onto this realization early in his career. "I was lucky enough to have several mentors early on," he says, "and it was a tremendous support. They taught me how to increase my skills and helped me to become more willing to take risks. Then, after my career had progressed for a time, I realized I still needed the support of a mentor but for different reasons. At different points I ran into blocks, and if I kept the problem to myself, it always took longer to work it out. By taking a risk and making myself vulnerable to somebody else (a mentor), I received immediate feedback and always sailed through the problem faster.

"After a time, I began to notice a shift. I was in a graduate program in counseling when other therapists began talking to me about their problems, and I started to mentor them. I found that everybody had different needs, and I made a few mistakes along the way, just like the people who had mentored me. It's not a perfect science; it's all about support and respecting each other's boundaries. Sometimes we traded massage work on each other, and at other times it was just a counseling relationship. Mostly, it was friendship and a meeting of equals."

"This is where a word of caution is advised. Often I found that the most gifted mentors had their own agenda

(continues)

and were actually out to create groupies or clones. New therapists gave up their power to them. It's an interesting situation because these mentors really believe in what they do, but sometimes they believe too much and it becomes dogma—that's a disservice to the person seeking guidance and also to the whole profession. This is where the respecting of boundaries comes in, and it's why I wrote the book—to plant the seeds to facilitate group processes and mentoring of equals by equals.

"I foresee a graduate-level peer counseling program in massage schools to help people integrate into the workforce and grow naturally into their roles as therapists. Many therapists have gravitated toward this idea and understood its importance, but the majority still haven't discovered the importance of mentoring and peer counseling. It's a whole new paradigm, and my role is to present it in a way that makes sense to them. That's the goal that led me to write *The Healer's Journey.*"

Excerpt from **The Healer's Journey**

Ernesto Fernandez has developed a list of six "Competencies" for the massage and bodywork profession, with some suggested group activities for each category that are helpful to engage in with mentors and peers. The following is a list of those competencies, with just

one of the many suggested activities from each, as excerpted from *The Healer's Journey.*

1. **Self-promotion:** The skills and ability to attract and generate new clients. Suggested activity: Demonstrate, practice, and receive feedback on your phone skills.

2. **Massage therapy skills and professional identity:** The hands-on technical knowledge and skills to effect positive change in our clients. Suggested activity: Share and receive the bodywork you need to maintain your body.

3. **Business management:** The administrative knowledge and skills of running a business. Suggested activity: Help each other with federal income tax and sales tax issues.

4. **Therapeutic relationships:** The human relationship skills to effect positive change in our clients. The application of professional ethics. Suggested activity: Debrief each other on issues that came up while working with your clients or referral sources.

5. **Social support:** Relationships and social activities that are recharging and supportive for the therapist. Suggested activity: Create and perform meaningful rituals for each other.

(continues)

Ernesto J. Fernandez (continued)

6. **Personal empowerment:** The knowledge, skills, and experience to perceive one's self and behave in a manner that is life-affirming. Suggested activity: Discuss challenges with prosperity, and practice exercises to improve your prosperity.

For more information or to order *The Healer's Journey,* contact Ernesto Fernandez at (813) 977-2832.

Conversely, the mentor will most likely feel a similar bond with you, or the situation won't be profitable to both partners. The mentor may see a youthful version of himself reflected in you and be inspired by the image. In any case, the relationship works as a two-way street and should always remain so or it will become unbalanced.

The best way to initiate a relationship with a mentor is by giving something, not asking for something. One natural gift to give is a massage, of course. Offer a free treatment to someone you think may be mentor material. Tell them you're doing so to get feedback on your technique and, frankly, to be in their presence and open a dialogue. I had the opportunity to offer Dr. Andrew Weil a massage at his home in Tucson once, and in return I got the honor of spending a couple hours with him and having a tour of his organic garden.

A relationship with a mentor may last just two hours, or it could last many years. If you come to the relationship in the spirit of giving and mutual exchange, you'll automatically be lifted up to a new level through the sharing of ideas, motivation, experience, and commitment. Finding a mentor is definitely worth the temporary embarrassment you may feel at first when approaching experienced therapists you don't know. Go for it.

4 Discovering Your Ideal Workspace

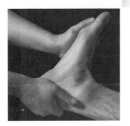

Now that you've seen what a dynamically growing field massage therapy is and you've determined that there is definitely a healer inside of you who is worthy of being trained as a professional at the school of your choosing, it's time to learn about the many different ways in which you can get started in the business. As the number of salons, spas, clinics, and private practices grows, so too does your potential to earn a respectable living working as a therapist. You'll need to be prepared, though; each work environment has its own set of duties and special requirements. This chapter is meant to familiarize you with the demands and rewards you can expect to find when you start your new career working in one of these settings.

STATUS: INDEPENDENT CONTRACTOR OR EMPLOYEE?

At many of the establishments listed in this chapter, you may have a choice of whether you'd like to receive your pay without deductions and without benefits (independent contractor) or as a regular employee subject to state and federal withholding, social security taxes, and possibly insurance and pension fund deductions. Should you remain footloose and fancy free or begin right away to create an established, secure position? The answer, of course, is up to you. Weigh the benefits of each option at whichever establishment you are applying to. And take a serious look at your own situation. How important is security to you at this stage of your life? And how important is freedom and flexibility? Remember, taking home more money and having more control over your schedule may feel better most of the time, but when April 15th rolls around and you have to pay Uncle Sam, you might wish you'd been forced to put away those tax payments after all. (See "Taxes" in chapter 6 for more information.)

Salons

Many therapists are forging working relationships with salon owners across the country. Often these owners see their competition creating extra revenue by offering massage therapy, and they figure out ways to include massage in their salon even if it means turning a closet or changing room into a massage room. At other times an enterprising therapist will approach the salon owner and suggest ways in which they can develop a working relationship, perhaps through a referral setup whereby the salon refers clients requesting massage to a particular therapist, and this therapist pays the salon a one-time referral fee. Usually these situations work out extraordinarily well; therapists feel like their own boss and yet have an ongoing source of new clientele, and salon owners have added value to their business. Salons and massage can be a perfect match. However, problems can also arise. I worked at a salon in Miami once, and as a result I ended up in the Dade County Courthouse.

It was partly my fault. When the salon owner called me to ask if I was interested in doing massage on his premises, I was flattered. He has one of the busiest upscale salons in town, and I knew him personally from a former association at a spa. It seemed like the perfect next step as I continued to branch out on my own. When I asked him if his salon had a State of Florida Massage Establishment License, he said, "Yes." Since I knew him and trusted him, I didn't ask that he show me the physical license; instead, I just took his word that it existed.

You guessed it. Mistake. One day several months later, after already building up a fairly affluent and consistent clientele at the salon, I received a call from an agent of the Florida State Department of Professional Regulation. "I need you to come downtown tomorrow," he said in a cold, ominous voice. "I can't tell you why." Click.

I was afraid. Had I done something that was going to get me in trouble? I spent the rest of the day in a depression, trying to figure out what that could be. The following morning, at the department offices downtown, I learned that the salon owner had lied to me—he had not applied for a massage establishment license, and I therefore was working illegally. "Cooperate," the man in the gray suit told me, "and we might be able to keep this off your record."

I ended up having to go to court and testify against the salon owner to keep my own good record intact, an experience that any massage therapist can do without. I was upset about the incident, but there was nobody to blame but myself. In those states that require a massage establishment license, it is *your* responsibility to find out that the license definitely exists.

All was not lost, however. As a result of the connections I made during just those few months working at the salon, I met some excellent clients.

Hospital/Hospice Work

Some of the most satisfying work you ever do as a therapist may not be for pay. In Miami, we are fortunate enough to have the Touch Research Institute at the University of Miami Medical School. This organization, run by Dr. Tiffany Field, a pediatrician and psychologist, conducts research in a clinical setting to prove the effectiveness of massage and allied therapies. At any given time, a dozen or more studies are being conducted. Subjects are tested for stress, blood counts, hormone levels, psychological profile, antibodies, and more. Then they undergo a series of controlled, codified massage treatments under the supervision of a study coordinator. The therapists who perform the treatments are all volunteers who receive no compensation for the massages—but the rewards are high on a spiritual basis. The institute's research is fundamental in proving to a skeptical medical community just how viable massage therapy is as a means for healing. In the future, their findings may be the cornerstone for a new paradigm in which massage is billed to insurance companies and used at large corporate headquarters as part of their employee wellness plans. This is already starting (see "Third-Party Billing" in chapter 6 and "Corporate Headquarters" later in this chapter).

I worked as a therapist for a number of Touch Research Institute studies. The experience was always rewarding on a personal level, and sometimes it was even good for business in a very tangible way. When a massive hurricane hit this area, we did a program for kids who suffered from post-traumatic stress syndrome after seeing their homes blown away. I also worked on a study for depressed teenaged single mothers and another for neglected grandparents. All of these experiences benefited me greatly in my ability to help varied types of clients. When I worked on an HIV study, however, the rewards were also monetary. Gary, one of the men who received massage from me in the study, liked the experience so much that he signed up as a paying client after the study was over. As a regular client, he became a boon to my business, and the continued massage helped his condition as well. The results of the study proved that serotonin levels, essential for aiding the immune system in its battle against HIV, were raised by receiving massage.

Some hospitals have massage therapists on staff, and the number is growing. Call your local hospital's personnel or human resources director to find out if positions are available. In many cities, organizations have been formed that offer free massage to hospital patients, especially AIDS victims, and people in hospices. Working in this setting can be one of the most fulfilling experiences of your life. Ask any therapist who's done it.

To find out about hospice or volunteer hospital work in your area, contact your local massage school, usually found under vocational/technical schools in the yellow pages. The telephone number for the Touch Research Institute is (305) 243-6781. They also have a newsletter available called *Touchpoints.* See the appendix for information.

The National Center for Complementary and Alternative Medicine at the National Institutes of Health is also actively studying the effects of massage in several clinical tests and compiling much data on the subject. They can be reached at (888) 644-6226.

Another resource that may be of some help to you if you are searching for work in this field is the *Hospital Based Massage Network Newsletter,* c/o Information for People, Inc., PO Box 1038, Olympia, WA 98507-1038; (800)754-9790; http://www.info4people.com.

Chiropractors

More and more commonly, chiropractors are finding a happy symbiosis by having massage therapists work with them in their offices. The two modalities go hand in hand. The usual way this works is for the massage therapist to spend a short period of time—20 minutes or less in most cases—working on the patients before the chiropractor performs the adjustment. This benefits the patients because adjustments of the joints are easier once the surrounding tissue is warmed up. It benefits the chiropractor because he makes more money and his patients are happy with the added level of service; and it benefits the therapists because it's a good form of income plus a way to gain experience in a clinical setting.

In some cases, therapists can earn a good living because the treatments they give are billed to the patients' insurance under the auspices of the chiropractor. A full day of 20-minute treatments can really add up. If you're lucky enough to find a chiropractor who shares an equitable portion of his insurance billing with you, the rewards can be substantial. However, in other cases, the chiropractor pays only a low hourly wage to the therapist and takes the rest of the profit for himself. It all depends upon the arrangement you work out at the commencement of your working together. Be wary of chiropractors who appear to have a thriving business but say they can only afford to pay you $7 an hour.

Another way to work in a chiropractor's office is to set up your own concession and perform full-hour massage therapy sessions. Many of your clients will come from the chiropractor's pool of patients, and you will compensate him for this, usually in the form of rent paid for the room you work out of in his office. Sometimes a per-patient referral fee is paid, as well. This arrangement is a little more daunting at first because it requires the massage therapist to put money out up front plus actively seek out a clientele instead of being supplied one. In the long run, though, the therapist may end up doing better with this scenario and feel a greater sense of freedom and self-reliance (see the profile of Julia Cowan in chapter 7).

The key here, as with all working situations, is *communication.* Start with a good understanding, work out the details in writing for both parties to sign, and you're likely to have a positive relationship.

Doctors' Offices

The situation here is similar to that in a chiropractor's office. The doctor will probably not have you work on as large a percentage of his patients, though, because many of them may not have musculoskeletal problems. With the right doctor, you can gain a large number of referrals and build up a loyal following quickly. If the doctor's attitude is not conducive to your success, however, you may find yourself struggling. Most physicians who include massage therapy in any way in their office do so because they personally believe in it. A few may be experimenting with massage because they've heard it's a way for them to bring in more revenue.

The phenomenon of "medical day spas" started in the mid-1990s and promises to keep growing. In these physician-owned facilities, a full staff of therapists, as well as aestheticians and spa technicians, work with the doctor, offering a more holistic approach to health and a more medical approach to beauty than previously available. The majority of physicians who own day spas are plastic and reconstructive surgeons. Many opportunities will be available in these spas, especially for people who have been cross trained in massage and cosmetology. See the section on spas later in this chapter for more information.

Offices, Malls, and Airports: On-Site Massage

Every weekend, somewhere in the country, another "on-site" massage workshop is being taught. On-site massage is performed at the workplace, at public kiosks in busy places like malls or airports, and in storefronts. The client sits in a special massage chair that supports the body's weight comfortably, allowing the therapist to effectively apply massage to the back, shoulders, neck, and arms. The client does not have to disrobe, which makes this form of massage especially attractive to shier clients and those without much time on their hands for a complete massage. See Figure 4-1.

On-site massage is growing rapidly. Several companies have already been formed to fill the public demand for this type of massage, and you'll find them in cities everywhere. The Great American Back Rub, for example, has opened several stores across the United States.

David Palmer is the man credited with starting the massage-chair phenomenon back in 1982 when he began giving on-site massages in the

Figure 4-1 | On-site chair massage offers many opportunities for the therapist to promote her business.

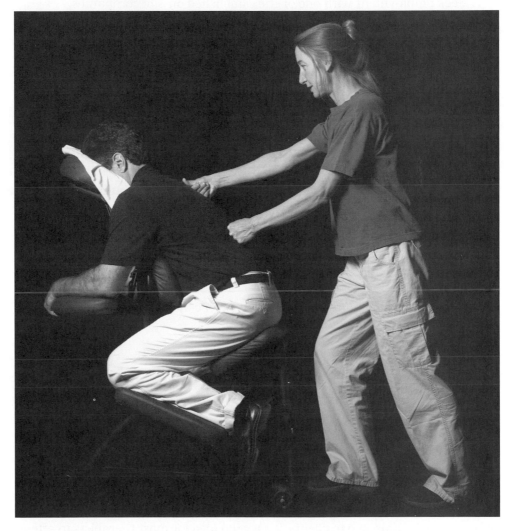

offices of Apple Computer Corporation. In 1986 he developed the first specialized chair to be used for this purpose (see "Equipment" in chapter 7). He also created TouchPro seminars to train therapists in the technique and how to market it. The Seated Massage Experience is another well-known seminar on the topic. See the appendix for details.

Many therapists use on-site massage as an addition to their regular practice. They find it's a good way to generate extra income and make contacts with prospective new clients.

There are several ways that you can work as an on-site therapist:

1. Seek employment with one of the established on-site companies.

2. Find work in a salon or day spa that offers on-site massage to its clientele in the lounge or waiting area.

3. Work in a spa or on a cruise ship that offers on-site massage to its guests. I trained therapists to do chair massage at a spa in Jamaica, and they offered it to guests on the beach.

4. Buy your own massage chair and offer your services privately in office buildings or similar settings. The price of a massage chair is similar to that of a massage table, so if you go out on your own, you'll have to make an extra investment up front. Some massage schools and retail outlets rent the chairs, which might make more sense if you are just beginning or experimenting with the idea of chair massage.

Some of the interesting places you can set up your own massage chair include:

- A health fair at your local mall, where you can pass your business cards out
- In the lobby of the salon where you work, to help entice prospective customers who haven't tried massage before
- By the pool at the country club or health club
- In a health food store
- At the farmers' market
- The waiting room at the chiropractor's office where you work

Regardless of the avenue you choose, or even if you don't think you'll be offering on-site massage to clients, it's a good idea for most therapists to attend one of the weekend workshops that will familiarize them with the techniques. You never know when the opportunity may come up to perform massage in this unique manner.

Corporate Headquarters

Some of the larger corporate headquarters have a health and fitness department on their premises. I know of two in Miami. Both Ryder and

Burger King have space that massage therapists work in. I'm sure there are other such offices in Miami—and perhaps in the town where you live, too. If you feel drawn to work for a particular company but want to retain the independent status of a massage therapist, approach that company and inquire about its facilities. If you wind up with a job there, it will be a good networking situation for future clients and you may meet people who can offer good business advice. If they don't already have a massage facility on the property, perhaps you can convince the owner to build one!

Private Practice in Your Home

This is the type of massage that most beginners envision giving when they are attending massage school—a separate space set aside in their own home, a sanctuary where people can come for peace and healing. The benefits of this type of setup are obvious and many.

1. You don't even have to leave your home to work.

2. You have complete control over the environment.

3. You make your own schedule, seeing as many or as few people as you like.

4. You keep *all* the money—no need to share the profits with business owners, doctors, or anyone else.

5. You have total professional independence, nobody to tell you what to do or when to do it.

This type of work is very tantalizing; and if you can manage to build up a private clientele quickly enough to support yourself, it may be the only type of work you ever need to do in order to make a good living as a therapist. Beginning therapists tend to overestimate their ability to build up a clientele, though, and it's probably a good idea to prepare for other types of work before relying solely on your private clients.

Also, there are a few concerns to be aware of when you're working out of your house:

1. You'll want to check the zoning regulations in your neighborhood. Many areas don't allow for the operation of a small business. Of course, this

may not be an issue if you simply see the occasional lone client. However, if you have a steady stream of clients parking on the street, traipsing up to your front door, and exchanging money for services inside, you'll want to check into any operating licenses you may need before a nosy neighbor calls the local authorities on you.

2. In some states, you'll need an establishment license. Check with the office that regulates massage in your state.

3. You'll have to keep records and pay your own state and federal taxes. (See chapter 8, "Day-to-Day Realities.")

4. In some cases, you may have a stranger come into your home.

Regardless of the challenges, many therapists still regard a private clientele arriving at their doorstep as the ultimate in a massage therapist's lifestyle. It's what they dream of, and they will keep working toward that goal until it becomes a reality. But until it occurs, treat all your other employment experiences as important learning tools, and you won't be overly frustrated if the dream doesn't come true as quickly as you'd like it to.

Private Practice in a Separate Studio

If you choose to lease or buy a space outside of your home for use as a massage therapy studio, you'll face certain challenges that you wouldn't face while building a private clientele at home. First of all, there's the expense. Leasing is not cheap, and you'll have to come up with a deposit before you can move in. Other expenses can include property taxes, utilities, repairs, and maintenance fees—on top of your monthly rent.

Why, then, would you want to go to the trouble to open your own massage studio? Some of the advantages are:

1. People will respect your professional working environment.

2. Some clients will prefer an office environment, and you can build a larger client base.

3. You can hire other people to work in the space with you.

4. You'll definitely be in compliance with zoning laws.

5. You'll have a place to "get away to" to do your work; and, at the same time, home will feel like a place of relaxation rather than a work/living environment. You may be able to divide your work life and home life more effectively.

Some people just plain like the idea of going to work, and they would be dissatisfied staying at home all the time. You'll have to weigh the pros and cons yourself before deciding. One way to help you make up your mind is to seek out a colleague who already has a massage studio and offer to work there part time. See for yourself how it feels to head into the office each day.

For more information about running your daily business in a massage office, see chapter 8.

Private House Calls

A popular option for massage therapists is the house call (see Figure 4-2). Many clients love house calls because they can receive the massage in the comfort of their own home, at their own convenience. Often this is the only option certain clients will entertain, especially more affluent clients. This is good for you, because you can charge the clients for the convenience; therapists usually charge more for house calls to make up for the time spent commuting and the extra money in gas and car upkeep. For example, during a period of several years, I charged my clients $50 for a massage in my studio and $60 for a house call. Some therapists add a slightly larger "trip charge" to their normal fee when they travel, asking their clients to pay an extra $20 or $25 for each trip, regardless of the number of massages given. So, if two or three people receive massages at one location, the trip fee can be split among them.

On the downside, you'll have to lug your portable massage table around with you from house to house in the back of your car; you'll spend more time in traffic; and you'll have to deal with clients' families, including their kids, pets, and other distractions. In spite of this, many therapists, including myself, enjoy giving house-call massages. I think I prefer it because I'm making the clients feel as comfortable and cared for as possible by taking the trouble to travel and set up my portable office at their home. Many clients have ended up as dear friends over the years, and they've made me feel as if I'm at my home away from home when I pay them a massage visit.

Figure 4-2 | Private house-call massages can be given outdoors.

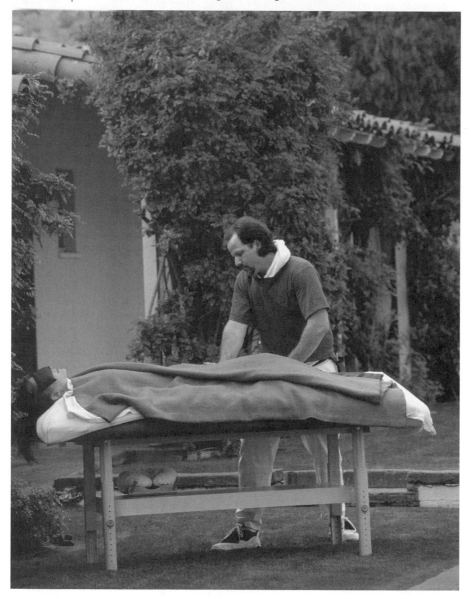

Chapter 4

Hotel Calls

To drum up business in hotels, visit some in your area and pass out your business cards and brochures. Usually the best person to speak with is the concierge. He or she is in charge of guest services and satisfaction. You'll usually be paid through the hotel's accounting department, and you'll be expected to give the concierge a tip. Make sure this tip is generous (in the $10 range each time you are called in for a massage) because the concierge usually has several other therapists on his or her list. Most hotels will prefer that you have a pager or cellular phone so that you can be contacted at a moment's notice. When one of their guests wants a massage, the concierge goes down his or her list, and the first therapist to answer gets the massage. The more quickly you respond, the more often you'll get work. Another good person to get to know is the hotel's meeting planner.

Some hotels have spas or fitness facilities on the grounds. For work in these environments, refer to the section about spas later in this chapter.

Be careful about the clientele in hotels; make sure they are ethical customers interested in therapeutic massage before you give out your business card with a home phone number on it.

Working for a Massage Network

Some enterprising therapists have started their own massage networks. They advertise a central toll-free number that customers or hotels can call directly. When a call comes in, it is referred out to an on-call therapist. Usually a massage therapist is guaranteed to show up at the client's door within the hour, so these businesses prize therapists they can quickly and easily get in touch with. After the massage, the therapist is responsible for turning in a specified percentage of the fee—usually 30 to 40 percent—to the network, keeping the rest plus any tips.

The advantage of this system is that the network does all the advertising for you and handles all the phone calls. Usually a network is quite good about screening customers. Some outfits tell all callers that the massage is therapeutic and nonsexual, just to clarify the point.

On the downside, you often don't know when you are going to be working; it's hard to make plans to do other things if you're waiting for your pager to beep, trying to keep yourself open for potential business. Plus, of course, you have to split the profits. Occasionally, there have been reports of unethical massage network owners who encourage their therapists to engage in sexual massage to increase business. Inquire about a network's reputation from therapists who have worked with it before you start yourself.

A SPECIAL FOCUS ON THE SPA INDUSTRY

I am writing this special section on the spa industry not just because I have been working in this field myself for the past 20 years but because spas represent for you the single largest source of potential job opportunities.

Oh yes, I can hear what some of you are thinking right now. "Spas? Me? No thank you. When I graduate from massage school, I am going to go directly to an outback third-world medical massage post where I will utilize my skills diligently to save the world within three or four years. Of course, it may take a little longer than that and I may have to upgrade my skills once or twice, but it can be done. At least I will be heading in the right direction and *not* wasting my time catering to rich housewives with nothing to do with their time except pamper themselves. That's not for me."

How can I know so precisely what it is that you're thinking? Because I thought the same exact thing myself when I was in massage school and we went around the room the week before graduation and everyone had to say what they planned to do with their newly acquired skills. I, like many of my classmates, was going to save the world and attain inner peace. When one woman said she wanted to work in a spa, you could hear an audible groan in the room, and I remember thinking, "I will *never, ever* work in a spa."

Well, here it is 20 years later and I make my entire living working in the spa industry in one capacity or another. The private clients I have I met through spa connections. I teach spa startup seminars. I write columns about spas for industry publications. I write books about spas. I hire and train new spa staffs. Life has become, for me, spa-centric. How did this complete reversal take place?

Of course, a lot of it had to do with money. When I graduated with my second massage therapy certificate (from the Suncoast School in Tampa, Florida—I needed more hours to practice in that state after moving there from California), I found myself looking in the want ads for a job. Any job. At that particular time in that particular place, the classified section was not what you'd call jammed full of ads looking for new massage graduates. So I was happy to see that the Safety Harbor Spa just 20 miles away needed people for the upcoming season. I raced over there in my beat-up Toyota with no air conditioning and got the job. I was paid $8 an hour for giving old-fashioned mega-oil 25-minute full-body rubdowns in a big room with 20 massage therapists working side by side. The octogenarian clientele loved to tell ribald jokes after stubbing out their stogies in the ubiquitous ashtrays found throughout the spa. If we therapists were lucky, we'd get a dollar or two in tips from each client, netting us a whopping $10–$12 per hour total. I used to give 13 of these full body massages per shift.

My, how things have changed. Almost all spas today are modern beautiful facilities, as shown in Figure 4-3. I now find myself jetting all over the country, giving classes, consulting, training, and covering events as a spa correspondent. I have even been a spa "secret shopper," traveling for free to top resorts, receiving luxurious treatments, and reporting on the service to management. It is quite a life.

As far as saving the world goes, I have tempered that zeal into something a little humbler. Now it is my mission to help the people I can help; and, as it turns out, the people I am equipped to help are the ones (perhaps you?) who are looking into spas and other possibilities to shape and advance their careers in massage therapy. I hope that by helping these people I am also helping the people they touch.

Spa Industry Growth

I am lucky to have specialized in a field that has been growing so rapidly over the past two decades, offering opportunity to so many people. Spas have experienced a huge mushroom cloud explosion kind of growth right up through 2003, and now it has begun to even out to a more reasonable level of growth that is still quite healthy. It is also more sustainable. An industry can't keep exploding forever or it will burn itself out.

Between 1999 and 2004, the spa industry saw a cumulative growth of 128 percent. That means that the number of spas more than doubled in this short time span. Total annual revenues are $11.2 billion dollars, which means spas take in more money than movie box offices or amusement/theme parks. That's right; spas are bigger than Disney World. In fact, Disney World knows this and has built several spas on its own properties.

As of June 2004, there were 12,102 spas with a combined total of 87 million square feet of operating space. Consumers make about 136 million spa visits each year. That's a whole lot of spa going. So, assuming that you come to peace with the idea of working within this industry (see the "Beyond

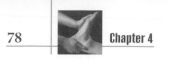

Figure 4-3 | Spas offer an incredible work environment! (Courtesy of Roosevelt Baths, Saratoga Springs, New York.)

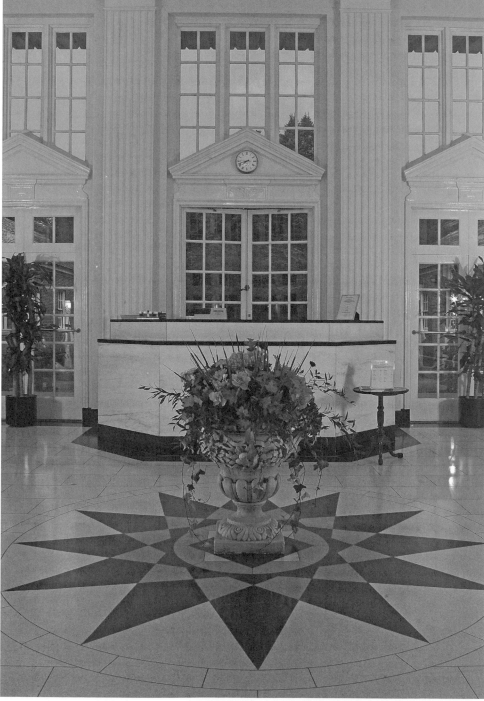

Pampering" section just ahead), it is here that you may find your best chance at building a good clientele quickly.

These statistics are courtesy of the ISPA 2004 Spa Industry Study. *ISPA* stands for International Spa Association, a group that has been around for over 15 years. The first annual ISPA conference was held in Miami, with 125 people in attendance. The 2004 conference in Las Vegas had over 3,000 attendees. Many people are wanting to get on this bandwagon.

Beyond Pampering

Let me just say it straight out right here. I hate the "P" word. When people utter the "P" word, all the high-quality work done in spas around the world by well-trained therapists using multiple modalities is completely negated. "Oh, you're going to a spa? How wonderful to be *pampered* for a day!" Yuck! I hate the sound of this. In my workshops, I playfully forbid the use of the "P" word.

It is of course true that some poorly managed spas have offered and continue to offer run-of-the-mill treatments given by uninspired therapists, but this is more a function of a lack of vision and training on the part of a particular establishment than it is an industrywide phenomenon. You may be tempted to think that the very nature of spas, with their time constraints and customer volume, is anathema to quality massage work, but you would be wrong. Oh yes, sorely mistaken. In actuality, it is through the vehicle of these constrictions that some of the best-quality work can be done, in the same way that high-quality artistic performances are created through thousands of hours of disciplined practice. One of the best ways to hone your skills as a therapist, in fact, is to walk into a room hour after hour after hour and perform one massage after another and to make them all different, all good.

The truth is that today many therapists are doing fine, nonpampering, therapeutic work in spas. Spa menus feature items such as CranioSacral Therapy, Thai Massage, Myofascial Therapy, Shiatsu, Reiki, Polarity, Trager, and others (see Figure 4-4). It is a great disservice to yourself, and to these skilled therapists, to refer to the work done in spas across the board as "pampering."

Even if you are performing a simple, body-exfoliation procedure in a spa, it is still possible to make it therapeutic, intentional, and deeply beneficial—even meaningful. What it comes down to is the quality of the work you are doing,

Figure 4-4 | Spas today offer advanced modalities and high-quality massage services. (Copyright Canyon Ranch. Reprinted with permission.)

CANYON RANCH SpaClub
AT THE VENETIAN
Las Vegas, Nevada

Menu of Services

	Tuesday through Thursday	Friday through Monday
SPACLUB™ PASSPORT		
• One day	$35	$35
• Three days	80	80
• Five days	115	115

A one-day SpaClub Passport is just $15 with purchase of any spa service (excluding the Salon) and complimentary with the purchase of any health & wellness service.

	Tuesday through Thursday	Friday through Monday
NUTRITION		
• Lifetime Nutrition Consultation 50 minutes	110	110
• Power Lunch 80 minutes	195	195
• Diabetes Meal Planning 80 minutes	160	160
• Healthy Weight Tune-Up 50 minutes	110	110
• Healthy Weight In-Depth 80 minutes	160	160
• Healthy Weight at Home 30 minutes	50	50
PHYSICAL THERAPY		
• Back Care 50 minutes	150	150
• Balancing the Body – Ergonomic & Posture Assessment 50 minutes	150	150
• Sports Injury Prevention & Treatment 50 minutes	150	150
• Physical Therapy Assessment for Orthopedic Problems 50 minutes	150	150
COMPLEMENTARY MEDICINE		
• Acupuncture 50 minutes	150	150
EXERCISE PHYSIOLOGY		
• Body Composition Analysis 25 minutes	50	50
• Basic Fitness Assessment 80 minutes	160	160
• Exercise for Weight Loss 50 minutes	110	110
• SpaClub Exercise Prescription 50 minutes	110	110

	Tuesday through Thursday	Friday through Monday
MOVEMENT THERAPY		
• Pilates 50 minutes	$110	$110
FITNESS		
• Personal Training 50 minutes	90	90
• Rock-Wall Climbing 25-minute individual	50	50
50-minute individual	95	95
• Team-Building and Private Group Exercise Class	fees vary	fees vary
SIGNATURE SPA SERVICES		
• Euphoria™ 100 minutes	300	310
• Canyon Stone Massage 80 minutes	245	255
• Canyon Ranch Mango Sugar Glo 50 minutes	150	160
100 minutes	300	310
MASSAGE THERAPIES		
• Canyon Ranch Massage 50 minutes	135	145
80 minutes	220	230
• Head, Neck & Shoulders 50 minutes	135	145
• Shiatsu 50 minutes	135	145
80 minutes	220	230
• Ashiatsu – Deep Barefoot Massage 50 minutes	150	160
80 minutes	245	255
• Canyon Ranch Sports Massage 80 minutes	245	255
• Thai Massage 50 minutes	135	145
100 minutes	270	280
• Neuromuscular Therapy 100 minutes	270	280
• Deep Muscle Soother 80 minutes	245	255
• Reflexology 50 minutes	135	145
• Hydromassage 50 minutes	150	160
• Aromatherapy Massage 50 minutes	150	160
80 minutes	245	255
• See the Difference 50 minutes	150	160
• Prenatal Massage 50 minutes	135	145
• In-Suite Massage 50 minutes	170	180
80 minutes	250	260

	Tuesday through Thursday	Friday through Monday
TWO-BY-TWO THERAPIES		
Prices listed are for two people with two therapists.		
• Canyon Stone Massage 80 minutes	$490	$510
• Shirodhara 50 minutes	340	360
• Ayurvedic Rejuvenation 80 minutes	490	510
• Aromatherapy Massage 50 minutes	300	320
80 minutes	490	510
• Canyon Ranch Massage 50 minutes	270	290
80 minutes	440	460
• Ultra-Moisturizing Treatment 100 minutes	590	610
ENERGY THERAPIES		
• Tibetan Bowl Healing 50 minutes	135	145
• Reiki 50 minutes	135	145
• Craniosacral 50 minutes	135	145
BODY TREATMENTS		
• MY Body Treatment 80 minutes	245	255
• Lulur Ritual 100 minutes	300	310
• Rasul Ceremony 50 minutes – single	165	175
50 minutes – per couple	290	300
• Royal King's Bath 80 minutes	245	255
• Sea-Estal 80 minutes	245	255
• Body Boosters 50 minutes	150	160
• Conditioning Body Scrubs 50 minutes	150	160
• Deluxe Conditioning Body Scrub 100 minutes	300	310
• Self-Tanning Treatment 50 minutes	150	160
CANYON RANCH BODY COCOONS		
• Cocoon 50 minutes	150	160
• Body Thermal 50 minutes	150	160

Rates and services are subject to change without notice.
Detailed descriptions of all services are in the SpaClub Guide to Services.

1039 – 12/04

the connection you are making with the person on the table, and *not* some preconceived notion of what is real massage work and what isn't.

Unfortunately, there are still some teachers in massage schools who have this "P" word mentality, and they infect their students with it unwittingly. I believe this attitude is a holdover from earlier decades when some spas were not much more than assembly lines for poor-quality massage work. Also, it is partially a factor of the "entitlement mentality" that some folks in the massage community share. Some massage school owners and faculty, either consciously or subconsciously, convey the message to their students that spa work is "beneath them" because it does not offer the same immediate monetary rewards as private practice or some clinical work. You will have to watch out for this when you are making the rounds at prospective massage schools. This attitude is definitely changing rapidly, and you will find it more and more rare to run into people who look down upon spa work. In fact, many massage schools are incorporating a spa curriculum into their core programs. I am writing a text on precisely this topic because there have been so many requests for it in the industry.

I hope you agree with me that spa work represents much more than just pampering. It is often high-quality therapy, and this becomes more true every day as the spa industry matures. There are, indeed, several distinct advantages to working in spas, especially when you are just starting out on your massage therapy career:

- ✻ You can quickly build a clientele with no overhead investment.

- ✻ You can develop your skills by working on a large number of "bodies" in a short period of time.

- ✻ You do not need to focus on anything else (marketing, products, rent, fixtures, equipment, and more), as the spa takes care of this for you.

- ✻ During slow periods, you can still work at the spa in allied capacities if you are a full-time employee.

- ✻ Employees receive benefits such as health insurance and 401Ks.

- ✻ You will meet a lot of interesting clients.

- ✻ You will enjoy the camaraderie offered by fellow employees as compared to working alone in a private practice.

- ✻ Often, spas will pay for your continuing education after you have worked there for a specified period.

Sharing the Profits

Spas employ nearly 300,000 people, most of whom are interchangeable to one degree or another with personnel in the hotel, restaurant, and fitness sectors; but *you,* my friend, are something entirely different and represent the single biggest asset *and* the single biggest thorn in the side for spa owners because without you the spa cannot exist yet you also receive the lion's share of the income at any given property. That's right. The amount of compensation paid to the hands-on staff in spas is the single most important factor in determining that spa's ultimate success or failure. This is because spas have to pay a huge portion of their income to the therapists and aestheticians. It may not seem like it to you, but it's true.

What I would like to do for you in this very short section on sharing the profits is to convince you that it is a good idea not to complain about your pay in a spa. Believe me, lots of therapists do complain. Their major line of reasoning goes something like this: "The spa owner is charging over $100 for this wrap I'm performing, but I only get paid $28 for the hour it takes me to perform it. That's not fair because I'm doing *all* the work!"

This kind of reasoning is immature, unrealistic, and the product of a pampered personality (and you know how I feel about the "P" word). Somehow, therapists who graduate with their few hundred hours of training believe the world owes them at least $50 an hour. In my opinion, you have to earn that level of income through disciplined application of your skills over an extended period of time. In my case, it took several years.

Yet, many therapists continue to make the mistake of somehow equating the cost charged for the service with the rate they get paid. Make no mistake about this—there is no direct correlation. I'll repeat this: There is no correlation between what a spa charges and what you are paid.

A spa owner is free to charge whatever he or she deems appropriate for a service in his or her spa. Just because the spa owner raises the price on a given treatment does not mean that he or she must therefore raise the amount paid to the therapists for performing the treatment. What you may notice is that your tips go up in the spa if the services cost more, because clients will be more likely to leave a larger tip for a more expensive service. The spa owner, on the other hand, is doing everything in his or her power to eek out some profit from a business that costs an arm and a leg to run. You will discover this for yourself if you open your own spa business one day.

If you end up working in a spa, do yourself, your spa director, the owner of the spa, and your fellow therapists on staff a big favor and do not complain about your pay. Instead, think in terms of sharing the wealth. Do the best work you can, and know that part of your efforts go toward supporting the receptionist, managers, spa attendants, landlord, marketing staff, PR experts, and everyone else it takes to make a successful spa. You are the lynchpin, the key, and your attitude will flavor the entire enterprise. An attitude of gratitude will serve the spa—and you—best.

Where to Work

There are a multitude of options today when it comes to working in the spa environment. No longer are you limited to the "fat farm production line" system of decades gone by. Your choices include destination spas, resort/hotel spas, day spas, cruise ship spas, club spas, medical/dental spas, and a private practice incorporating spa services. The following descriptions will give you a brief idea regarding what the work conditions are like in each of these environments.

Destination Spas

Destination spas are what many people think of when they think of spas. These are the Canyon Ranches and the Golden Doors, the facilities that are dedicated to the spa lifestyle and nothing else. They are, by definition, destinations unto themselves, and everybody who visits them is there for one main reason—health and wellness. These spas include accommodations; and all the guests stay overnight, many for a week or more at a time, in an attempt to make noticeable changes in lifestyle, fitness level, diet, and perhaps even state of mind.

There are 191 destination spas in the United States. That may seem like a large number to you, and it certainly represents a variety of choices when it comes to work environments, but you should keep in mind that these "queen bees" of the spa scene account for just 1.5 percent of the total. Statistically, you stand a better chance of finding work in the day spa sector, which is by far the largest in the industry. But, like many therapists, you may have your sights set on the goal of working in one of these premier facilities. I certainly did, and I found the experience to be quite rewarding.

The truth is that only a small percentage of the world's population can afford to stay for any length of time at a destination spa, which can cost thousands of dollars per person per week. The people who can afford it are often quite demanding, but they are also an interesting bunch. They've been around. They've been educated. They've made things happen, and they have been part of current events. Often, they are celebrities, industry titans, or well-known performers or sports personalities. It can be fun to get the chance to work with them.

Destination spas are likely to offer some form of benefits package, so you as an employee can enjoy perks like health insurance, paid vacations, and subsidized education. You'll enjoy the intangible benefit that comes with working at a prestigious address. Future employers will take note of your experience at one of these high-end facilities, and it will look very good on your resumé.

For these reasons, therapy positions in destination spas are highly sought after and not always easy to come by. If you have your mind set on working in a particular spa, make yourself as attractive as possible to your prospective employer by following some of the suggestions in chapter 9, "Creating a Professional Image." Apply at the beginning of the spa's busiest time of year, as many of these facilities are seasonal. Be persistent. If there are no positions available the first time you try, continue to hone your skills and then reapply the following season. Although the overall destination spa sector is smaller than some of the other sectors, the potentials for advancement here are greater as there are many paths to follow as you move up through the ranks at these larger facilities. This has happened to thousands of therapists, many of whom are now spa managers or even spa directors.

Resort/Hotel Spas

Resort spas are located within the confines of a larger resort facility where not all (or even a majority) of the guests are there for spa services or the spa lifestyle. These include the Marriotts and the Hiltons of the world, among many others. These days, a modern resort of any quality cannot be built without a spa if it expects to compete with other properties, and there are over 1,700 such spas in the United States alone. This creates another huge opportunity for therapists seeking employment.

Some therapists consider work in a resort/hotel spa as less desirable than a destination spa because the guests do not usually have the same dedication to health and wellness as do destination spa guests. They are there, most likely, on holiday, and the spa is referred to officially as an "amenity." You may rebel at the idea of working in an amenity, dedicating your efforts toward a goal that some guests dismiss as a frivolity; and it is true that the occasional guest will arrive on your table with nothing more therapeutic in mind than sipping another margarita and heading back out to the pool. However, an increasingly large number of travelers are becoming quite sophisticated about bodywork, and you may just run into someone who is looking for serious therapy.

The advantages of working for these large corporations are obvious. Many offer health insurance, vacation benefits, and even the opportunity for travel and/or relocation to another property. If you want to find work at one of these resorts, the normal procedure is to apply through the human resources department. While this is totally appropriate, you may give yourself a better chance at success if you also make a personal contact of some kind with the spa director or some of the other therapists. Interfacing with them at a job fair or at the local massage school, for example, is a good way to do this. There are some extremely nice resort spas around that, in fact, deserve to be categorized as destination spas, but they cannot be because the property also caters to nonspa guests. The Ojai Valley Inn & Spa in California is one example, as is Enchantment in Sedona, Arizona.

Day Spas

Day spas include those businesses that offer spa services but no accommodations. Guests come in just for the day. This type of spa is the bread and butter for thousands of therapists all across the land. There are over 9,000 of these facilities in the United States, and those are just the ones that can be counted. Countless other small places that perhaps do not meet the true stature of "day spa" nonetheless employ a great number of massage professionals in one capacity or another. Probably the majority of these practitioners are considered contract laborers, as compared to full employees.

It is completely up to you, of course, as regards what kind of day spa you would like to work in. There are fast-paced urban day spas filled with glitz and glamour and the sound of hair dryers whirring in the background as part of a big salon complex. There are day spa retreats in small towns and in rural settings, day spas in people's homes, bed and breakfast day spas, dude ranch day spas, clinical day spas in office buildings, strip mall day spas, and a hundred other kinds. They range from elaborate, multimillion-dollar facilities to one-room operations. So, how do you choose? Often, the decision is left up to chance, or fate, and that may be the best thing in the long run. For example, you may run into someone who is thinking about opening a small spa in a barn on her back lot and you work together in creating that goal; or you may speak to the owner of the salon where you have your hair styled, suggesting she may benefit by the addition of spa services; or you could go the traditional route and apply to an established local spa.

Some therapists use their time working at a day spa as an opportunity to build experience, widen networks, and work toward opening up a private practice of their own. While this may be a good idea for some people, you should also keep in mind that day spa owners will be more likely to hire dedicated employees who have the spa's best interests in mind first and foremost.

Cruise Ship Spas

Cruise ships are being constructed at a tremendous rate, and they're getting bigger every year. The record was broken again in 2006 with the launching of Royal Caribbean's 3,600-passenger *Freedom of the Seas*. Every one of these ships has a spa on board, and some liners are even slated especially as "spa ships." Many of the passengers are unfamiliar with massage, and a cruise is the first opportunity they have to experience one. This makes for some frustration among shipboard therapists, who would rather deal with clients who know what they are looking for. By far, the majority of therapists aboard ships are European, and they are used to dealing with customers on an "assembly-line" basis. I have known several U.S. therapists who became disenchanted quite quickly because of this atmosphere and because the massage rooms on board are usually smaller than those on land. Plus, they're rocking back and forth!

I'm not trying to discourage you from seeking employment aboard cruise lines; I am just giving you a realistic perspective on this somewhat romanticized part of the business. In a moment, I'll give you a Web site URL for the company that provides the spa concession aboard almost all the ships. They are actively looking for U.S. therapists, and opportunities aboard are very real. Several advantages exist to working at sea, and I'll list those, too. But first, consider a few more reasons to think twice before taking your massage skills out to sea: (1) cramped living quarters, usually with one to three strangers; (2) restricted access to many of the "fun" decks, where all the passengers hang out; (3) spending all your money in the crew lounge on alcohol, like everyone else does; (4) everybody knows everybody else's business; (5) very limited time allowed off ship in the ports; (6) greasy, unhealthy food in the crew cafeteria; and (7) the general feeling that you're a peon and a cog in the wheel of a gigantic floating hierarchical structure.

For these reasons, it's a good idea to go on board with a friend or a mate. I know one U.S. couple, both therapists, who did quite well as a team at sea; but even they were ready to jump ship after nine months.

In spite of the hardships, working the cruise ships can definitely present a fun and different opportunity for a therapist who possesses a chunk of free time and the ability to travel light. Some of the good points about working on a cruise ship include: (1) plenty of travel to exotic destinations; (2) adventure and new friendships with fellow crew members; (3) lots of experience under your belt, which is especially attractive to new therapists; (4) the ability to sock away some money in the bank if you're careful about partying and visits to the ship's casino; (5) short-term commitments, usually six months at a time; (6) meeting and networking with some wealthy, interesting passengers who may become important to your career back on land; and (7) escape from wherever you are now.

I worked on a cruise ship myself for seven months, but it was on a Windjammer Barefoot Cruises sailing ship, and I was a deckhand. Several years after that experience, I was working at a spa in Miami and I happened to massage the owner of Windjammer, Captain Mike Burke. He offered me the opportunity to go aboard for a one-week cruise, gratis, in exchange for massaging his passengers. This points to another possibility for therapists with an entrepreneurial spirit: Actively seek out business owners (especially owners of exotic sailboat cruise lines!) who may be willing to trade for your services. You'll discover several opportunities for cut-rate vacations this way. (For more about bartering massage, see chapter 8.)

Here's that Web site URL. If you're interested in employment on the cruise ships, visit http://www.steinerleisure.com. Good luck!

Club Spas

Many larger health clubs, wellness facilities, YMCAs, training centers, and gymnasiums offer massage to their clients; and some have even incorporated a spa environment into their facilities, complete with body wraps and facials. These can be good locations for a massage practice. On the upside, you have a constant stream of potential clients coming through the door, most of whom are aware of their bodies and have sore muscles on a somewhat regular basis. They are quite likely in need of massage. The trick in health clubs is to get people to *realize* that they need the massage. For many unaccustomed to the "luxury" of massage therapy and spa services, the idea of actually paying for one doesn't often enter their minds. They'll walk by you a thousand times on the way to the treadmills and the weight machines, figuring that your livelihood is assured by fellow gym members who have more disposable income.

The key at health clubs is education. The therapists who do well are aggressive in their marketing, often setting up signs and posters offering special deals, especially when they are first beginning at a club. Some offer free demonstrations, lectures, or seated chair massages in the entryway, juice bar, or some other well-trafficked area.

Each club has its own arrangements as far as payment goes. That depends on the owners. Some of the best opportunities come at new clubs or at established clubs that have just recently decided to add massage services or a full-fledged spa to their repertoire. If you get in at just the right time and impress the owners sufficiently, you may be able to set up a *concession* for yourself—renting the space for a certain amount and hiring your own therapists to work for you, keeping a piece of the action for yourself.

On the downside, most health club architects don't appear to be aware of or sensitive to the specific needs of a massage space. Either the treatment room is tacked on as an afterthought in an unventilated cinder-block closet or it's sandwiched between the locker room and the aerobics studio, with pounding music seeping through the walls on both sides. If you're the type who can take a challenging environment and make it work to your advantage, this scene may be for you.

An optimistic note: Recently, the trend seems to be toward providing better and more well-thought-out rooms for massage and spa treatments in some of the newest upscale health clubs and university wellness centers. If you can land a spot in one of these, you may find it a bit cushier than what therapists have had to deal with in the past.

Medical/Dental Spas

I recently attended a medical spa conference in Miami and sat in on a discussion that featured dentists and doctors debating the merits of medical spas. During this discussion, one thing became clear very quickly. Medical spas are big business. In fact, with 471 facilities and a 45 percent annual growth rate, they represent the hottest segment of the overall spa market.

There is a debate regarding what a "medical massage therapist" really is, and you may think that would have some bearing on your chances at landing a job at a medical spa. But that is not necessarily the case. Those therapists who practice medical or orthopedic massage often end up working in more clinical environments. For the most part, what the doctor/owners of medical spas are looking for are therapists who can work with their patients to perform top-notch relaxation and restorative therapies. They need therapists who are good "people people," with excellent bedside manners and the ability to put patients at ease through their touch and their presence. Also much in demand are practitioners with abilities in more than one area, such as those with training in massage therapy and aesthetics or paramedical aesthetics.

If the trend can be judged by the level of enthusiasm exhibited by the attendees at that recent spa show, it looks like dental spas will be the next big thing, even bigger than medical spas. Why? Believe it or not, spas and dentistry seem to be a natural fit. Most people associate a trip to the dentist with painful or unpleasant procedures. By incorporating a spa environment and simple spa procedures, dentists can calm some of the apprehension that often accompanies these procedures. "It's a natural fit," says Susie Ellis, president of Spa Finders. "People are eager to trade some of their anxiety for the relaxation that spa services and a spa environment can offer."

Private Practice Incorporating Spa Services

Many therapists are finding that they prefer the flexibility and independence of a private practice but still want to benefit by the popularity of spa services. For these individuals, offering spa services in their massage rooms or even taking spa services into the homes of clients is an excellent option. (See the profile of Kara Mathenia.)

PROFILE: Kara Mathenia
Spa Specialist

Kara Mathenia of Sonoma, California, has developed a unique way to add value to her service as a massage and spa therapist. She brings the spa to her clients' homes during out-call visits, and she has created a minispa environment in her own home for clients who visit her there. With the help of some lightweight equipment, she provides spa treatments as well as traditional massage. To create luxurious moist heat, for example, Kara uses the Steamy Wonder—a little domed nylon tent that fits over the massage table and holds in the steam generated in a small unit on the floor.

Kara now feels that the biggest challenge massage therapists face is knowing how to set boundaries about how much and when they will work. "At one point I found myself working seven days a week, eight- to twelve-hour days," Kara says. "This is not the type of work in which you can do that. It takes a real toll on the body."

Having too much work was not always Kara's problem, though. As with so many therapists, first building up a successful business was a challenge. "I had moved to a new town and was working for the local newspaper selling advertising. I liked my job but knew it wouldn't be a fulfilling long-term career. At that time a girlfriend took me for a surprise massage at a school in the Berkeley area. I was so impressed with the school and the quality of the massage, I inquired about becoming a student. With help from a student loan I finished massage school while still working at the paper. It was hard for two years. I worked part time selling ads, part time at a spa, and built my private practice, as well. Then I worked mostly at the spa for a time. Now after five years I've been able to leave the spa and work completely on my own, and it's great. I have all the private clients I can handle!"

Spa treatments are usually easier on the therapist's body than a full hour of giving massage. The minor cost of certain spa supplies can be figured into the price of the treatment. And people absolutely love to be cared for and nurtured in this luxurious way right in their own home!

It is not overly difficult to take spa equipment and supplies with you on house calls. These items weigh no more than a massage table and include a heating unit such as a hot towel cabbie, a roaster or small Crock Pot™, several extra towels, body muds, scrubs, and seaweeds. Performing these services in your own massage room is even easier because you won't have to transport any supplies. In fact, there is a growing number of therapists who consider it essential to offer at least some basic spa services to their clients. Of course, in order to offer these spa services, you will need to be trained in the appropriate modalities. Many therapists get this training while on the job at a spa, but you can also take spa training classes on your own (see the appendix for training options), and a growing number of massage schools are offering spa curricula as part of their program.

You may think that offering spa treatments to your private clients (and charging those premium spa prices) is a way to enjoy the best of both worlds. On the one hand, you retain your autonomy; on the other hand, you reap the rewards of the spa boom. It almost seems too easy, doesn't it? Hmmm . . . as in all areas of life, if it seems too easy, there is probably something wrong with the picture. In this case, you have to be aware of the effort it will take to switch clients over to the thought of home spa services or massage-office-based spa services. They are used to the idea of going to an actual spa for their body treatments, and there are many good reasons for that. Spas are great. People love spas. It's a special treat for them to go to one. So, you have to be prepared to offer something special, to create moods, and to meet expectations when you attempt to bring the spa experience to your clients directly. It is not enough to simply bring some sea salt along and rub it into their skin. See chapter 7 "Creating the Perfect Space," to get some more ideas in that regard.

Opportunity in the Spa World

There are perhaps more opportunities for therapists in the spa industry than in any other. Because of its rapid growth and the need for qualified personnel to fill the positions created along with that growth, the industry is always experiencing a void at the top, a void that is often filled with folks who move up from within. If you have hands-on skill and the understanding of clients that comes with it and you have even the tiniest bit of organizational capability, you may find yourself rising quite rapidly into a position of leadership.

This is exactly what happened to me. Within two years of starting at a large destination spa in Florida, I was the supervisor in charge of the entire massage and spa treatments department. I found that I did not particularly like management tasks, but I loved the training aspect of the job; so, over time, I evolved a position that included more training and less paperwork. There are so many niches in this market today that each therapist can find a role suited to his or her particular strengths and proclivities.

So, how do you prepare yourself for this rapid-advancement track? What political games must you play? Whom should you get to know? My advice is to be yourself and to develop those skills that make you most satisfied in your job situation. There are many ways to fit into this varied industry and make a meaningful contribution. Why not be happy while you're doing it?

A SPECIAL RESOURCE FOR JOB SEEKERS

If you are looking for a job as a massage therapist in the fast-growing spa market, there is a Web site made especially for you. Called *BestSpaJobs.com,* this site lists both employers looking for therapists and therapists available for employment. It can prove invaluable, especially if you are someone who is looking for a little adventure and willing to relocate for a new position. Visit the site for postings, advertising, and further information: http://www.bestspajobs.com

JOB INTERVIEWS AND TEST MASSAGES

I have received over a hundred test massages from therapists applying for jobs at spas where I was in charge. The dynamics of this particular situation are quite unique. There I am, lying on the table, trying to relax, and the therapist is trying to relax me; but at the same time, we both know that a job is at stake, so we're both slightly tense. The therapist wonders how I'm feeling, and I wonder if I'm receiving the therapist's best work.

A massage is a very personal offering, like an artist's painting or a writer's story. The test-massage recipient never wants to criticize the person giving the massage, only specific techniques if necessary. He or she has to be at least partially critical to hire the best staff for his or her business. There's always going to be a little tension in this situation. It's unavoidable. However, there are certain tips you can follow to make the experience as painless as possible—and hopefully help land you a job, too!

Tips for giving a test massage are:

1. Forget that it's a test massage if at all possible.

2. Remember all the basics: Wash your hands beforehand, use proper draping, inquire about sore areas or physical problems, respect boundaries, be polite.

3. Dress similar to the therapists who work at the establishment where you're applying.

4. Give an entire massage if it's requested. *Don't* say, "Well, it's been five minutes. You must know if you like me by now. Do I have the job or not?"

5. Use conversation sparingly. After the first couple minutes, only respond to the interviewer's remarks instead of talking first yourself.

6. Only give a test massage if you're already confident and comfortable with your technique. This is not a time for practice.

7. At the end of the massage, step quietly out of the room and wait. *Don't* ask how you did.

8. When you say good-bye, shake hands firmly. Looking your interviewer straight in the eye, smile and say, "Thank you for this opportunity." Then leave your resumé and business materials behind and walk confidently out the door as if you had already gotten the position.

9. Remember that if this is the first test massage you've given, the next one will be much easier.

TALES FROM THE TEST-MASSAGE TABLE

Being the recipient of a test massage is not always fun. In fact, it can be quite stressful. Over the years, as I've received test massages at various spas, I've learned some lessons the hard way about what it takes to get hired—and what will certainly keep you from getting hired. Here are three instances that may give you some insight into what it's like to be on the other end of the test massage:

1. I received a test massage from a young blind Indian man from Peru. He came to the grand luxury spa wearing a colorful poncho, a white cane extended before him. My heart went out to him for his bravery and self-confidence. He did not speak much English, and he had taken an hour-long bus trip alone to arrive at the spa. I knew that in Korea, for example, the majority of professional therapists are blind. And I thought we could make it work at the spa. I truly wanted to offer him a job. Eagerly, I awaited his touch. But when he finally started the massage, it was horrible, fumbling, and amateurish. As much as I wanted to help him, it

(continues)

would have been a disservice to the spa's clientele to hire him. Regretfully, I had to suggest that he practice more, improve his skills, and perhaps come back in the future. I never heard from him again.

2. One young man came back twice to give a test massage after failing to secure a position the first time. The only reason he received a second chance was because he had a friend who already worked at the spa. During the second massage, as he had in the first, the fellow banged my limbs around without skill, sometimes even smashing my own hand into my face, causing discomfort. I should have listened to my own better judgment rather than go through another experience that was painful to both of us.

3. One job applicant gave me a very proficient, enjoyable massage. In fact, it was almost too automatically good. And during the massage he spoke the whole time about how he had worked at so many spas that he was really not that inspired about the work anymore. It was obvious to me that he wanted to move on to the next phase of his career, and he was holding himself back by doing what came easy. Our spa guests wouldn't have received the best service from someone with his attitude. Still, when I declined to offer him a position, he phoned me and sent me an angry letter, questioning my skill as a manager.

WORKING WITH MASSAGE THERAPISTS: A MANAGER'S GUIDE

If you think that one day you may end up as a salon or spa owner, the manager of a doctor or chiropractor's office, or the director of a destination spa, you may receive the singular opportunity of working with one of the most truly unique groups of people to be found anywhere on the planet—unique and, at times, difficult.

Massage therapists taken as a group have a tendency to be a little on the demanding side, viewing themselves not so much as technicians as performers. They are artists, magicians, and channels of healing energy who really cannot be disturbed by the mundane realities that you, unfortunate one, have to deal with on a daily basis. Yet, even though they may seem "airy" or "on another plane," you'll find that when it comes to receiving their paycheck or getting the schedule they want, somehow they manage to come back to this plane very rapidly, and they will let you know in no uncertain terms how displeased they are with you if you haven't made them utterly happy.

In addition, some therapists are under the illusion that, somehow, they are members of the one group that does not have to pay their collective dues and climb the ladder of success. They expect to be earning top dollar immediately out of school. Exactly why this sentiment has been promulgated is not entirely clear, but rest assured that if you find yourself managing a group of 7 or 12 or 45 therapists, you will run head on into this mindset.

So what can you do if you find yourself in charge of other therapists? I'll offer some advice from my own experience and that of others I've known who faced similar challenges. At one point for over a year, I was the manager of approximately 40 massage therapists at a large spa in Miami. During my term as a manager, I learned a few secrets that will help you deal with your own staff. These ideas have been echoed by fellow managers and owners I've known over the years.

1. **Be distant but kind. Be kind but distant.** Therapists are often party animals, especially the younger ones, and it's a good idea to be on friendly terms with your staff socially. But there is a line that should be drawn. Your authority should be soft and compassionate, yet undisputed. Show the staff that you are totally committed to them by winning concessions from the owners, investors, doctors, or whoever it is who holds the purse strings (even if that someone is yourself), and you'll have a group of people staunchly on your side. Then when you have to do something that's unpopular, they'll respect you for it and know it's a necessary responsibility.

2. **Try to be one of them, even if you're not.** At the very least, take a one- or two-day course in the basics of massage therapy and show your employees that you have an interest in their work—in its sublime aspects as well as its mundane realities. They'll appreciate it if you have at least heard the terms "energy work" or "deep muscle therapy." And they'll feel that you care if you demonstrate an understanding nature about choices in oils, creams, sheets, and tables. Therapists take their lingo and the tools of their trade very seriously; and you should, too.

3. **Be fair.** Most facilities with several therapists on staff have instituted a "seniority" system that rewards employees who have worked there the longest by giving them first choice in hours, rooms, clients, and the like.

Although this may be the easiest way to offer an incentive to stay longer with the company, it's often not the most effective way to keep the best therapists. What if, for example, you hire someone who turns out to be absolutely top notch and guests clamor for her services, but you can't give her the hours she deserves because several other therapists have been working there longer?

Eric Chesky, spa director at a first-class resort in Napa Valley, California, has one possible solution. Instead of working with a strict seniority system, Eric factors in the variables of guest feedback and employee attitude. Every time guests receive a massage, they fill out a quick form, and employees are reviewed by management on a bimonthly basis. Their ranking then changes periodically, and the most popular, hardworking therapists with the best attitudes are rewarded.

I used a similar system at the spa in Miami. Once your employees get over the initial shock of its implementation, you may find yourself with a more cooperative, dedicated staff. Don't worry too much about those therapists who complain and bemoan their fate if you try something like this. They are probably the lazier ones, content to rest on their laurels or their longevity. They probably need the stimulation. Besides, it's the customer who is number one, after all, and the customer's satisfaction counts more than anything.

4. **Consider encouraging friendly competition.** Offering a prize or monetary reward to the therapist who garners the most guest compliments works well at times. Therapists soon learn that soliciting positive feedback forms usually backfires. The ones who do the best job inspire guests to write without being asked to. If product sales are involved in your facility, offering rewards above and beyond whatever commissions are earned is good way to keep employees motivated.

5. **Encourage continuing education.** One of the best things you can do for your massage staff—and something that's sure to be greatly appreciated—is to provide some type of advanced education for them on premises. Most therapists have to take continuing education to renew their license, and they enjoy this aspect of their careers. If you can sponsor a popular trainer to come give a workshop after hours, you'll be helping your staff fulfill a professional requirement, upgrading the skills offered to your clients, *and* building good will among everyone involved. It's certainly worth the investment.

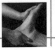

WHEN CLIENTS ORIGINALLY MADE IN YOUR BUSINESS ARE CO-OPTED BY YOUR THERAPISTS

If you own a business that offers massage to a local clientele, you should be prepared for the eventuality of your hired therapists going to a client's home and offering private sessions. As much as you may want to avoid this reality, it *is* going to happen, as experience has shown time and again. Often the practice is tolerated but never spoken of. In most spa and salon environments, for example, managers know that their therapists occasionally do house calls for their clients, but they turn the other way and pretend it's not happening. Some businesses even have their therapists sign a noncompetition agreement. This makes things uncomfortable for guests and therapists alike, who have to surreptitiously exchange phone numbers or business cards while nobody else is looking.

You can offer strict rules against the practice, but they are usually counterproductive and serve only to foster a hostile work environment for everyone involved. It's better to face the facts; if your therapists are the best around, your clients will call on them when they want a massage in their own homes. It's better to keep the best therapists instead of forcing them away from you by restrictive work policies.

A more positive and realistic approach, in my opinion, is to actually encourage therapists to work privately with clients. It may hurt at first, when you see that income going out the door, but in the long run the practice will pay off both in customer and employee loyalty and morale.

Many customers will keep coming back to your establishment for massages, as well, especially if you make them comfortable by not frowning upon private house calls. Help create an environment in your facility that they want to return to. Entice them with services that therapists don't usually offer at home, such as steam, sauna, hair care, wrapping, and others.

5 | Massage Clients: Finding Them and Treating the Whole Person

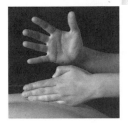

The time may come in the near future when you will meet a woman for the first time and be able to know, just by looking at her, how she is feeling inside her own body. For many massage therapists, no words need be spoken for this empathetic bond to begin forming. Your hands become sensors to other people's pain; your fingers immediately fly to the problem areas and sore spots of your clients—and even those of people whom you meet in more casual environments.

This happens to many people as they gradually develop their intuitive skills along with their proficiency in massage techniques and maneuvers. This phenomenon has to do with question number 2 in "The 10 Traits of a Born Therapist" at the beginning of chapter 2: Do you feel sympathetic pain someplace in your own body when someone else tells you about his or her own pain?

Physicians have experienced the same phenomenon. Even though most of them want to be known as "scientific" and "unbiased," and they carefully avoid any suggestions of this "hocus-pocus" from their dealings with patients, many have reported experiencing sympathetic pain or an intuitive awareness of their patient's condition without the need for any verbal communication whatsoever.

The truth is, we are connected to each other. All human beings have the potential to become empathetically aware of their environment and of the other people in it *if* they take the time to slow down and *focus* on that environment. When you study and practice massage, you have no choice but to slow down and become acutely aware of those around you, especially the ones who end up on your treatment table. This focusing of attention on other people is what helps cultivate an intuitive awareness of their pains, discomforts, and states of mind.

You will relate to your massage customers in ways that you've never related to any other people before. You'll form bonds with them that you never experienced before. You'll enjoy a depth of communication and understanding that you perhaps had forsaken as you grew older and found fewer and fewer opportunities to spend quality time with others. Massage is quality time, an hour at a time, time after time; and your customers will become a big part of your life, for better or for worse. For many beginning therapists, one of the trickiest parts of starting out in their new careers is finding the right balance between personal and professional relations, between giving all that they've got and holding something back for themselves.

My intention in this chapter is to help you happily and successfully integrate this new circle of clients, friends, and acquaintances into your life. I'll show you how to find your clients in the first place; how to act when you first make contact with them; and how to maintain harmonious working relationships with them, forming well-stated boundaries when necessary. I'll also discuss several special types of clients and how to deal with them.

CLIENTS—WHERE TO FIND THEM

Many beginning therapists make the mistake of thinking that massage customers are going to magically materialize from surrounding neighborhoods and city streets, as if irresistibly drawn by the therapists' newfound skills and healing powers. You may recognize yourself as someone who is counting on a certain undefined personal magnetism to attract clients. While highly developed skills and a galvanizing physical presence may indeed help solidify your reputation, very few people are going to know about these qualities unless you *do something* to let them know.

Action is the key word here. A systematic, organized plan is what it will take to really get you up and going as a therapist. Let's start with those potential clients who will be easiest to approach first, the ones who will most naturally be interested in hiring you as you begin to develop your career. These include: (1) family and friends, (2) other people you already know, and (3) people you could easily get to know if you tried.

Family and Friends

Let's face it, the easiest people to approach when you first start selling yourself as a massage therapist are those who already care for you as a person. In fact, if you're like most of us, in the beginning you won't be "selling" your massages at all but, rather, giving them away. This is a good practice while you're still in school, but don't give away free massages to too many people outside your immediate circle of friends and family or they may never be willing to pay you real money once you're a professional. A good guideline to follow is to offer one free massage per customer when you're a student or recently graduated.

Keep in mind that in those states where licensing is required (see chapter 6 for a list), it is illegal to accept money for doing massage without a license. Even in other states where licensing is not an issue, practicing professionally without an official school certification may be severely frowned upon by your peers. This happens for two reasons: (1) Other therapists don't want the reputation of their profession diminished through the activities of unqualified practitioners; (2) Other therapists have worked long and hard for their own professional standing, and they don't want it threatened by some untrained neophyte bold enough to hang out a shingle.

Vermont, for example, is a state with many trained, qualified therapists, but there is no licensing required. Vermont is known for its rugged individualism, and many therapists there want to remain unlicensed because they don't want their livelihoods controlled in any way by a governmental body. Each state has its own quirks as far as licensing is concerned. For further information on this issue, take a look at chapter 6.

Now, assuming that you are duly licensed or certified, as the case may be, how do you go about getting other people to part with their hard-earned cash for a chance to lie on your table? Again, you can start with family and friends. But now that you've become a professional, it's time to do what professionals do: charge money. I personally don't charge my immediate family for massages, and I don't think many therapists do. Other relatives and friends, however, are fair game. Your cousin Bill is visiting from Kansas and has never had a professional massage? Here's his chance to experience one. Your great aunt Margaret is complaining of sciatica? You might be able to help. Friends at work are feeling stressed out? You're the person for the job.

Of course, you don't want to build a reputation as a money-hungry fiend who preys on his own friends and family. I suggest that you give these people generous discounts and not solicit their business constantly. Offer them your services once; then if they want more, they'll know whom to ask. Also, provide them one of your brochures with prices on it so they can see how professional you are *and* what a great discount you're giving them. Often, bartering works well with friends and family. Trade items and services—like a bag of Cousin Bob's fresh baby corn straight from the farm or a platter stacked high with Aunt Margaret's famous desserts. For more about bartering your massage services, see chapter 8.

Other People You Already Know

Where do you go when you've massaged every last long-lost relative and old high-school friend? When you run short on people you know well, move on to people you know just a little. If you work at a bagel restaurant, for example, pass out your cards to regular customers. Of course, only do this if your boss agrees that it's a good idea! (One way to assure this is to offer your boss a free massage.) On the other hand, if you are the regular customer at the bagel restaurant, give your cards out to the employees—your favorite waiter, the kid behind the counter, the owner. As I mentioned earlier, this approach will probably work better than simply tacking one of your cards to a bulletin board for customers and employees alike. For massage, the approach has to be personal.

Who else knows you? Here's a partial list:

- Repair people who come to your home (and may be excellent candidates to barter with, by the way)
- Your children's teachers
- The owner of the dry cleaners you use

✳ The people in your monthly yoga group, bridge group, or bird-watching group

✳ The clerks and cashiers at local stores

✳ Your dentist or orthodontist

✳ Your doctor, OB-GYN, eye specialist, heart surgeon, psychiatrist, or psychologist

✳ The butcher, baker, deli owner, or realtor in your town

✳ Your church congregation

✳ The owner of the local gym

✳ The fitness counselors and personal trainers at the gym

See how many others you can think of yourself. You may be quite surprised to realize how many people you already know without being aware of it. Every one of them could potentially become your client, and many of them will refer still other clients to you.

People You Could Easily Get to Know If You Tried

With massage, people often want to know you and feel comfortable with you before they'll purchase your services. Often just meeting you in person for a few moments is enough. But of course there are only a limited number of people you can personally meet in any given day, month, or year. How do you reach out to others with whom you may not get the chance to interact? How can you let them feel like they've already gotten to know you? Here are a few ideas that may help:

1. Write articles for local papers, magazines, and newsletters. This topic will be covered more fully in chapter 9, but I wanted to touch upon it here because it is an excellent way to meet new clients. Even if you think you can't write well, give it a shot; put your heart into your words, and let the editors take care of the rest. Many small publications are eager to receive new material. Make sure you can give your phone number or e-mail address at the end of the article. That way people can get in touch with you, and you'll be able to use it as a calling card of sorts, too. Have copies made for handing out. Print your logo, address, and other information on the blank side, fold it in thirds; and you have a ready-made brochure.

People feel they've gotten to know you when they read what you've written from the heart.

2. Appear on local health-related talk radio shows. There are plenty of these on smaller AM stations. Request a taped copy of the broadcast from the station and give it to prospective customers. People also feel they've gotten to know you if they hear you speak.

3. Give your hair stylist, your plumber, your car mechanic, your personal trainer, and anyone else you can think of a free massage along with a stack of your business cards. They will become your advanced scouts, finding new clients where you'd never think to look.

4. At parties, barbecues, picnics, and other social events, introduce yourself as a massage therapist. You'll be amazed how many positive responses you get. People will say, "I could sure use you about now"—and you'll immediately hand them your card. Do this in restaurants, nightclubs, at boat shows and air shows, and anywhere else you can think of.

PARTY PROTOCOL
HOW TO NETWORK YOUR MASSAGE SKILLS

Say you're at a party. You've just received your massage license the day before, and you're raring to go. The world is your oyster, and everybody in the Western Hemisphere is going to sign up for your services. Only problem is, you're deathly shy.

I know about this because it happened to me. Small talk is not my forte. Many customers slipped through my fingers, so to speak, because of an unwillingness to simply shoot the breeze. Years later, I've come to understand that people *want* to tell you about their problems and concerns; and by telling them you're a therapist, you're giving them permission to do just that.

If you're shy, just remember these few key words the first time you're faced with networking at a party: "Hi, my name is _____ , and I'm a **professional massage therapist.** What do you do?" Then listen. People will tell you everything you need to know about their stress, their anxiety, how tough their job is, and much more information.

Then, if they're at all familiar with the concept of massage, they will invariably ask this next question: "What kind of massage do you do?"

You answer, "I actually specialize in _____." And you fill in the blank with your potential client's problem, *not* your own particular massage

(continues)

expertise. For example, if the person is complaining about a stiff back, you say you specialize in helping people relax the tension in muscles that often causes stiff backs. You do this because people really want to know what's in store for *them* if they sign up for a massage from you. Most of them are not so much interested in your mastery of any particular techniques. However, *after* you've told them what you specialize in, *then* you say: "I accomplish this with the techniques I've learned like Swedish, shiatsu, neuromuscular, and _____." List whatever modalities you know. A good percentage of the general public is becoming more familiar with common massage terminology, and you may be surprised to find many people conversant with terms like trigger point therapy or Rolfing®.

Of course, you don't want to promise people something you can't deliver. Refer to the section later in this chapter, "Consultations and Evaluations: What You Can Realistically Hope to Accomplish and What Cases You Should Refer Out."

By simply listening to people and using a few key words like *professional* and *specialize,* you'll greatly increase your chances of attracting new clients. Remember, if you don't get good at attracting them, they'll never receive the benefits you have to offer and will therefore miss an opportunity to be good to themselves. By honing your networking and sales skills, you are helping your fellow humans. On the other hand, if you remain shy at parties, all you're doing is protecting an old self-image of yourself as a shy person. This image helps nobody.

GETTING REFERRALS AND INTRODUCTIONS

One important point to remember when you are giving a massage to anyone, whether it be your step-sister, a local lawyer, or your best friend, Michael, is to always ask them for referrals. A good time to ask for the referral is shortly after the massage, when your client has gotten up off the table and is about to leave but is still feeling completely relaxed and under the beneficent effects of your touch. If you ask, you may get one name or several names right on the spot. If your client can't think of anyone offhand, give him some of your business cards that he can hand out to friends and colleagues who ask about massage later.

Sometimes you'll be able to get referrals even if your client doesn't directly know the person he's referring you to. How does this work? As an example, one therapist friend of mine, Dianne, has developed an extensive practice at a large condominium complex. She started out with just a single client there, but soon other residents noticed her carrying her massage table to appointments. Meeting her in elevators and hallways, they asked her for her card, which she always had ready. In a single year, from clients in that one condominium alone, Dianne earned $19,800. The fact that she was in the building giving massage to another condominium owner, plus her professional appearance and demeanor, gave her the stamp of approval she needed to get in those other doors.

One way to help prompt referrals is to offer clients a free massage for every new customer they send your way. Note: In this situation, *always* insist on giving the free massage promptly and happily so that your client doesn't feel like it's a burden.

ADVERTISING

One of the easiest ways to spend yourself right out of business, especially at the beginning of your career, is to jump into heavy advertising expenses. The best advertisement is word of mouth, and that should definitely be where you put your focus—at least in the beginning. Actively seek the support of clients you already have. This kind of networking usually works best. However, if you do decide to advertise, here are a few basic rules to follow that may help you maximize your return on the investment and minimize any unwanted surprises:

1. Stick to highly targeted local publications. If you pay a lot of money to advertise in the Sunday newspaper, most of the people you'll reach are not likely to be very educated about massage. If, on the other hand, you advertise in the less expensive local organic food market's monthly newsletter, chances are much better that you'll reach the kinds of clients you're looking for.

2. Beware of advertising salespeople who insist you have to make "multiple impressions" before anyone responds to your ad. If you get very little response from a particular ad, cut your losses and pull out before you sink your own ship.

3. If you advertise in the local "new-age" directory, try to come up with an ad that's distinct from the rest. So many massage therapists advertise in these publications that it's hard to tell them apart at times.

CONSULTATIONS AND EVALUATIONS: WHAT YOU CAN REALISTICALLY HOPE TO ACCOMPLISH AND WHAT CASES YOU SHOULD REFER OUT

Eventually, if you stick to it, you are going to have *too many* clients, and you'll be turning some away. Even if you are not at that point yet, it's important to know whom you can realistically treat and which clients would be better served by another professional. Massage therapy is a wonderfully diverse field with room in it for many types of practitioners accomplishing greatly varying results treating a plethora of conditions. This does not mean you can "cure" everyone who comes to you, however. You have to take into account your level of experience, your training, and each client's particular complaint.

In the table on the next page, you'll find a list of conditions with recommendations for whether you should treat them or not. This reference is for beginning therapists with a basic massage certification and/or license and without advanced training in other modalities. Of course, as your expertise grows, so will the number of potential clients you can treat.

SPECIAL CASES

One thing you'll notice very quickly when you start working with the public is that there are many people with special needs. A good percentage of your clients may fall under one or another of the categories listed in this section. These are all people who will benefit from massage therapy, but you should make sure that you are confident and competent enough to treat any particular person or condition before you actually begin.

To treat many of these people, you will need "people skills" as well as your massage-related skills. I am not suggesting that you offer psychological counseling to your customers. But I am suggesting that you have to know a little bit about human nature to treat people gracefully. Your clients will appreciate your tact and understanding. (See the sidebar, "Massage Therapy and Psychotherapy" later in this chapter.)

Many excellent articles have been written in the massage publications about how to deal with "special cases." I recommend that you definitely subscribe to one or more of them (see the appendix). You can also request back issues that dealt with certain types of clients. Ask the people in the circulation and subscription departments at each publication for more information.

Here, then, are some of the people whom you may meet on your massage table one day. Getting to know them a little bit now may help you when you meet them face to face.

Conditions with Recommendations for Whether or Not You Should Treat with Massage

Condition	Treat	Don't Treat	Comments
Stress and tension	X		Massage was custom-made for these common problems.
Muscle aches and pain	X		For minor aches, massage is recommended.
Severe back/spine pain		X	Best left to chiropractors, trained neuromuscular therapists, or physicians
Tiredness	X		Even "chronic fatigue" reacts well to massage.
Immediately postsurgery		X	Don't treat without a physician's OK and only after waiting an appropriate time for healing.
Temporary headache	X		Often caused by tension.
Chronic headache		X	Could be more serious; refer to physician.
Athletic fatigue	X		Massage is great after sports events, races, etc.
Nervous or psychiatric disorders		X	Massage may be beneficial in some cases, but you should initially refer to a physician.
Pregnancy	X		Be extra careful positioning clients, take blood pressure, avoid pitting edema and stay away from certain areas (you'll learn in school).
Heart conditions		X	Always consult with a physician first; and, if massage is OK, avoid overly stimulating maneuvers.
Wounds and sores		X	Wait until healed.
Skin conditions		X	Some conditions (psoriasis, for example) are fine, while others, like some rashes, may spread through contact; consult a physician.
Cancer		X	There has been controversy on this point; some fear spreading cancerous cells through the lymph system while others do not; treat with care and consult a physician.

People with Disabilities

People who are immobilized or have a limited range of motion benefit greatly from massage therapy. If you sit in a wheelchair all day long, circulation can become sluggish and muscles weak.

By using your new massage skills, you can reach out to these people and make a positive impact in their lives. Massage will make a connection between them and you, a connection of touch and communication.

Whenever you can, take the opportunity to offer massage to those who have any kind of disability. You will be making a difference in ways that really count.

People with Disfigurements

People whose bodies have some disfigurement (massive burn scars, for example, or a ravaging skin condition), need massage for two main reasons. One is to help the condition; the other is to help a person feel better about having a flawed body. Study after study has shown that bringing an increased blood supply to affected areas increases microcirculation, lessens pain and sensitivity, and sometimes even improves the outward appearance. What's inside the person, however, can improve more.

People need to know that they are cared for, no matter what they look like. By massaging a person and touching him or her on areas other people are reluctant to even look at, you are sending a message deeper than words saying, "You're OK just the way you are."

You may have to develop some strength of character you didn't know you had to treat people who are disfigured in one way or another. You will be directly facing the fragility of the human body, which is something most of us would rather not think about unless it is absolutely necessary. This makes it doubly important to work with such clients at some point in your career; it greatly helps the client, *and* it helps you become stronger, more compassionate, and probably a better therapist all around.

Emotionally Needy People

Somehow, people who are especially needy often get drawn to strong, giving massage therapists. You know the type: They have a thousand questions, most

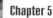

of which have obvious answers. They want you to tell them, step by step, how to become as healthy and vibrant as you are. With every question they ask, you get the sinking feeling inside that no matter what you tell them, they are not really listening. They are just being needy, and it seems they will always be this way.

In the massage and spa workshops I've taught all over the country, there was usually one person in every group of 20 or 30 who demanded extra attention, especially from me but also from the entire group. I had a special method for dealing with them.

Quite simply, I would put them at the center of everybody's attention and then ask the equivalent of the following question: "Is this what you really want?" Invariably it was. And the second they realized that they were at the center of attention and everybody was looking at them, wondering what message or insight they were going to share, they quieted down.

This method is a little harsh, but I learned from experience that if I continued to answer their questions one by one, constantly catering to their every need, the rest of the class would suffer.

You can use a similar method for dealing with needy clients. Usually they'll be asking you questions, putting you up on a pedestal, while all along slipping in subtle jabs to your character. My suggestion: Sit them up on the massage table, look them in the eye, and say, "You are a fascinating, complex person, and you have my complete attention right now. What do you have to tell me?"

Usually a shift will happen in their attitude. They will be quiet and grateful—at least for a while. Chances are, you'll have to be constantly vigilant with these clients to make sure they don't drain you of all your good intentions and positive healing energy. Refer to "Establishing Boundaries" later in this chapter to find out where you should draw the line in such situations.

Obese People

People with a poor body image caused by being overweight have to make a special effort to go see a massage therapist. Many simply will not. They make excuses like, "I don't want anyone seeing my body looking like this, much less touching me. I'll get a massage when I look better." And, of course, they often never get to that point of looking better.

Overweight clients are making themselves vulnerable by coming to you, and you have to respect that. By coming to you, they may in fact be taking the first step in really changing their body image, whether or not they ever lose weight in the future.

You can do several things to make an overweight person more comfortable on your table. I remember one client who, as he turned over, actually cracked the wooden frame of my massage table beneath the padding. A look of embarrassed terror spread across his face, and I quickly said, "That wasn't caused by you. It's been making that sound all week." I then bought some reinforcing braces for my table.

Once I massaged a 450-pound man at a spa in Jamaica. He was one of the most grateful clients I've ever worked on. The secret? *Massage the person inside the body.* Everybody, regardless of weight, has the same number of muscles and bones. They can be worked on in much the same way. Fat can be moved aside so simply; it's the image in the person's mind of being fat that is difficult to move. You can help with that.

People Who've Suffered Sexual Trauma

People who were sexually abused present a special situation for the massage therapist because sexual trauma always involves touch. In fact, it is a violation of the sacred trust that each child seems to come into the world with—the trust that they will be touched appropriately, especially by those who care for them.

For you to be trusted to touch, the abuse survivor must relax and release a huge amount of fear and stored tension. You will have to be especially sensitive and nonintrusive when dealing with these clients, *and* you will have to receive some in-depth education on the subject to make sure your treatment is appropriate.

Sometimes, though, people are not aware that they were abused early in life. The memories of abuse may begin to surface when they end up on your massage table and they are touched. What do you do in that situation? Be on the lookout for signs of this such as: increasing unexplained anxiety during the massage, a sexual response to clearly nonsexual touch, and crying or sobbing that the client cannot explain.

When it becomes apparent that your female client is experiencing a flashback to an earlier traumatic experience, break physical contact and completely cover her with towels, sheets, or blankets so that she feels protected. Using her name, make physical contact with her once again, reestablishing the immediate reality of the room you are in. For example, you can say, "Suzy, are you here with me now? It's Steve." Slowly and gradually bring her back and then make sure she is safe to drive home. Perhaps she'll need a friend to come be with her.

Do not try to play psychotherapist and heal your client's wounds with soothing touch and words of wisdom. This may only aggravate the situation further, putting the client—and you—at potential risk.

A number of trainings can help massage therapists learn how to cope with abuse survivors. Some interesting literature exists on the subject, as well. I highly recommend a helpful series of five articles by a well-known therapist and teacher, Ben Benjamin. His articles are entitled "Massage and Bodywork with Survivors of Abuse," and they begin in the summer 1995 issue of *Massage Therapy Journal* and conclude in the summer 1996 issue. They are filled with important information.

As suggested further reading on the topic, you can check out the following books. For complete information on these titles, refer to the appendix.

❋ *The Compassionate Touch* by Clyde Ford.

❋ *Trauma and Recovery* by Judith L. Herman.

❋ *Boundaries: Where You End and I Begin* by Anne Katherine.

People with AIDS

I was involved in two different programs to massage people with HIV and AIDS. The first was a blind study at the Touch Research Institute. It involved some HIV-positive and some HIV-negative men, and they were all given a standardized massage over a period of weeks. Neither the therapists nor the scientists measuring blood, T-cell, and hormone levels knew who was who. The results were overwhelmingly encouraging, with the HIV-positive men having significantly altered T-cells and increased levels of serotonin, which contribute to healing.

The other experience was not as encouraging, but it was one of the most deeply moving of my career. I helped in a hospital AIDS ward by volunteering to massage the patients. The people there were frightened, in pain, and without hope. Many of them had only days to live. One of them died moments after receiving his massage.

In spite of the pain and incredible challenges they were facing, each and every patient was extremely grateful for his or her massage, especially considering that AIDS patients are sometimes shunned like lepers and not touched as much as they need to be. The level of appreciation that those patients expressed really taught me about the importance of touch.

You can make a difference in the lives of people going through similar challenges. Touch others in a way that matters. Working with AIDS patients is not easy, but do yourself and them the favor of reaching out in this way. The rewards for both you and the patients will be unutterably valuable.

Check with your local massage school for programs in your area that do work with AIDS patients. Or start a program yourself by contacting the local hospital or AIDS support network (see chapter 4 for more information about working in hospitals).

Athletes

Has it always been your dream to go to the Olympics one day? Many massage therapists have made that dream come true, thanks to their skill and perseverance (Figure 5-1). At the 1996 Summer Games in Atlanta, approximately 130 U.S. therapists worked on the athletes, and it was the first time that massage was officially recognized as an offering by the Olympic committee. Any of the therapists lucky enough to have participated in any Olympics since then always mention the experience as one of the most uplifting, fulfilling, and important moments in their careers.

Perhaps one of the few things more fulfilling than working as a therapist at the Olympics is working at the Paralympics. These special games are held immediately after the regular Olympics and feature athletes with disabilities who, even with their handicaps, turn in some performances that are truly astounding. The massage therapy community plays an active role in the Paralympics. For example, in Atlanta, one of the biggest massage table manufacturers, Living Earth Crafts from Santa Rosa, California, supplied special commemorative edition tables for the Paralympics, and a team of therapists used them to work on many of the athletes.

Figure 5-1 | Nancy Dail giving massage to an athlete at the Olympic Games.

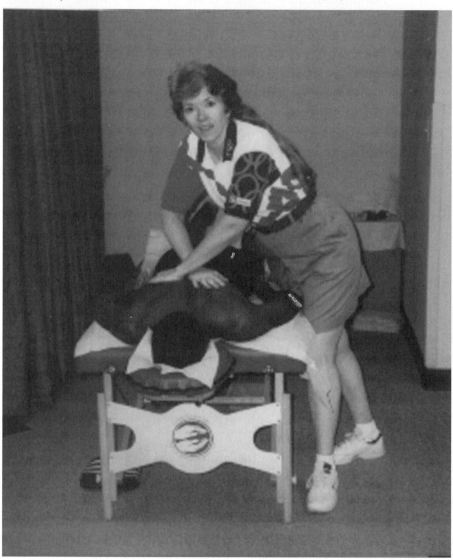

Of course, weekend athletes enjoy and benefit from massage therapy as much as Olympic or professional athletes. The majority of sports massage specialists work privately or in clinics, and their clients range from aerobics instructors to jai alai players to the third baseman on the company softball team. People are more active than ever these days, and the services of a sports massage specialist are often in high demand. Demographically, there has been a shift in the types of injuries sustained by the average working American. Whereas 30 years ago,

In his previous life, Brian Glotsbach would never have dreamed he was headed for the Olympics. Brian was an engineer for eight years until he made a midlife career switch to massage therapy, eventually becoming a co-owner of *Body Mechanics Sports Massage Therapy* in Atlanta, Georgia. Prior to and during the Summer Olympics in 1996, Brian ended up playing a pivotal role in helping U.S. massage therapists become a part of the sports therapy team that worked on the athletes.

With the enthusiasm typical of people who are doing the one thing they most want to do with their lives, Brian recounts the events that became a focus of his life for much of a year. "I was part of a group chosen by the Atlanta Committee for the Olympic Games to be responsible for assembling the massage team at the sports medicine clinic in the Olympic Village. It was exciting because it was the first time that massage was officially sanctioned at the Olympics."

Prior to 1996, massage was conducted off official Olympic grounds at a hotel or other nearby venue. The therapists in Atlanta all wanted the Olympic community and the sports medicine community to take massage therapy seriously, so they put a lot of effort into building a great team. Brian, besides being a therapist and an engineer, has a degree in sports medicine and athletic training, making him eminently qualified to be part of the selection committee. He says that selecting the therapists was a daunting task.

Over 3,000 applications were received and screened for only 130 positions. "One hundred therapists working at the games were assigned to work a particular sport," he recalls. "The other 30 therapists were chosen to work in the sports medicine clinic in the Olympic Villages where massage was available for all the athletes. They had to be highly recommended and have good credentials to be taken seriously. We ended up choosing people who had a lot of experience and who were dealing with athletes on a fairly consistent basis.

"Since massage was new to many athletes and new as an official service at the games, it was slow going at first. The clinic was open two weeks prior to the opening ceremonies and remained open through the duration of the games. For the first week, just a trickle of athletes came in. But then by the middle of the second week we really started to pick up, and soon we were going full bore, working three shifts, giving a 150 20-minute treatments a day. Our therapists were arriving from all over the country. Some stayed for two or three weeks, some for all four, and we had six or eight therapists per

(continues)

Brian Glotsbatch (continued)

shift, three shifts per day working on the athletes from 7 AM till 11 PM. The only way we could be fair to the athletes was to offer massages on a first-come-first-served basis, and sometimes we had them waiting in line for two hours to get their treatments."

Brian, besides helping to coordinate and lead the team's effort, was right in the thick of things, too, working on a wide variety of athletes himself. He says the experience was more fulfilling than he had expected; it was an uplifting feeling to be part of something on such a large scale. Yet there was a share of frustration, as well—mostly about not being able to do as much as he wanted to.

"The only downside," he recalls, "was that since this was the first Olympics to officially sanction massage, a lot of the athletes didn't know it was available. Even some of the marathon runners, in the very last event of the games, didn't know they could receive free massage after running if they wanted to. It was a shame that some of the athletes couldn't take advantage of the free service just because of inadequate communications. For the next games in Sydney, we drafted an article mostly for the benefit of the Australian therapists to point out some of the challenges we faced."

In spite of the challenges, massage therapy was the most requested medical service in the history of the Olympics, a truly groundbreaking phenomenon. Due in part to that success, Brian was asked to speak at an International Massage Symposium in Barcelona, Spain. "Massage opened a whole new avenue for me," he says. "There were over a thousand people at that conference, and many were interested in what I had to say. I've only been a therapist for five years, and already I've had such inspiring events happen directly related to massage. In the future I see myself getting a PhD in biomechanics (the study of human movement) and applying it to massage work. I'm continually pushing forward in that way. But I insist on having fun while I'm doing it! That was part of my personal mission statement when I switched to massage therapy—it had to be fun or I wouldn't pursue it. So far, massage hasn't let me down."

heart attacks and coronary disease were the number one threat to health in the workplace, now joint and tissue damage is a more common reason for people to miss time on the job. The sports massage specialist can help.

To become a qualified sports massage practitioner, you'll need to get a certificate. This can be accomplished in three different ways: (1) You can sign up for an advanced training program in sports massage once you've graduated massage school; (2) You can choose a school that offers a curriculum that includes sports massage (the Downeast School of Massage in Maine, for example, offers a special course that combines Swedish and Sports Massage); and (3) You can take continuing education seminars in sports massage.

Sports massage is excellent if you are the type of therapist who likes to solve puzzles and focus closely on specific problem areas. Brian Glotsbach (see profile) spends an hour at a time on one shoulder or one hip, seeking the deeper interlocked causes behind the problems his clients have. With the ongoing dedication of people like Brian, this discipline will continue to grow and mature and sports massage will become increasingly recognized as an adjunct to the practice of medicine. Then many more intelligent, educated, dedicated individuals will get the chance to use their hands for the benefit of athletes everywhere.

Disaster Victims and Relief Workers

Most disaster victims experience some form of post-traumatic stress syndrome. Even people far from the epicenter of destruction can be deeply affected. The Red Cross and other agencies have often been aided by teams of volunteer massage therapists who work on-site to provide relief to the relief workers and others.

After Hurricane Andrew hit South Florida, I joined with dozens of other therapists who reached out to offer assistance. Three days after the storm, we were in Homestead, where the army had set up its headquarters. After massaging the general in charge of the operation, I was given permission to work on the troops. In a small basement room (one of the few rooms for miles around that hadn't been destroyed by the storm), a continual stream of hardworking disaster workers came down for 15-minute chair massage sessions. We also worked on the Red Cross volunteers, the county 911 operators, city workers, and assorted other stressed individuals as everyone pulled together. We even worked with grade-school children suffering from post-traumatic stress.

In spite of the circumstances, working in a disaster situation usually ends up becoming an uplifting experience and is often actually "fun." People cooperate and appreciate each other in new ways. When we're thrown out of our routines through the exigencies of nature, we recognize our common humanity, at least for a while, and therapeutic, stress-lowering touch between humans is more apt to be recognized for what it is—a great gift.

If you want to volunteer when disaster strikes, contact massage schools in the area and inquire whether there has been an organized relief effort started. The Red Cross has become accustomed to the sight of massage therapists during many of their operations, and they may be able to direct you, as well. Your help will always be appreciated.

The American Massage Therapy Association has developed a team of ever-ready practitioners who are specially trained to work in disaster zones treating responders and rescuers, not the victims themselves. They speak the same language and use procedures that are familiar to all emergency management personnel. Called the Massage Emergency Response Team (MERT), this elite crowd has pledged its willingness to work in challenging and potentially dangerous areas. In some instances, only these trained therapists are allowed on site; so, if you are potentially interested in volunteering, it is a good idea to contact the AMTA at http://www.amtamassage.org or at (877) 905-2700. To become a MERT volunteer, therapists need to be either nationally certified in Therapeutic Massage and Bodywork or an active professional member of the AMTA. They also need to be licensed and insured and have completed a MERT training course. All team members are unpaid. Often, they eat and stay for free when they are working at a site, but travel expenses still need to be covered out-of-pocket. Some therapists have held fund-raising events to help subsidize their efforts.

PROFILE: Bob Bottorf
Disaster Relief Massage—The Oklahoma City Bombing

It was a personal disaster that originally inspired Bob Bottorf to become a massage therapist, and he's had compassion for other disaster victims ever since. Several years ago, he was driving his motorcycle at approximately 45 miles per hour when he collided with a car. Bob is a big man, and gymnastics was not his specialty, but he did a full cartwheel as he flew through the air before experiencing the "culture shock" of the pavement.

Two orthopedic surgeons wanted to operate on his back, but Bob decided to go to a chiropractor instead. A massage therapist in the chiropractor's office massaged him over a nine-month period, after which he was pain free. Shortly thereafter, Bob enrolled in massage school.

(continues)

Bob Bottorf (continued)

He was at a massage convention in San Diego a year later when he heard about the Oklahoma City bombing. Knowing firsthand about the pain that was being suffered by people in such a catastrophe, Bob got in his truck and drove straight to Oklahoma City.

He arrived a few days after the blast to find a massage relief center already set up and running at the Civic Center downtown. People from the massage school in Tulsa were in charge. About 20 massage tables filled one part of the staging area, and Bob jumped straight into the action.

"We got there the day after the rescue team from Miami arrived, and they were just coming off their shift. They were the first people we worked on, and it was good to have something in common with them since we were from Miami, too. We worked on everybody: cops, emergency medical technicians, fire fighters, relief workers, government investigators. These people were extremely exhausted and frazzled. A lot of them just fell asleep on the table, and we just let them stay until they woke up.

"And it was good we got there when we did, a few days into it, to allow some of the other massage therapists to take a break. They were working 20 hours at a stretch."

Bob stayed in Oklahoma City for three days until the initial rescue operations began to wind down, and then he headed back to Florida. After that, living outside of Gainesville, he opened his own massage therapy center in a refurbished structure that he called Bob's Massage Garage.

Bob's story reflects a trait that many massage therapists share: caring. Most of us are ready and willing to jump up and help at a moment's notice, whether it be at the site of a national disaster or in the simple treatment of one client at a time in the garage behind your house. People will always need therapists, and if you're in tune with that need, your career in massage will take you places you can't even imagine right now.

"I can stand anything but being bored," says Bob. "And with massage, I don't think I ever will be."

Sometimes, perhaps more horrendously, it is not Mother Nature who causes us to bond together in this way but, rather, the act of a fellow human being. The bombing in Oklahoma City was such a case and, of course, 9/11. As usual, many massage therapists rushed to the aid of those in need. One therapist drove to Oklahoma a few days after the bombing there, and he vividly remembers the experiences he had (see the profile of Bob Bottorf).

Elderly People

At the Touch Research Institute in Miami, I was involved with a study testing the effects of massage on elderly people (see Figure 5-2). Plenty of blood samples, urine samples, and psychological profiles were taken; and, sure enough, we found that elderly people respond favorably to massage. More important than the physiological results, however, were the psychological ones. Elderly people, especially in our society, are often neglected; and the structured interaction of consistent massages was a great way for them to reconnect with other people. In fact, it was shown that older folks benefited almost as much from giving touch as from receiving it, and so a special study was instituted wherein grandparents massaged young people. The effects were always positive.

If you take the time to connect with some elderly people in your community and share with them through massage, you'll be amazed at the satisfaction you'll derive from it. Call local nursing homes, or simply network with people

Figure 5-2 | **Massaging an elderly person.**

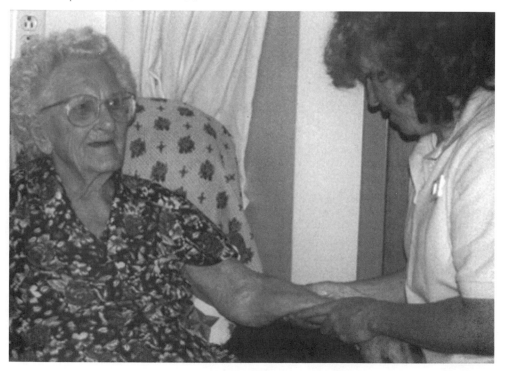

you know. Often, elderly people will be willing to exchange some baby-sitting or other useful chores for massage.

An excellent resource is the Daybreak Geriatric Massage Project, which offers training, correspondence programs, and videos on the subject. The founder, Dietrich Meisler, has a goal of getting massage into nursing homes and retirement homes around the country. You can contact him at 216 Pleasant Hill Ave. N., Sebastopol, CA 95472; telephone (707) 829-2798.

People with Serious Illnesses

People with cancer may approach you for massage services. People with all of their hair fallen out and unsightly scars on their scalps after brain surgery may want you to work on them, too. Fibromyalgia is a condition that resists every treatment science has thrown at it, but sufferers of the disease report great relief with massage therapy. Likewise, people with chronic fatigue syndrome have said that massage is one of the most important tools to help them prevail over the struggle with their own bodies. People with some forms of muscular dystrophy also respond well. Other conditions can be helped, too.

Sometimes the help you give will be mostly companionship and compassion, as in the case of some cancer patients. In other instances, you'll be providing the crucial hands-on therapy that will help a person to heal. Your most important goal in treating these clients should be to learn as much as you possibly can about their condition and to consult with their physician before undertaking any therapeutic intervention (see the table, "Conditions with Recommendations for Whether or Not You Should Treat with Massage," earlier in this chapter). You should also attend any training that may help you improve your skills in the required techniques.

People Who Are Dying

> *An understanding of death at any age is a must for all therapists because so many dying people truly need the loving touch of massage.*
>
> —Frances Tappan, *Healing Massage Techniques: Holistic, Classic, and Emerging Methods*

Once I was called to the house of a friend whose father had suffered a serious stroke. My friend had to help me turn his father over on the table because he was no longer in control of his own body. For an hour I tried the best I could to offer this man some relief from the obvious pain and fear he was experiencing. I didn't know if I was getting through until, near the end of the massage while I was working on his arms, he reached out, grasped my arm, and held onto it as if it were a life raft in a raging sea.

During the 30 seconds that he held me, a strong current of communication flowed between us. His silent touch told me about what was important in life and what was not. When I left, we made another appointment for two days later, but during those two days he left the world. I'll never forget the grip of his hand.

As a massage therapist, you will have the opportunity to offer something meaningful to people who are in the last days of their lives. When everything else is stripped away, the dying are left with only what's real—and that is the shared experience of life, which is love. You can *be* with people at those times, and they will appreciate it because the massage therapist, as much or more than any other person they will come into contact with, is offering his or her own being to the person going through the transformation of death. When you think of it this way, massage is simply a way to *be with* another person in a direct, tangible, bodily way. Refer to "The Spirituality of Touch" in chapter 2.

You can call your local hospice to find out more about working with dying people in your own area.

ESTABLISHING BOUNDARIES

When you become a massage therapist, many people will think that they know you really well. They'll believe that they know how you eat, how you drink, and even how you think; and sometimes they're going to call you up and request that you come massage them at midnight. Somehow, when you become a therapist, you become a knowable entity and people will slip you into certain slots in their minds: "Oh, he must be a health nut," or, "She must not drink alcohol," or, "He must care about people so much that he'll come try to help me at any hour." When you put on the persona of the therapist, it's like putting on the persona of police officer or chef or secretary. For better or for worse, you will be categorized.

When people assume a certain familiarity that you would rather not provide, the experience can be draining. Some clients, for example, may think that because you massage people all day, you're immune to nudity. They'll want to force their own nudity on you. Other clients will assume you're a vegetarian and try to make you feel guilty for eating a hamburger.

To keep from being tugged in too many directions at one time, you will have to learn how to erect some psychic fences around yourself. This will be necessary for two reasons: (1) to keep *out* the draining, invasive influences of certain clients who think they know you too well; and (2) to keep *in* your own helpful, positive, therapeutic energies that can only help other people if you are still in possession of them, *not* if they've been drained by overuse.

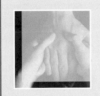

MASSAGE THERAPY AND PSYCHOTHERAPY: **A PROPER DISTINCTION**

In the course of giving massage therapy to a wide variety of clients, you are going to run across some who will ask your outright advice about relationships, personal problems, delicate family matters, and other situations. How should you react when someone is asking you something that would probably be better addressed by a social worker, counselor, or psychologist?

The first and best course of action for the massage therapist is to quietly, nonjudgmentally listen. A goodly portion of the benefit in any therapeutic exchange is derived from the therapist merely listening. If you're really *there* for your client, she'll feel it and trust you. You are not in a professional position to counsel people, but you are in a position to listen and to care.

As an example, imagine that a client tells you that she just found out her husband has been cheating on her. She is crying on your table, and she asks for your response. You definitely don't want to ignore her plea for commiseration, but you have to be careful about what you say.

Here are two responses, one wrong and one right:

Wrong: "You should confront Jasper with your feelings and tell him he has to change his ways or you'll leave him."

Right: "I understand why you're having these feelings. Let's work together to relax some of the tension that's been created in your body so that you can make proper, clearheaded decisions about the situation."

Of course, at some point, you may become friends with a certain client and see her socially. In that case, you can offer whatever advice a friend would normally give. But it becomes even more important then to separate your friendship from your professional relationship. While she's on

(continues)

the table, don't judge or advise; let her feel and process her experiences for herself.

If you take more advanced trainings in a modality like Rubenfeld Synergy or in certain breathing techniques, you'll learn how to deal with the emotional manifestations of your clients. After intensive study, you'll be qualified to guide emotional experiences rather than simply observe them.

In the beginning, though, just listen. If what your client is divulging makes you uncomfortable, you can always stop her at any time and tell her that. Don't make her feel that she is being inappropriate; rather, let her know that you are personally too "sensitive" to hear such stories or that it's against your personal code of ethics.

If you're a good therapist, you'll do everything in your power to help your clients, but you have to establish some boundaries to limit exactly how far that helping will go. In the sidebar, "Boundary Rules," you'll find a few simple rules that will help you maintain your own space and thereby also help you maintain your ability to help others through your work.

CLIENTS WHO BECOME FRIENDS

All this talk about boundaries is not meant to scare you away from becoming friends with your clients. There is no reason to create an impenetrable personal barrier between yourself and other people just because you do business with them. Boundary rules are there just for protection, to help shield you from the many unknowable forces you'll come in contact with in the course of your career.

Many of your clients, quite likely, will be people that you'd like to get to know better, people you could really care about, people you'd like to call friends. No ethical or professional constraints should keep you from getting to know your clients better and eventually forming friendships with them. However, there's a slight stigma that may always be there with certain customers, because initially they *hired* you and you'll always be thought of by them as an employee of some kind. With these people, you may have to *stop* massaging them to deepen the friendship. The same thing applies if you're thinking about starting a relationship with one of your clients. Many a therapist has had to decide whether gaining a friend or lover was worth losing a good customer!

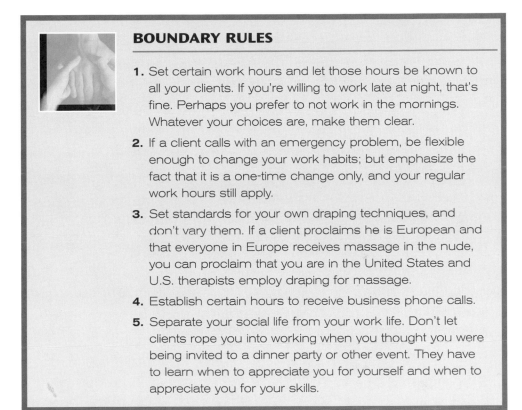

BOUNDARY RULES

1. Set certain work hours and let those hours be known to all your clients. If you're willing to work late at night, that's fine. Perhaps you prefer to not work in the mornings. Whatever your choices are, make them clear.

2. If a client calls with an emergency problem, be flexible enough to change your work habits; but emphasize the fact that it is a one-time change only, and your regular work hours still apply.

3. Set standards for your own draping techniques, and don't vary them. If a client proclaims he is European and that everyone in Europe receives massage in the nude, you can proclaim that you are in the United States and U.S. therapists employ draping for massage.

4. Establish certain hours to receive business phone calls.

5. Separate your social life from your work life. Don't let clients rope you into working when you thought you were being invited to a dinner party or other event. They have to learn when to appreciate you for yourself and when to appreciate you for your skills.

I personally have become extremely close to several massage customers, some of whom I still see as clients, too. People whom I've first met on my table are now my neighbors. I've gone hiking and camping with them, stayed in their homes, traveled across the world to see them, been present at the birth of their children, invited them to my wedding, gone to theirs, and in fact married someone whom I met through a client. For those who follow this profession as a path through the years, the connections between people and the rich variety of relationships formed becomes a treasured part of their lives. To rephrase an old saying, it's not just a job, it's a *massage adventure.* If you are persistent enough to develop a successful massage career for yourself, you will definitely discover some unexpected blessings along the way; and it's the unexpected that often turns out to be the most precious.

6

Touch and the Law

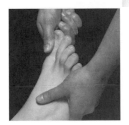

Touch between people is powerful.

Before we were born, we were constantly touching our mother's body from inside the womb, a process that culminated with a long, slow, sensuous and painful slide out through her body into a world where somebody else was waiting to touch us.

Often, when a crime is committed, one person touches another, invading personal boundaries; and, when two people are intimate, they reach across those same boundaries to touch each other. A physician may also touch you, probing your flesh to determine the health of your tissue and organs, which is something that may frighten you; and, of course, the dentist with his drill touches you. When we're riding the subway or being herded onto a jet, something about the oppressive touch of all those other bodies around us makes us draw into ourselves, cutting off our bodies from the outside world.

The whole world is "out there," and we are "in here"; and, for the most part, our touch boundaries are very tightly guarded. We choose to let in only a few other humans among the billions on the planet; and, when we do, the result is often a highly emotional moment.

Touch is powerful. Massage—the sustained intentional touching of one person by another—is one of the most powerful forms of touch in the world. Most massage therapists and massage recipients understand and respect the inherent dangers, as well as the benefits of that touch; but, because the medium itself is so powerful, it is only appropriate that massage should be regulated under certain widely understood and accepted societal guidelines—laws, in other words.

When you think about it, most laws govern touch in one way or another. Criminal laws govern the touching of other people's money, property, or bodies; other laws seek to regulate touch in the workplace, touch in public, even touch between intimate partners in the privacy of their own home. Touch between husband and wife or parents and children is also a concern; we hope to ensure that anger and frustration don't result in physical abuse or violent touch. On a worldwide scale, international laws determine who can touch whose fish or who can travel to which country, touching certain soil with their bodies or their shoes. The law is all about touch.

Touch and the law go hand in hand. The purpose of this chapter is to acquaint you with some of the more important aspects of the law as it relates to the practice of massage therapy.

THE PARAMETERS OF THE PROFESSION: WHAT YOU LEGALLY CAN AND CANNOT DO AS A MASSAGE THERAPIST

Some therapists, after they discover the wonderful healing powers of their own touch, can't resist the temptation to explore those newfound powers in an experimental way. They make claims they shouldn't make, they treat conditions they shouldn't treat, and they make promises they may not be able to keep. What's worse, they may even unintentionally cause someone harm. Don't let this be you.

When you're in massage school, you'll no doubt learn every indication and contraindication for massage. Your teachers and classmates will remind you about your boundaries, and they'll warn you about overextending your professional limitations. At the end of this section, I list 10 basic commandments about what you should and shouldn't do as a beginning therapist—but more important than that, I'm here to remind you that your ego will not listen to these admonitions. If you're like many therapists, you may feel you're on a mission of sorts to affect the world positively and anything that gets in your way is an obstacle to be righteously overcome.

To clarify for you some of the ways in which your ego/mind may try to inflate your sense of infallibility in the realm of healing, I've categorized four personality types that this inflated ego may assume as a way to convince you that what you're doing is right, no matter what anyone tells you. They are: (1) the crusader, (2) the philanthropist, (3) the fellow victim, and (4) the know-it-all.

❋ **The crusader:** This therapist is on a mission to "save" as many people as he can. He will not listen to anyone who suggests that his training and skill may not be adequate to treat *any* condition whatsoever, including the most serious and life-threatening ones. He is often an enemy of allopathic medicine and considers all Western techniques to be suspect and inferior.

Once, when I was the supervisor at a large spa, a highly recommended therapist came to work with us from out of state. He showed up one day carrying an armload of paraphernalia and tromped up to his assigned massage room as if he were a king arriving for a royal ceremony. Within minutes, he had transformed the room into a strange and exotic environment with six-foot posters, incense, statues, and flowing swaths of silk and velvet. He then took off to observe "the lay of the land," as he called it, returning with a timid client whom he proceeded to treat with some rough-and-tumble manipulations from the "Far East," irrespective of the fact that the client had not asked for such a treatment.

At the end of his first week, this therapist was fired.

❋ **The philanthropist:** The philanthropist will gladly work for free to ease the pain and discomfort of her fellow humans. While this is an admirable trait, it can sometimes backfire. The therapist may end up confusing some of her clients—and even herself—when trying to determine who gets free massage and who pays. Assuming she must make at least a part of her living through offering massage, this can lead to a common dilemma many therapists experience; they end up asking the perennial question, "Is it ethical for me to charge money for something that is basically an act of giving and love from my heart?" When that question is asked too often, the philanthropist finds herself in a bind, unable to help herself *or* her clients.

Also, not all clients are as upstanding and giving as the philanthropic therapist, and this may lead to someone being taken advantage of—usually the therapist. Sometimes the philanthropic therapist has to learn her lessons the hard way, at the expense of some precious illusions she's cherished all her life.

Instead of being philanthropic as a therapist, be excellent—and charge accordingly. Then, in a separate offering, give your services for free to specific people or causes that need them. You will make everyone happier, and this will clear up a lot of confusion between what's good or bad, ethical or economical, service or self-serving.

✳ **The fellow victim:** This therapist has been hurt in the past, either emotionally or physically or both, and he easily bonds with the clients he treats, based on shared pain. Although certain amounts of empathy and understanding are appropriate for the client-therapist relationship, the fellow victim goes too far and actually fosters an environment of codependence that only perpetuates and deepens the wound.

Don't be like this. It may hurt you at first to distance yourself from your clients to some degree, especially if they've gone through some trauma similar to your own, but in the long run you will be doing them a favor through this objectivity. Sometimes if you get too close, you can't tell if the hurt you're seeing is yours or your client's, and this confusion will lessen your ability to help. To be effective, stay objective.

✳ **The know-it-all:** The know-it-all just cannot say no, even if she knows nothing about the condition of the person she is treating or the specific type of massage the person is asking for. The know-it-all will gladly oblige a client who asks for Hawaiian Lomi-Lomi technique, even though she's only read one article about that type of massage in a magazine two years ago. The know-it-all will say something like, "A little of my specialized energy work will help you feel better about that grapefruit-sized lump in your abdominal wall." The know-it-all will forever be running around offering bits and pieces of secondhand medical information and nutritional advice to her clients, entirely missing the fact that she may be doing them a disservice through this partial information rather than truly helping them.

Sometimes, as the saying goes, you have to be cruel to be kind. You may have to tell a client point-blank that you can't help her, that you have not been trained sufficiently to answer her questions, that she really needs someone in another field to offer his or her professional opinion, and that you do *not* know it all.

If any of these descriptions sound even remotely familiar, *watch out!* Instead of marching off on a massage crusade, it's better to be humble and realistic, especially when you're starting out. Build your skills and your understanding one step at a time, remembering the motto, *Promise less, deliver more.* Although it may surprise you, people will respect your honesty and day-to-day diligence more than the pyrotechnics of your spectacular healing gift. If you find, as many therapists do at one point or another in their careers, that you've facilitated some "miraculous" sort of recovery or healing, accept it with a grain of salt; explain that the phenomenon was due to the power of touch therapies, not your own personal power; and then move on to the next client. You may quite likely find this kind of experience happening at the very beginning of your massage career because at the outset you are trying especially hard, paying very close attention to every detail of your client and your own techniques, and you haven't yet built up the impediment of too much knowledge. You don't yet know what doesn't work.

Be amazed and inspired by such occurrences, but don't get stuck in them. Soon enough, you're sure to encounter another client who does not heal so easily, who presents a completely different problem, and who challenges you in a new way. The massage business is a one-day-at-a-time way of life. You'll learn much more than you can realize now, but you have to give it time. Go easy on yourself.

As a quick reference to help keep you on track when you're first starting out, I've included here a list of the 10 commandments you as a beginning massage therapist should definitely never break, regardless of your personality type and no matter how strong the temptation:

1. **Thou shalt not make any chiropractic adjustments.** Manipulating spinal vertebrae and other bones is definitely *not* your field. Chiropractors go through intense advanced training to safely and effectively adjust the skeletal structure. Your expertise is in the *soft* tissues. I've heard of therapists who've caused injury to clients by trying to "crack" their necks. Even if you are not trying to cause an adjustment, be extra careful while working on the spine, especially the neck. Never apply traction and twist the head at the same time, for instance. Always be much more safe than sorry when it comes to anything remotely approaching chiropractic.

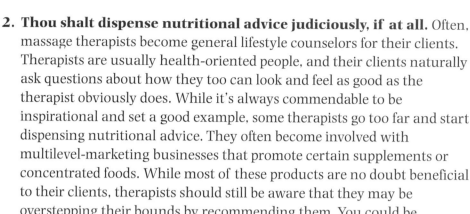

2. **Thou shalt dispense nutritional advice judiciously, if at all.** Often, massage therapists become general lifestyle counselors for their clients. Therapists are usually health-oriented people, and their clients naturally ask questions about how they too can look and feel as good as the therapist obviously does. While it's always commendable to be inspirational and set a good example, some therapists go too far and start dispensing nutritional advice. They often become involved with multilevel-marketing businesses that promote certain supplements or concentrated foods. While most of these products are no doubt beneficial to their clients, therapists should still be aware that they may be overstepping their bounds by recommending them. You could be stepping on the toes of the registered dieticians in your area and perhaps even breaking the law. Check the laws in your own state to make sure you're within your rights when offering any guidance regarding diet or supplements.

3. **Thou shalt not offer diagnoses.** A client may come to you with a specific set of problems that you recognize from a previous client. If, for example, the previous client was eventually diagnosed with muscular dystrophy, do not tell your present client that he probably has muscular dystrophy as well. You have not been trained to recognize all the different parameters of any particular disease pattern. If people come to you with problems that you suspect may be of a serious nature, suggest that they visit a physician to find out for themselves.

4. **Thou shalt honor the requests and objections of the client.** Even if they seem off the wall, complaints and concerns coming from a client, especially while they are on your treatment table, should be immediately honored. If someone says she's uncomfortable with your draping techniques, acknowledge this and ask what you can do to make her more comfortable. If a client says she thinks your new-age music stinks and that she prefers golden oldies while receiving massage, go break out the Elvis Presley. "The customer is always right" applies doubly to massage therapists because we are dealing with people on such a personal level.

5. **Thou shalt not speak disparagingly of thy fellow therapists.** Make no mistake about it; there is some degree of competition between therapists in most if not all communities. As massage becomes more accepted, enrollment at massage schools continues to grow and more practitioners fill the market. The temptation exists for some of us to tout our own skills

while either subtly or not so subtly knocking those of our neighbor. Perhaps you've heard of a therapist who did something unethical. It may be right for you to report him, but to the proper authorities, not to your clients. Judgmental and abusive talk about other therapists only lessens the perception of massage in the eyes of the public. Be kind whenever you can, and the favor will come back to you in ways you can't understand. In fact, if you talk *up* the competition, you will probably do better in your own business. Winners are helpful. Those afraid of losing guard their own territory fiercely. Act like a winner and you'll be one.

6. **Thou shalt pursue advanced education.** Don't let early success as a therapist make you smug or early challenges make you despair. Massage is an ongoing, ever-developing process fueled by the periodic inflow of new ideas, techniques, and influences. Make a commitment to yourself and your continuing education right at the beginning of your career, and never waver from it. Take classes, read books, and trade techniques with other therapists. You do your clients a disservice if you are not constantly growing as a therapist.

7. **Thou shalt put thy own health first and foremost.** If you don't take care of yourself, you won't be well enough to take care of others. Massage requires the expenditure of a lot of energy, much more than it would appear on the surface. It's easy to overextend yourself and perhaps even cause yourself physical damage. We'll touch upon this in more depth in chapter 8 in the section on burnout. For now, just remember to take this commandment seriously. Working too hard to help your clients to the point of neglecting your own well-being is doing harm to yourself *and* your clients.

8. **Thou shalt endeavor to learn as much about business as about massage.** Tragically, many gifted therapists just can't seem to make a career out of massage, and they end up out of necessity working for their uncle Bill at his poultry processing plant in Maryland. This shouldn't be you. Make a commitment to yourself to spend conscious, focused energy on the real-life details of your massage business. Buy as many books as you can, and attend seminars that talk about those dreaded words *profit* and *money.*

9. **Thou shalt become a member of a like-minded community.** Nothing is more discouraging than thinking you're the only one out

there who feels the way you do, but other therapists have walked where you are walking now. Form strategic alliances and meaningful bonds with people who've decided on a similar path. These bonds will probably begin to form in massage school, but you may have to remind yourself to keep nurturing them once you get out into the busy workday world. Continue to develop relationships, and remember that two minds together create a third and more powerful mind that will help you both grasp new concepts and solve problems. To recoin a phrase for massage therapists, "No hand is an island."

10. **Thou shalt receive massage as well as give.** A tense therapist is a handicapped therapist. To stay inspired, you periodically have to remember how good you're making everyone else feel. Do yourself the favor of receiving regular treatments; and when you get too busy or too self-denying to do this (as every therapist does at one time or another), forgive yourself. Then pick up the phone and call for an appointment.

LICENSING

Many practitioners of massage therapy consider what they do more of a healing "art" than a science. Feeling that way, they may experience some justifiable confusion when it comes to getting licensed to practice their art. After all, did Picasso need a license to paint? Or Van Gogh? Did Michelangelo require a permit to sculpt David?

As it turns out, even these great artists, like all artists everywhere, have had to pay homage to the powers that be. In fact, they and their art were in large part shaped by the social and political environment in which they worked. Nobody—no matter the chosen profession—works in a vacuum. Massage artists are no exception.

You will find that licensing regulations for massage vary widely from state to state, from county to county, and from city to city. I strongly encourage each of you to become familiar with the rules in your own community. However, I can present you with the general outline of some situations that apply in most locations.

To license or not to license is a hotly contested issue in many areas. As I mentioned earlier, many therapists in Vermont are not in favor of licensing massage because it would impose regulations on the free-spirited, independent attitude they have about their profession. There may be a correlation between the rugged individualism of the state's population and the license-free practice of massage there. In some respects, this may be a good thing, perhaps even an "American" thing. We were founded, after all, on ideals of freedom of expression and the entrepreneurial spirit. Because so many therapists care deeply about doing the best work possible in whatever manner they see fit, they have unfortunately come to perceive licensing as a restriction rather than a boon. As Deane Juhan said so eloquently in *Job's Body*, the therapist's hands are more like "flashlights in a darkened room" than scalpels or drugs. How do you regulate light? How do you impose rules on the healing energy that awakens self-awareness?

Therapists have reasons for wanting to keep their talents and energies unrestricted, and most of those reasons are very noble. However, a majority of people in the profession agree that licensing and regulation are an important part of the future of massage therapy in this country, even in Vermont. Without it, we won't be able to grow in both reputation and size. Other professionals in the medical and rehabilitative industries won't consider us serious partners to work with. Insurance companies won't pay us for the work we do. To optimize our importance as professionals and to help as many people as possible, licensing and other regulations, while they may at times feel restrictive, are definitely necessary.

In many communities across the country, the licensing laws have been written to keep massage therapy and prostitution apart. While this is a worthwhile effort, the effect has often been to create a hostile environment for ethical massage therapists to practice while actually limiting the practice of prostitution very little, if at all.

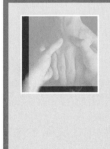

STATE BOARDS
ADMINISTERING MASSAGE PRACTICE
Alabama Massage Therapy Board
660 Adams Ave. #150
Montgomery, AL 36104
Phone: (334) 269-9990
Fax: (334) 263-6115
http://www.state.al.us

(continues)

Arizona State Board of Massage Therapy

1400 West Washington, Suite 230
Phoenix, AZ 85007
Phone: (602) 542-8604
Fax: (602) 542-3093
E-mail: info@massageboard.state.az.us
http://massagetherapy.az.gov

Arkansas State Board of Massage Therapy

PO Box 20739
Hot Springs, AR 71903
Phone: (501)623-0444
E-mail: asbmt@hsnp.com
http://www.state.ar.us

Connecticut

Massage Therapy Licensure
Department of Public Health
150 Washington Street
Hartford, CT 06106
Phone: (860) 509-8373
http://www.dph.state.ct.us

Delaware Board of Massage and Bodywork

Cannon Building, #203
861 Silver Lake Blvd. #203
Dover, DE 19904
Phone: (302) 739-4522 x205
Fax: (302) 739-2711
http://www.state.de.us

District of Columbia Board of Massage Therapy

Department of Health Professional Licensing Administration
825 N. Capitol Street NE, 2nd Floor
Washington, DC 20002
Phone: (202) 442-4774
http://www.dchealth.dc.gov

Florida Board of Massage Therapy

Florida Department of Health, Medical Quality Assurance
4052 Bald Cypress Way
Bin #C09
Tallahassee, FL 32399-3259
Phone: (850) 488-0595
Fax: (850) 487-9874
http://www.doh.state.fl.us/mqa/massage/ma_home.html

(continues)

Hawaii State Board of Massage Therapy
Department of Commerce & Consumer Affairs
PO Box 3469
Honolulu, HI 96801
Phone: (808) 586-2699
http://www.state.hi.us/dcca

Illinois Department of Financial & Professional Regulation
320 West Washington Street
Springfield, IL 62786
Phone: (217) 785-0800
Fax: (217) 782-7645
http://www.idfpr.com/dpr/who/masst.asp

Iowa Department of Health
Massage Therapy Advisory Board
Lucas State Office Bldg, 5th Floor
321 E. 12th St.
Des Moines, IA 50319-0075
Phone: (515) 242-5937
Fax: (515) 281-3121
http://www.idph.state.ia.us/licensure

Kentucky Board of Licensure for Massage Therapy
PO Box 1360
Frankfort, KY 40602
Phone: (502) 564-3296 x240
Fax: (502) 696-4818
http://finance.ky.gov/ourcabinet/caboff/OAS/op/massth/

Louisiana Board of Massage Therapy
12022 Plank Road
Zachary, LA 70811
Phone: (225) 771-4090
Fax: (225) 771-4021
E-mail: admin@lsbmt.org
http://www.lsbmt.org

Maine Board of Massage Therapy
Department of Professional and Financial Regulation
35 State House Station
Augusta, ME 04333-0035
Phone: (207) 624-8624
Fax: (207) 624-8637
http://www.state.me.us/pfr/led/massage

(continues)

Maryland Board of Chiropractic Examiners
Massage Therapy Advisory Committee
4201 Patterson Ave., 5th Floor
Baltimore, MD 21215-2299
Phone: (410) 764-4738
Fax: (410) 358-1879
http://www.mdmassage.org

Mississippi State Board of Massage Therapy
PO Box 12489
Jackson, MS 39236-2489
Phone: (601) 856-6127
Fax: (601) 853-0336
E-mail: director@msbmt.state.ms.us
http://www.msbmt.state.ms.us

Missouri Massage Therapy Board
Division of Professional Registration
PO Box 1335
Jefferson City, MO 65102
Phone: (573) 751-0845
Fax: (573) 751-0878
http://pr.mo.gov/asp

Nebraska Massage Therapy Board
Health and Human Services
Credentialing Division
PO Box 94986
Lincoln, NE 68509-4986
Phone: (402) 471-2117
Fax: (402) 471-3577
http://www.state.ne.us

New Jersey Board of Nursing
Massage, Bodywork & Somatic Therapy Examining Committee
124 Halsey Street
Newark, NJ 07102
Phone: (973) 504-6430
Fax: (973) 648-3481
http://www.state.nj.us/lps/ca/medical/nursing.htm

New Mexico
State Board of Massage Therapy
PO Box 25101
Santa Fe, NM 87504
Phone: (505) 476-4870
Fax: (505) 827-7095
http://www.rld.state.nm.us/b&c/massage

(continues)

New York State Board of Massage Therapy
Cultural Education Center, Room 3041
Albany, NY 12230
Phone: (518) 474-3817 x27
http://www.op.nysed.gov

North Carolina Board of Massage and Bodywork Therapy
PO Box 2539
Raleigh, NC 27602
Phone: (919) 546-0050
Fax: (919) 833-1059
http://www.bmbt.org

North Dakota State Board of Massage
PO Box 701
Grand Forks, ND 58201
Phone: (701) 872-4895
http://www.ndboardofmassage.com

Ohio State Medical Board
Massage Licensing Division
77 South High St., 17th Floor
Columbus, OH 43266-0315
Phone: (614) 466-3934
Fax: (614) 728-5946
http://www.state.oh.us/med

Oregon Board of Massage
3218 Pringle Rd. S.E. #250
Salem, OR 97302-1596
Phone: (503) 365-8657
Fax: (503) 378-3575
http://www.oregonmassage.org

Rhode Island Department of Health
Division of Professional Regulation
3 Capitol Hill, Room 104
Providence, RI 02908-5097
Phone: (401) 222-2827
Fax: (401) 222-1272
http://www.health.ri.gov/hsr/professions/massage.php

South Carolina Department of Labor, Licensing and Regulation
110 Center View
PO Box 11329
Columbia, SC 29210
Phone: (803) 896-4494
Fax: (803) 896-4484
http://www.llr.state.sc.us/POL/MassageTherapy

(continues)

Tennessee Massage Licensure Board
Cordell Hull Building 1st Floor
425 Fifth Ave. N.
Nashville, TN 37247-1010
Phone: (615) 532-3202
(888) 310-4650
Fax: (615) 532-5164
http://wwwz.state.tn.us/health/Boards/Massage

Texas Department of State Health Services
Massage Therapy Program
1100 West 49th St.
Austin, TX 78756-3183
Phone: (512) 834-6616
Fax: (512) 834-6677
http://www.dshs.state.tx.us/massage

Utah Division of Occupational & Professional Licensing
Board of Massage Therapy
160 East 300 South
Salt Lake City, UT 84145
Phone: (801) 530-6628
Fax: (801) 530-6511
http://www.dopl.utah.gov

Virginia Board of Nursing
Dept of Health Professions
6606 W. Broad St., 4th Floor
Richmond, VA 23230-1717
Phone: (804) 662-9909
Fax: (804) 662-9943
http://www.dhp.state.va.us

Washington State Department of Health
Massage Therapy Program
PO Box 47867
Olympia, WA 98504-7868
Phone: (360) 236-4866
Fax: (360) 664-9077
E-mail: hpqa.csc@doh.wa.gov
http://www.doh.wa.gov/massage/default.htm

State of West Virginia
Massage Therapy Licensure Board
200 Davis St. #1
Princeton, WV 24740-7430
Phone: (304) 487-1400
http://www.wvmassage.org

(continues)

Wisconsin Department of Regulation and Licensing
Massage Therapy Board
1400 E. Washington Ave.
PO Box 8935
Madison, WI 53708
Phone: (608) 266-8609
Fax: (608) 267-0644
http://www.wisconsin.gov

PROFILE: Dan Ulrich
Licensing and Regulation

Over the years, Dan Ulrich has been a therapist, a massage school owner, an entrepreneur, and an advocate of positive legislation for massage therapists. He and his wife Telka were the original owners of the Suncoast School of Massage in Tampa, Florida; and, from 1987 until 1995, Dan was the chairman of the Florida Board of Massage. He has worked hard to gain recognition for both the profession and his fellow therapists.

"The most profound initial changes for us as a profession came when we officially changed our name from 'masseuse' or 'masseur' to the more professional sounding 'massage therapist,'" recalls Dan. "Also, we got legislation passed requiring any form of advertising for massage services to include the massage license number of the advertiser. Those two things seemed to really turn the corner for us. It was like a magic change overnight,

and it was sorely needed. It's what seemed to spark the beginning of the profession's turning around even more than it already was."

This level of attention paid to such legislative details is an example of how massage therapists care for their clients through improving the standing of their profession. In addition to the hands-on therapy offered in traditional therapist-client relationships, practitioners have branched out to use their other skills in the promotion of massage. Dan, for instance, found that he needed every bit of the business and academic training he received in college to be an effective voice for the needs of massage therapists in the State of Florida. He was one of the people instrumental in setting guidelines for the number of hours massage therapists need to study to be certified, and he helped make sure therapists were required to periodically upgrade their skills and the

(continues)

services they offer through continuing education.

"When I was president of the Florida State Massage Therapy Association, I had a vision," states Dan. "If we can just continue informing the public, that's the most important thing. There's no substitute for education. All massage organizations have to get speakers out there and reach out to other groups. We've had to take a somewhat aggressive attitude, but we were tired of getting held hostage by unethical advertisers. As a profession, we've held on for a long time, trying to teach people what massage is really about, and now this education has started to pay off."

This kind of work on the intellectual and legislative levels is an extension of the therapy that goes on in every massage room across the country. Our heads, as well as our hands, need to care. With regulations that support us, we can both prosper and help our clients more effectively.

Sometimes the laws seem made to *promote* prostitution. For example, in Santa Monica, California, where I first graduated from massage school, to get my license to practice in that city I had to pay a visit to a county health clinic and be tested for VD, as if the city assumed that anyone who wanted to practice massage was going to come into sexual contact with a lot of people and that they should be checked out. This was both time-consuming and embarrassing; and, to add to the frustration, I was forced to *lie* to the people at the clinic because they were tired of new therapists coming in for tests to get their license and they refused to admit any more of them. I had to tell them I thought I really had VD in order to get the test and eventually receive the license. I'll never forget what the examining doctor said as I left the clinic. Even though, of course, he had been unable to find any trace of venereal disease, he looked at me with old, tired eyes and said, "Next time, wear a condom."

I didn't want to be treated like that. That was not what I went to massage school for. Anger and resentment against prostitutes welled up in me for a short time, but then I realized that it wasn't their fault. It was nobody's fault in particular. Our society as a whole still has fears and inhibitions about its collective body. People who are paid to touch the collective body, whether for sensual pleasure or therapeutic relief, are still looked on with a bit of trepidation by lawmakers and good citizens who have not yet and will probably never take that step of becoming a touch professional of any kind.

In a way, we therapists scare people with our willingness to actually touch a stranger, *any* stranger. The most common negative comment you'll hear from people who find out you've become a massage therapist will most likely be, "How could you touch all those strangers? Fat ones, skinny ones, old ones, ugly ones? I could never do it. Yuck."

That "primal yuck" stems from the essential disconnection that many people feel from all other people. We, as therapists, have set ourselves the task of reconnecting ourselves to other people, reconnecting those people to their own bodies, and perhaps even helping people reconnect to each other. We have to remember, with some humility, that this is a task that many people don't feel capable of—at least not at this point in their lives. They may learn to expand their connectedness to other people eventually, and you may be the one to teach them, but we have to understand and forgive their fears right now because that's all we can do, and it's the only way to help people overcome those fears in the long run.

My advice now is to bite the bullet and do whatever it takes to become legally licensed in your area, even if that means saying you forgot to use a rubber.

Certification

In many parts of the country, you still don't need a license to practice massage; in that case, it's important to become certified. Certified therapists have attended a recognized massage training facility and have proven their level of skill by passing a course and/or an exam.

Many beginning therapists still encounter some confusion when it comes to differentiating between licensing and certification. A *license* is the piece of paper you may or may not need to legally practice massage therapy in your state, county, or city, and it will be issued by that governmental body. A *certificate* is the piece of paper you receive after graduation from an accredited massage school or passing a particular exam. No matter where you practice, you'll need some kind of certificate before you are allowed to apply for a license.

National Certification

National certification of massage therapists is overseen by the National Certification Board for Therapeutic Massage and Bodywork (NCBTMB). The

NCBTMB was formed in 1992 and has since grown into a strong voice for the profession. You can take the national certification exam after you've graduated from massage school with 500 or more hours of training *or* if you can prove a certain degree of professional experience equivalent to 500 hours. Many states have adopted the national certification exam as their official licensing exam, and some require it in addition to their own state examinations.

Although it is a positive step forward toward the professionalization of massage, some people feel that the National Certification Exam is over-restrictive and does not take into account the experienced, highly qualified practitioners of different massage techniques such as Rolfing® and Trager® who may not necessarily have the skills and knowledge about Swedish massage needed to pass the test. The NCBTMB has recognized this and has researched plans for more advanced testing capabilities that will allow practitioners from various fields to receive certification. There has also been talk of varying levels of certification for practitioners with differing degrees of skill and education.

It's now extremely simple to take the National Certification Exam in most parts of the country, and it's becoming ever more accepted as a standard everywhere. You'll be doing yourself and your profession a favor by becoming a nationally certified therapist, even if you have plenty of other documentation to prove your competency. To find out more, contact the National Certification Board for Therapeutic Massage and Bodywork at 1901 South Meyers Road Suite 240, Oakbrook Terrace, IL 60181, telephone (800) 296-0664 or (630) 627-8000; Website: http://www.ncbtmb.com.

Continuing Education Units

Once you've reached your goals of becoming certified and receiving a license, the educational component of your massage career is by no means over. Every time you renew your license or your certification status (or even your membership in one of the massage organizations), you will be required to show that you have earned a certain number of continuing education units (CEUs). The number of CEUs required is not high, usually just 12 per year, which can be earned in one weekend workshop or during one massage convention. If you're like many therapists, however, you will far exceed your quota of education for any particular time period. The range and volume of choices available are just too enticing to pass up. You could continue to take interesting, useful classes every month for the rest of your life and never come close to running out of options. Massage truly is a lifelong learning process.

Licensing, CEUs, and certification are a way of life for massage therapists now, as they are for many other professionals, but it wasn't always this way. Until quite recently, massage therapists had to struggle to attain the level of professionalism they now enjoy. In many ways, this struggle is still going on. What most therapists want is simple recognition; they want people to know that what they are doing is helpful, that it is corrective in some circumstances, that it is a viable adjunct to health care, that it matters. Licensing and certification help the public understand that all these things are true.

ZONING

If you plan to set up your own massage business, zoning regulations may play an important part in determining exactly *where* that business will be set up. Have you found the perfect old Victorian house that's just begging to be converted into the massage studio of your dreams? Better check with the zoning board first.

Ask your town clerk to show you a zoning map that details where certain types of businesses may and may not be opened. You'll also have to determine what kind of business your community considers therapeutic massage to be, because this can differ in different areas.

If you want to do massage on a consistent basis from your own home (and especially if you want to advertise that fact), you should contact the zoning board for approval. You may even have to go before the board for a hearing. What you'll want to stress to them is the low impact that your massage business will have on the neighbors and the neighborhood. If it's just you practicing, mention the fact that only one car at a time will be parking in front of your house, one person walking up to your front door, and so on.

ESTABLISHMENT LICENSE

Besides your own personal massage license, if you are starting a place of business, you may also need an establishment license. This is a separate document that must be paid for (and renewed) separately. To acquire it, you'll have to show proof that your facilities meet certain standards. In most areas, you'll need a shower available for clients, for example. You may also need handicapped-accessible facilities. The rules for establishment licenses vary from region to region, just like the personal license, and you'll have to check with your local governing organization to make sure you are in compliance (see the list earlier in this chapter).

LIABILITY INSURANCE

Even though you'll be spending 99 percent of your time as a therapist making people feel better, there is always the chance that someone might find cause to sue you for making him or her feel worse in some way. As you are aware, you need to be extra careful about this issue. People in the United States have been lawsuit-happy in recent years. You might be the victim of a suit that was completely unfounded, but you'd still be liable for damages. That would not be your fault, but it would be your fault if your career and perhaps even your life were ruined because of it. It's easy to attain the kind of insurance that will protect you against such claims.

Two million dollars per occurance and six million dollars aggregate in liability insurance are included as one of the benefits of membership in the American Massage Therapy Association, for example. Dues are only $235 per year, and that includes other benefits as well. Other professional organizations such as Associated Bodywork & Massage Professionals and the International Massage Association also offer similar policies. Don't make the mistake of being unprepared for one of the ugly potentialities of *any* business. Get covered.

If you are working at a spa or other large establishment, any potential lawsuit would most likely be directed toward the deeper pockets of the institution. However, there are two good reasons for still making sure you have some form of liability protection: (1) The person filing the suit may not care if your pockets are shallow and, therefore, proceed against you regardless; and (2) the spa or other institution may require you to be insured as a condition of employment. In fact, going into any job interview with your association membership and insurance already covered shows prospective employers how serious you are about working in this field.

SAFETY CONCERNS

You're probably more likely to have someone sue you for falling down your front steps than for receiving a harmful massage. It pays for you, then, to cover your bases and make sure your practice is as safe as possible both for yourself and your clients. I've included a few commonsense guidelines here, some of which apply specifically to massage and some of which should be observed with any business.

1. Apply rough-textured adhesive strips to any steps or slick surfaces, especially those that get wet.

2. Make sure you have sturdy handrails next to any stairs.

3. Provide adequate lighting so clients don't slam their shins into furniture or walls. Remember to turn the lights back up, at least a little, after giving a massage so that clients can see when they get off the table.

4. Make sure the floor directly to the side of the massage table is covered with a nonslip rug or that the client wears some kind of slipper when he or she stands up. Massage oil on the soles of feet makes them slippery on slick tile, which could lead to an accident.

5. Provide handicap rails and ramps if you are going to see any disabled clients. Check with the zoning board to see if this is a requirement for opening an office.

THIRD-PARTY BILLING

During the past decade, the massage business has grown to become a recognized, insurance-eligible member of mainstream health care. This important change came through the efforts of many hardworking, determined therapists and professional organizations. Many insurers, even preferred provider organizations (PPOs) and health maintenance organizations (HMOs), include the massage profession in their eligible provider pool. This means that you can receive reimbursement for your services.

However, the insurance company still dictates what types of health conditions it will pay for and who can provide the service. A lot of work is being done in the massage community *and* in the medical community to demonstrate to the insurance companies the cost-effectiveness of touch therapies. If the insurance companies can be convinced that massage will save them money, they will pay for it. Studies to prove exactly this are being conducted by such respected organizations as the Office of Alternative Medicine at the National Institutes of Health. The University of Miami Medical School's Touch Research Institute is bringing forth much supportive evidence as well.

If you want to join the growing number of massage therapists who increase their practice and income significantly by working with doctors and chiropractors and make insurance billing a part of their practice, you will be wise to invest in some insurance reimbursement education to help you through the process. You will be successful only if you understand how the system works and how to use it in your practice. See the profile of Vivian Madison-Mahoney for more information about insurance billing.

PROFILE: Vivian Madison-Mahoney, LMT
Insurance Billing and Reimbursement for Massage Professionals

Vivian Madison-Mahoney was the first therapist to ever bill and be reimbursed for a workers' compensation case in the State of Florida. The judge of compensation claims there found that massage therapy services were indeed medically necessary and ruled for the patient to continue to receive this physician-prescribed service at Vivian's establishment. It was Vivian's tenacity, determination, diplomacy, and knowledge of Florida law that helped set the precedent for massage therapists to be recognized as health-care providers in the state's workers' compensation system.

Vivian was also among the first to successfully bill and be reimbursed for personal injury cases and major medical cases. These experiences led her to begin instructing other massage therapists on how to successfully bill and be reimbursed by insurance companies. Over the years, she has become a treasure trove of knowledge and information on the topic, keeping all interested therapists updated on the latest changes, regulations, rules, and other insurance issues (all for no charge) through her articles in many massage publications and via e-mails and phone calls. Her popular manuals and insurance home study courses include the 2004 edition of *Manipulate Your Future: Practice Building and Insurance Billing* and her *Comprehensive Guide to Insurance*

(continues)

Vivian Madison-Mahoney, LMT (continued)

Billing for Massage Professionals, which is continually updated. This was the very first insurance billing manual written for massage therapists, back in 1989.

Vivian is rightly proud of her work and the fact that a growing number of insurers are reimbursing therapists directly for prescribed, medically necessary massage therapy services. But she says our success is all due to the hardworking, dedicated massage therapists who are willing to take chances to help those in need while accepting insurance for payment.

Vivian states that workers' compensation and personal injury cases are now reimbursing massage therapists in almost every state. "More and more therapists," she says, "are realizing the satisfaction of working with injured, ill, and disabled patients. They realize too that accepting insurance helps to increase physician referrals. When working with medical cases, though, therapists cannot just randomly write down a medical code here and there and expect to become successful billing insurance. Working with medical cases means working with legal cases, and you need to be well prepared."

Unlike when she first started several years ago, Vivian says insurance companies now are thoroughly monitoring claims and documentation when massage therapy is involved. She councils therapists to have all of their *i*s dotted and *t*s crossed in order to prevent delays and denials of payment. Therapists who go into the medical/insurance territory fully prepared know to be careful and avoid accepting the types of cases that will ultimately either not pay or that will request monies back at a later date.

"Massage therapists can accept auto accident, personal injury, and workers' comp cases in most states," says Vivian. "However, we still have a long way to go with federally related programs or coverage such as Medicare and Medicaid, with the exception of the State of Washington that has what is known as the 'Every Category Provider Law.' While a couple of other states have what is known as 'Any Willing Provider Laws,' I am not sure to what extent massage therapists are taking advantage of this if at all. We need to continue research, gather articles, and use case studies that communicate the benefits of our manual therapy techniques to employers as well as insurance companies. Surveys continue to show that consumers use massage and body therapy services regularly and want their insurance companies to reimburse when the services are determined by their physicians to be medically necessary."

Vivian believes that we need to work hard together, continue research,

(continues)

maintain proper documentation that proves functional improvements due to our therapy, avoid arrogance and egotism, and retain our humility. "We always need to remember who we are," she says, "and to never forget how we achieved successes in the massage therapy field in the first place. It has been our effective work, caring attitudes, fair and ethical fees, and the extra time we spend with our clients/patients that have helped them to improve when all else failed. To forget this or to veer too far from our own path as massage therapists can cause us to lose ground very quickly. When working with insurance and medical referrals, it is important to do it fairly, ethically, and accurately from the beginning. Though it is not necessary to be certified in 'medical massage' in order to bill and be reimbursed by insurance (and I hope it never comes to that because many therapists as well as patients would be more limited in their choices), we have to be knowledgeable enough to work

with the physicians, insurance adjusters, and other professionals involved in the process."

Vivian earned her reputation one patient and one referral at a time, with more than 175 physicians referring to her massage therapy establishment at one time or another and patient visits averaging 28 to 32 per day over several years, and she has now become a leading authority on the topic. She is happy to hear about your own successes as well as your problems with insurance billing via phone or e-mail. For more information or to order manuals or approved home study courses, you can visit her Web site. To enroll in her "Insurance Updates, Tips, and News Program" mailing list, scroll to the bottom of her Web site order page and register.

Vivian Madison-Mahoney
http://www. massageinsurancebilling.com
E-mail: vivianmadison@aol.com
Phone: (865) 436-3573

TAXES

If you aren't working in a spa or doctor's office or health clinic, chances are that you receive a lot of your income directly from the customer. You'll have to be careful about that because you are still liable for taxes on that money even though it isn't coming to you in the normally recognizable, taxable form: a paycheck.

The first year you start out as an independent therapist, you won't know exactly how much you'll make. Since no money is being withheld, you'll probably end up with a nasty surprise at the end of the year when you figure out how much you owe Uncle Sam. Not only will you owe your personal income tax (plus state income tax if it applies), but you're also responsible for the social security tax that wasn't withheld. This will now be called your self-employment tax, and it's around 15 percent of your total income. Make sure to save some extra money on the side during your first year of independent status to cover these eventualities. Thereafter, you can make quarterly estimated tax payments based on what you paid the previous year. On the 15th of June, September, January, and April, you'll be responsible for sending in one-quarter of the total you owed the year before. This makes it easier for you because you won't be stuck with a large expense all at once.

It pays to keep track of your expenditures and then write them off as deductions later. If you are not sure about how to do this, follow this simple rule: get a receipt for *everything* and save it. Classify your receipts according to the type of expenditure. Automobile, transportation, meals, lodging, entertainment, and so on each get their own file into which you deposit the receipts. At the end of the year, add them up and fill in the appropriate blanks in the Profit or Loss From Business part of your tax return (see Figure 6-1). It's especially important to keep track of any big business purchases like a computer; any constant expenses like advertising, phone calls, postage, and the like; and *all* the miles you travel. Wear and tear on your vehicle can also be deducted.

Deductions are your greatest ally as an independent operator. With them, you can significantly lower the amount you have to pay in taxes. Cultivate your awareness of deductions until the whole world seems to be filled with deductions everywhere you look. Focus on them. Make them a part of your life.

Here are some examples of things that can be deducted:

- Your massage table
- The computer you do your accounting on
- Sheets, towels, oils, and creams
- Paper, rubber bands, pencils and pens, letterhead and business cards, and anything else you use in your daily business activities
- The cost of your massage license

Figure 6-1 | CIRS Schedule C, Profit or Loss From Business.

SCHEDULE C **(Form 1040)** Department of the Treasury Internal Revenue Service	**Profit or Loss From Business** (Sole Proprietorship) ▶ Partnerships, joint ventures, etc., must file Form 1065 or 1065-B. ▶ Attach to Form 1040 or 1041. ▶ See Instructions for Schedule C (Form 1040).	OMB No. 1545-0074 **2004** Attachment Sequence No. **09**

Name of proprietor | Social security number (SSN)

A Principal business or profession, including product or service (see page C-2 of the instructions) | **B** Enter code from pages C-7, 8, & 9 ▶

C Business name. If no separate business name, leave blank. | **D** Employer ID number (EIN), if any

E Business address (including suite or room no.) ▶ ....
City, town or post office, state, and ZIP code

F Accounting method: **(1)** ☐ Cash **(2)** ☐ Accrual **(3)** ☐ Other (specify) ▶ ....

G Did you "materially participate" in the operation of this business during 2004? If "No," see page C-3 for limit on losses ☐ Yes ☐ No

H If you started or acquired this business during 2004, check here .... ▶ ☐

Part I Income

1	Gross receipts or sales. **Caution.** If this income was reported to you on Form W-2 and the "Statutory employee" box on that form was checked, see page C-3 and check here .... ▶ ☐	1
2	Returns and allowances	2
3	Subtract line 2 from line 1	3
4	Cost of goods sold (from line 42 on page 2)	4
5	**Gross profit.** Subtract line 4 from line 3.	5
6	Other income, including Federal and state gasoline or fuel tax credit or refund (see page C-3)	6
7	**Gross income.** Add lines 5 and 6 .... ▶	7

Part II Expenses. Enter expenses for business use of your home **only** on line 30.

8	Advertising	8	19 Pension and profit-sharing plans	19	
9	Car and truck expenses (see page C-3).	9	20 Rent or lease (see page C-5): a Vehicles, machinery, and equipment	20a	
10	Commissions and fees ...	10	b Other business property ..	20b	
11	Contract labor (see page C-4)	11	21 Repairs and maintenance ...	21	
12	Depletion	12	22 Supplies (not included in Part III)	22	
13	Depreciation and section 179 expense deduction (not included in Part III) (see page C-4)	13	23 Taxes and licenses ... 24 Travel, meals, and entertainment: a Travel	23 24a	
14	Employee benefit programs (other than on line 19).	14	b Meals and entertainment		
15	Insurance (other than health) .	15	c Enter nondeduct-ible amount in-cluded on line 24b (see page C-5) .		
16	Interest:		d Subtract line 24c from line 24b	24d	
a	Mortgage (paid to banks, etc.)	16a	25 Utilities	25	
b	Other	16b	26 Wages (less employment credits) .	26	
17	Legal and professional services	17	27 Other expenses (from line 48 on page 2).	27	
18	Office expense	18			

28	**Total expenses** before expenses for business use of home. Add lines 8 through 27 in columns . ▶	28	
29	Tentative profit (loss). Subtract line 28 from line 7	29	
30	Expenses for business use of your home. Attach **Form 8829**	30	
31	**Net profit or (loss).** Subtract line 30 from line 29. • If a profit, enter on **Form 1040, line 12,** and also on **Schedule SE, line 2** (statutory employees, see page C-6). Estates and trusts, enter on Form 1041, line 3. • If a loss, you **must** go to line 32.	31	
32	If you have a loss, check the box that describes your investment in this activity (see page C-6). • If you checked 32a, enter the loss on **Form 1040, line 12,** and also on **Schedule SE, line 2** (statutory employees, see page C-6). Estates and trusts, enter on Form 1041, line 3. • If you checked 32b, you **must** attach **Form 6198.**	32a ☐ All investment is at risk. 32b ☐ Some investment is not at risk.	

For Paperwork Reduction Act Notice, see Form 1040 instructions.   Cat. No. 11334P   **Schedule C (Form 1040) 2004**

Figure 6-1 | continued.

Part III   Cost of Goods Sold (see page C-6)

33   Method(s) used to value closing inventory: **a** ☐ Cost   **b** ☐ Lower of cost or market   **c** ☐ Other (attach explanation)

34   Was there any change in determining quantities, costs, or valuations between opening and closing inventory? If "Yes," attach explanation . . . . ☐ Yes   ☐ No

35 Inventory at beginning of year. If different from last year's closing inventory, attach explanation . .	**35**	
36 Purchases less cost of items withdrawn for personal use	**36**	
37 Cost of labor. Do not include any amounts paid to yourself	**37**	
38 Materials and supplies	**38**	
39 Other costs	**39**	
40 Add lines 35 through 39	**40**	
41 Inventory at end of year	**41**	
42 **Cost of goods sold.** Subtract line 41 from line 40. Enter the result here and on page 1, line 4 . .	**42**	

Part IV   **Information on Your Vehicle.** Complete this part **only** if you are claiming car or truck expenses on line 9 and are not required to file Form 4562 for this business. See the instructions for line 13 on page C-4 to find out if you must file Form 4562.

43   When did you place your vehicle in service for business purposes? (month, day, year) ▶ . . . . / . . . . / . . . .

44   Of the total number of miles you drove your vehicle during 2004, enter the number of miles you used your vehicle for:

a Business . . . . **b** Commuting . . . . **c** Other . . . .

45   Do you (or your spouse) have another vehicle available for personal use? . . . . ☐ Yes   ☐ No

46   Was your vehicle available for personal use during off-duty hours? . . . . ☐ Yes   ☐ No

47a   Do you have evidence to support your deduction? . . . . ☐ Yes   ☐ No

   b   If "Yes," is the evidence written? . . . . ☐ Yes   ☐ No

Part V   **Other Expenses.** List below business expenses not included on lines 8–26 or line 30.

. . . .	
. . . .	
. . . .	
. . . .	
. . . .	
. . . .	
. . . .	
. . . .	

48 **Total other expenses.** Enter here and on page 1, line 27	**48**	

SAMPLE

✳ Professional association membership dues

✳ The sound system for your massage room

✳ The George Winston CDs you play on the sound system

✳ Mileage to and from massage appointments (but not commuting from your home to your massage studio and back, which is considered nondeductible)

✳ Meals you eat with prospective clients (partially deductible)

✳ All advertising for your massage business

✳ The seminar you took to learn new massage techniques

✳ The turkey sandwich you ate at the seminar

✳ Your hotel room facing the beach at the annual massage convention

✳ Books and videos and CD-ROMS related to massage

At first, you'll be amazed at how many expenditures you can actually deduct. Be careful, though. Some therapists might find the inherent deductibility of many of their activities to be a license to deduct activities that fall into a gray area or are perhaps an outright attempt to fool the IRS, which is not a good idea—especially when it comes your turn to be audited. The IRS has gotten stricter lately about those amorphous "entertainment" expenses. Even business meals can only be partially deducted now. You have to be careful.

Examples of claims that push the limits of plausibility include:

✳ The stereo system for your living room that a massage client can hear from the studio in the back of the house, but only if the doors are open and the stereo is turned up full blast (if you do claim something like this, at least make sure you have an establishment license for your house and the proper zoning approval)

✳ The tai-chi classes you take to strengthen your back for the practice of massage therapy (this might be justified if you had a note from your doctor documenting your debilitating back pain)

✳ The gardening gloves you wear to protect your hands while weeding in your backyard

Examples of claims that are fraudulent include:

- ✳ Your long-distance girlfriend's round-trip air fare from Topeka to come receive a massage from you

- ✳ Phone bills for the calls you made to the friend you went to massage school with and who later moved to Hong Kong

- ✳ Expenses for your weekend trip to the coast, where you massaged your wife and your children in the evenings after a day on the beach

If you work out of your home, the part of your house in which you do massage and conduct your business can be deducted. You'll need to file a special schedule with your tax return for that. Note: Sending in a deduction for "business use of the home" is a red flag to the people at the IRS, who may then send one of their helpful, meticulous workers out for a personal visit. Calculate your savings from such a deduction first and then determine if it's worth it to you.

When it comes to taxes, you'd be wise to find an accountant who can help you. He may know some creative ways to reduce your taxes to the minimum and maximize your income. Accountant services can be less expensive than you might think. You might want to follow the lead of several other therapists who have offered massage services in exchange for accounting. This is an area where bartering works great: You save on your taxes, and your accountant cuts down on his stress at what is, for him, the most hectic time of the year. See the section on bartering in chapter 8.

7 Creating the Perfect Space: How to Set Up and Maintain the Optimal Environment for Your Massage Therapy Practice

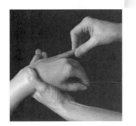

Even if you don't consider yourself an artist, you will probably find yourself, like most therapists, putting quite a bit of thought into the creation of a beautiful, tranquil environment that's conducive to your work. The reason for this is simple: Massage is the focused, *conscious* application of touch for the purposes of enhancing life; and the environment into which you invite people to experience this conscious touch is an extension of your intentions. The room you practice massage in can touch your clients, just like your fingers and your palms. Clients feel your influence simply through being in the place you have created.

CREATING YOUR SPACE: POINTS TO KEEP IN MIND

Thousands of other therapists have gone before you in the quest to provide their clients with an outer ambience that mirrors an inner state of peace, relaxation, and healing. How can you best achieve this goal for yourself? In my opinion, you should take into account these three points when you first start thinking about the setup and decoration of your massage area:

1. First, realize that the environment you perform your massage in is *not* the most important element involved in the success of your practice or the happiness of your clients—not by a long shot. The psychological or emotional atmosphere of safety, nurturing, and care that you provide means much more than the appropriate color scheme or pieces of expensive Native American sculpture. This doesn't mean that you shouldn't fill your space with beautiful art and creative designs. However, you should focus on your skills (both massage and business) before you begin investing much in your decor.

2. Choose a design theme that reflects who *you* are. The environment you create for doing your massage will be completely unique and personal. Each step you take in the creation process is a reflection of how you feel about your work and your life, and it is better to be true to your own vision than do something just because you think it's what other people expect. If all the other therapists you know paint clouds on their ceilings and fill their massage rooms with huge, glittering crystals from Brazil, this doesn't mean you have to. If you are an Egyptophile, for instance, and everything about that civilization fascinates you, you might consider painting a mural of the great pyramids on your treatment room walls (I've seen this done in a spa, and it made an impressive effect). Perhaps you could use some soft Egyptian music or essential oils imported from the bazaars of Cairo. Use your creativity to come up with your own signature atmosphere. Of course, you shouldn't go overboard with this; if your favorite hobby is miniature electric trains, you probably shouldn't have them chugging around the room while a treatment is in progress.

3. Create your perfect environment one piece at a time, fully appreciating each step along the way. Like most therapists, your massage space will probably be an ongoing production. You will, quite likely, never reach a point of being done with your creation. There will always be one more piece of art or one more useful tool you can add to your collection. Therefore, don't worry about rushing things at the beginning, just so you can get it "right." Your environment will continue to grow and change just as you yourself will continue to grow and change as a therapist through the years.

The types of rooms you are likely to do massage in (apart from rooms in your clients' own homes) can be broken down into four basic categories:

❋ An entire room or studio in your home

❋ One part of a room in your home

❋ Your own place of business in a clinic or office setting

❋ In somebody else's business, either a salon, spa, medical practice, or health club

Each of these environments calls for a distinct set of considerations in order to be set up appropriately. You'll need to pay attention to the mood or feeling you create while at the same time taking into account all practical realities. If you are designing your own work space within a chiropractor's office, for instance, the challenge will be to balance a clinical cleanness with your own personal touches. Here are some tips for each type of situation:

1. **A separate room in your own home.** This is where you'll find the most freedom to conceive of and execute your own personal statement. With a separate room and a door that closes behind you, you'll be free from the influences of other opinions, tastes, and concerns. It is somewhat of a luxury to have a space in your home dedicated solely to your massage work. If you are lucky enough to have one, you owe it to yourself and your clients to make it special. Your only guidelines, then, will be a faithfulness to your own vision and an objective concern for your clients' tastes and sensibilities. In your home studio, you may, for example, create an altar that holds objects that you think are conducive to positive healing experiences. These can be artifacts; pieces of nature (stones, feathers, crystals, bones); fabric; ceremonial instruments; or photographs of spiritual teachers, healers, or loved ones. In my home, I have a set of small bells from Tibet that fill the air with a peaceful high-toned sound when struck together. I'm not suggesting that you need to make your massage room into a shrine. The most important thing is to just be yourself. Your altar may include a snapshot of Joe DiMaggio if he is an idol of yours and his photo reminds you to always strive to do your physical best. You don't have to be New Age to be a good therapist (see the sidebar, "Massage Therapy and the New Age").

2. **One part of a room in your home.** You will have to make certain concessions to practicality if your massage room is also your living room or guest bedroom. However, those concessions often lead to some unexpected resourcefulness. When faced with turning almost any spot

MASSAGE THERAPY AND THE NEW AGE

Some people have an image of massage therapists as hippies wearing tie-dyed clothes and living in a world hazy with incense smoke and resonating with sitar music.

However, the truth today is that most of us are conservative, professional folks who feel more natural wearing polo shirts, lab coats, or suits than multicolored muumuus or flowery tunics. Regardless of our political or social orientation or choice of clothing, though, all therapists owe a certain debt of gratitude to those flower children who helped keep massage therapy alive during the 1960s and 1970s when it suffered a low point in its reputation. The New Agers were the ones who kept intentional, conscious massage from disappearing and laid the groundwork for the thriving therapeutic practice we see happening today. Much of this sustaining work took place in California, particularly at the Esalen Institute, but it was certainly not limited to this area. Pioneering practitioners across the country kept the message alive.

One reason that massage and the New Age seem to go hand in hand is that all serious massage therapists consider their work therapeutic, yet this therapy has not been fully accepted by the mainstream medical establishment, and it is thus categorized as "alternative." Being alternative is not bad. In fact, it may be quite beneficial. As noted in chapter 1, Americans spend billions of dollars a year on alternative therapies, creating a big market. Ironically, many of these so-called new therapies—massage and acupuncture, for example—are actually quite ancient, and it is Western allopathic medicine that is new on the scene in terms of human history.

We therapists can use the label "New Age" to our advantage and the advantage of our clients. If we carefully and with *good taste* make use of certain New Age writings, videos, music, and other tools, we can gradually turn alternative therapies into preferred therapies. Certain organizations have developed over the past several years to aid us in this process.

into a massage area, most therapists surprise themselves. I received a massage once from a woman who lived in a studio apartment in Miami Beach. The room was truly cramped, and when I first walked in her door, I wondered where she could possibly set up her table. Furniture and plants (lots of plants) filled the tiny space. A few minutes later, I watched in amazement as she scooted her futon into one corner and pushed two chairs back toward the kitchen. Then she lifted a couple of the plants off of their perches and hung them from hooks on the ceiling. Voila! A beautiful space was created just big enough for her massage table to fit into. The view looking up from that table was like being inside a tropical greenhouse. She had a big refracting crystal hung over each window that filled the room with rainbows. When she flicked on a tape player, bird calls sounded, intermingling with music. It was one of the most delightful massages I've had.

You can employ similar ingenuity when it comes to using part of your living space for your massage. The important thing is to make your clients feel that the time they spend with you is special and that the space they are in is especially made for massage, though in reality it may simply be an unused corner of your rumpus room. Try creating the illusion of a separate area by positioning plants and furniture. Room dividers and hanging beads or silk sheets also work well.

3. **Your own place of business.** Once again, because the business is your own, you have a large degree of freedom when it comes to setting it up. However, the public may expect something a little more toned down if they think of your office as a clinic. White walls and a no-nonsense reception desk will put people at ease if that's what they have come to expect. If, on the other hand, you set up your office as a spa (Figure 7-1), you'll have a good deal more artistic license when it comes to the ambience of your business. For some specific ideas about floor plans and layout guidelines for a massage business, see the next section, "Setting Up A Professional Space."

4. **Somebody else's business.** In this situation, you'll be the most severely restricted, and in many cases you may not be able to make any changes at all to your assigned work area. There are a few little secrets that can help you, though. For example, try bringing your own altar with you to work every day. This should not be anything large or obtrusive, perhaps just a small picture of your mate or child placed discreetly on a countertop. Most clients recognize and appreciate it when you add something of yourself to an impersonal environment. Make sure not to do anything that angers the owners or the management of the establishment; you don't want to jeopardize your job. You can also change the lighting by draping a silk scarf over lamps or under ceiling lights, taking the scarf with you when you leave each day. Try placing a few drops of some essential oil on a lightbulb before your client enters; this will fill the room with your chosen therapeutic scent without leaving the lingering odor and smokiness of incense.

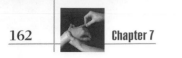
Figure 7-1 | Day spa interior. (Roosevelt Baths lobby, Saratoga Springs, New York. Courtesy of Xanterra Parks & Resorts.)

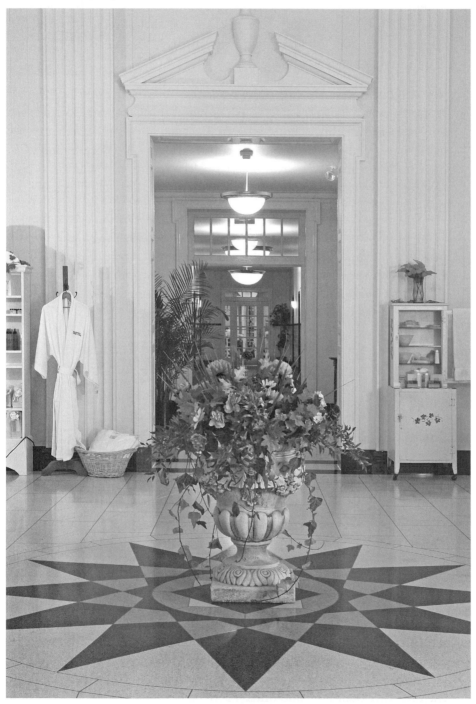

SETTING UP A PROFESSIONAL SPACE

Nobody can tell you where the best place to begin your massage business is going to be. A storefront or a free-standing building? An abandoned gas station or a refurbished Victorian mansion? One room, two rooms, ten? You have to listen to your own inner guidance, follow your heart, and do what feels right. *Plus,* you have to pay a lot more attention to the reality of your monetary situation than you might want to. ***This is extremely important!***

The biggest single reason therapists go out of business when they first get started, no matter whether they go into it with $100 or $100,000, is "undercapitalization." This is a fancy polite word that business experts will use to tell you that, basically, you're *too poor* to be running the business you had envisioned. You see, the old saying is true: It takes money to make money. And when you first start out, you should have cash reserves on hand equal to at least six months' living expenses so that if you don't see a profit from your business during that time (which is quite likely), you won't have to shut down and go work at McDonald's.

But there's a catch. However reasonable it may sound in theory, in reality very few new therapists have an extra six months' worth of capital lying about at their disposal. The answer to this dilemma is to take the route that so many therapists have taken before you. I call it sustainable undercapitalization, or, more commonly, eking by.

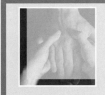

MEDITATION AND YOUR MASSAGE SPACE

Regardless of whether you work at home or at somebody else's property, you will want to infuse the room you work in with your own particular positive thoughts and feelings, your "energy." You can do this through a ritual, a ceremony, or simply by being still. If you are at all inclined to practice meditation, as many massage therapists are, I strongly urge you to meditate in your own massage area, perhaps right on top of your table. This is a technique I've often used, with some rather concrete results.

"I always feel so calm when I come here, like I can drop everything from the outside world and have no worries for a little while," clients often tell me when they come for an appointment. "You must lead such a peaceful lifestyle. I can feel it in the air here."

(continues)

Little do they know that just 20 minutes earlier I was rushing in from the post office or the gym, playing back my messages, returning important calls, and jumping into the shower for a two-minute rinse. My lifestyle is anything but peaceful. But then, as the time for the appointment approaches, I drop the need to be actively engaged in the minutiae that make up the bulk of everyone's life. Instead, resisting the temptation to keep rushing, I take a seat cross-legged on my massage table, take a few deep breaths, and just *be*.

There are hundreds of schools of meditation, and the contemplative arts form a vast, ancient, complex way of life practiced by adepts for millennia; but meditation really needn't be any more difficult than sitting on your table and breathing. If, in fact, you make the time to do this, you will be more relaxed and more resourceful than 99.9 percent of the people who will ever come to see you. Regardless of how popular it is in some circles, sitting still and not doing anything but breathing is an incredibly rare act. If you do it, other people will feel it.

It's particularly important to engage in meditation when you are "christening" a new massage space. Before you accept your first client into your new massage area, spend half an hour there just breathing. Focus on pulling your own positive healing intentions into the environment and purging any leftover molecules from previous tenants. If you feel comfortable doing so, burn some sage or juniper to aid in this process, as Native Americans have in purification ceremonies for centuries. You may be amazed by the effectiveness of the process. Some undefined, invisible energy seems to linger in rooms when people have left them after long inhabitation.

The following is a simple, nondenominational, 10-minute meditation meant to be used specifically by therapists who are about to receive a client into their room. If you consistently take these few minutes to calm and center yourself, you'll be surprised at what a difference it makes to your practice.

First, here are a few guidelines to help you in your meditation:

❋ Sit erectly on your massage table or somewhere nearby, using a cushion beneath you to help keep your spine straight.

❋ If you are stressed or wired, try lying down on your massage table for the meditation, but don't lie down if you're feeling tired because you will probably end up asleep just when your client is arriving.

❋ If your appointment time has already arrived, don't decide that you have no time to meditate and then spend the next several minutes both rushing *and* feeling guilty about not meditating. Clients are sometimes a few minutes late. Start your relaxation even if it's the appointed time. Just 60 seconds to focus and relax will help you a lot. Don't waste those precious moments.

(continues)

Ten-Minute Premassage Meditation

1. Whatever it is you're doing, *stop*. Make a conscious choice to move from your daily nontherapeutic mode into a stilled, intentional attitude.

2. Sit on or near your massage table or lie down on your back. Loosen any tight clothing.

3. Take one *really deep* breath when you first start out. As you exhale, shake your hands and arms. Make funny noises with your lips. Move your head in circles. And, in general, shuck off the accumulated tensions of your day.

4. Starting with that one first big breath, change your breathing pattern so that it is strong and deep and slow. Feel the air filling you up from your belly, through your diaphragm, and into your lungs.

5. With each exhalation, let a specific area of your body progressively relax, starting with your feet. This will only take 10 slow breaths: feet, legs, hips and pelvis, abdomen and lower back, chest and upper back, hands and arms, shoulders, neck, face, and head.

6. With each inhalation, try thinking of *nothing else* but that breath. Make the breath audible as it comes in through your nose so you have something to concentrate on.

7. Focus on your hands, feeling them warming up.

8. Focus on your heart area, feeling it grow soft and warm, as well.

9. With each inhalation, take warmth and vulnerability and openness into your heart. With each exhalation, send those feelings up over your shoulders, down your arms, and into your hands until you have a circular flow going. Concentrate on the breathing and the feelings, letting stray thoughts float in and out of your mind but not following them.

10. When you feel ready (or when you hear a knock on your door!) slowly open your eyes and go to greet your client.

This meditation is especially helpful on those occasions when you have a no-show or an exceptionally late client. Instead of stressing about your client being late, you'll end up relaxed and resourceful.

There is a famous quote by Goethe: "What you can do, or dream, begin it. Boldness has genius, power, and magic in it." This holds especially true for massage therapists because so much of what we do and what we create starts out as such a fragile dream in our hearts and our hands. If you don't take decisive action and initiative at some point, you may never get past working for an hourly wage.

That said, let's look at the reality of your situation. Do you have no money? You shouldn't let that stop you, but you should let it caution you and keep you from overextending. Be real. With $1,000, you are *not* going to open the massage clinic of your dreams. However, with that same amount, you can purchase supplies and start your own business within an already existing business like a salon or clinic and launch yourself toward success.

All you need is a room, really—just four walls to contain your vision. If you have enough depth in your pocketbook for a waiting area and reception desk, so much the better. But the real magical, income-generating square footage is all packed into that one room, the treatment room. Find a way to create it, and you may be on your way to fulfilling your life's ambition.

The following sections address the concerns you'll have when forging your massage room from the raw material found in salon or day spa settings, in clinics, or in your own private massage office.

Massage Rooms in Salons or Day Spas

If your treatment room is in a day spa or salon, you'll need to keep a few points in mind. First, ask yourself this question: If you were receiving a massage, would you want the whine of hair dryers and the odor of hair-perming chemicals to be invading the room? Of course not. So it's up to you to take whatever creative steps are necessary to devise a room free from those distractions, even though they may be just a few feet away outside your door (see Figure 7-2 and Figure 7-3).

Of course, most good day spas have been planned with the awareness of these problems in mind; if you open your business in one, you stand a fair chance of finding good working conditions. However, many day spas started out as salons first; because the owners had to build the treatment area around the styling area, more often than not they ran into challenges of this nature. You can help them provide a more pleasant experience for their clientele with some of the following suggestions.

❋ The answer for many situations is some heavy-duty insulation. For instance, make sure the space at the bottom of your treatment room door is completely sealed off. If you are involved in the planning stages, ask the contractor to make the treatment room walls a couple inches thicker and put insulation inside.

Figure 7-2 | Massage room in salon environment. Notice the placement of the massage room farthest away from the hair dryers as possible, and with extra insulation in the walls and door.

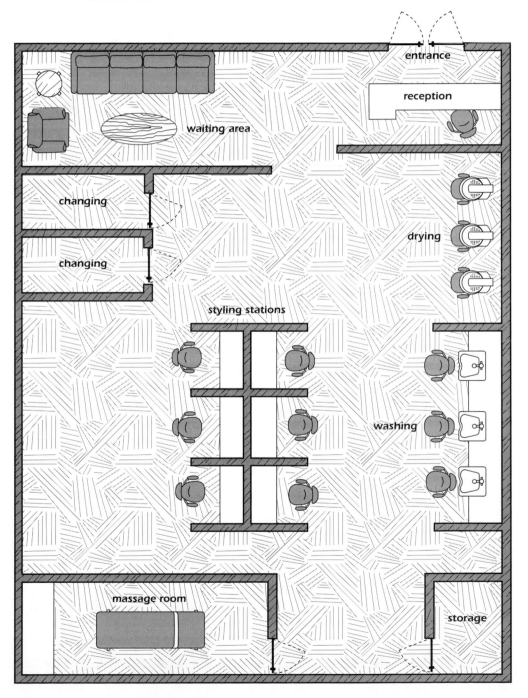

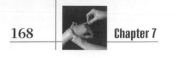

Figure 7-3 | Massage room in salon environment. Perhaps a more ideal setup, if the receptionist's phone is set to ring low.

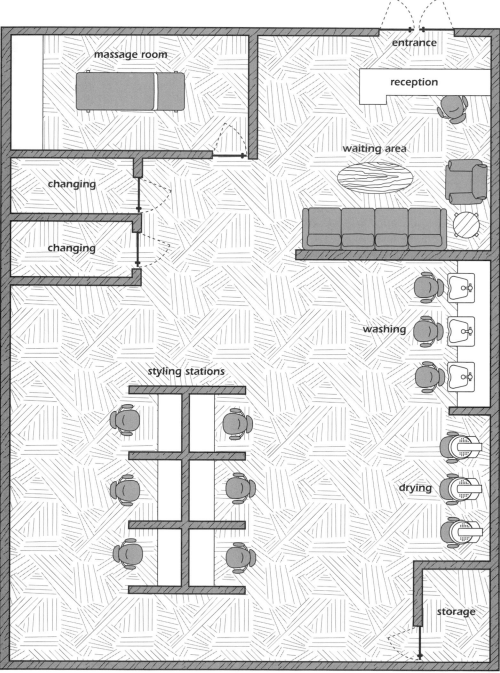

✳ If possible, install separate ventilation and climate control for your treatment room.

✳ When you are negotiating with the salon owners for your space, try to get the area farthest away from the hair dryers and manicure stations.

✳ Hang tapestries on the inside walls of the treatment room as sound buffers.

✳ As a last-ditch effort to drown out distracting noise, you can supply headphones for your clients so they'll hear the sound of ocean waves and Vivaldi rather than the incessant ring of the receptionist's phone.

✳ Try using aromatherapy or incense to overpower the odors common to hair salons, but be careful not to asphyxiate yourself or your client.

Massage Rooms in Clinics

Chiropractors' offices and sports medicine clinics are increasingly popular venues for massage therapy. When you work in a clinic, you'll have to adjust to the somewhat cold atmosphere found there, as compared to the warm feeling you may be accustomed to providing for your clients.

If you set up a practice within a chiropractor's office, you will probably be quite restricted as to the decor you can use as well as the clothes you can wear. A room will be provided for you, or you may even have to move from room to room to work on different patients. Massages often last only 15 minutes, and it's more challenging to feel grounded. You shouldn't feel that you'll have to forsake every ounce of individuality if you work in a clinic, though. Some therapists have been successful in making the switch to clinical work while still maintaining all the personality of their personal massage practice.

Your Own Office

The ultimate goal of many massage therapists is to open a private office, putting a stamp of individuality on a place and calling it their own. It is becoming ever more feasible for therapists to start up their own business as the general public becomes increasingly aware of the benefits of massage. However, opening your own office can be a somewhat risky move, especially in the beginning of your career.

PROFILE: Julia Cowan
Massage in a Chiropractic Clinic

Julia Cowan is a therapist whose experience working in chiropractic offices has ranged from painful to blissful. She is now a member on the management board at the Atlanta School of Massage. As director of education for the wellness, massage, and spa therapies program there, she spends a lot of time helping students get the most out of their education. Along with her management and human resources skills, what helped her get to that position was her background as a therapist in chiropractic offices.

"I always intended to work for a chiropractor," recalls Julia, "ever since I first started in massage. In fact, I had already heard from one chiropractor in Tennessee who offered me a job while I was still in school in Atlanta, and I was planning to go work for him, but then I ended up staying in Atlanta after graduation and seeking other employment.

"I worked at my first job with a chiropractor for just three months. He scheduled me for 10 hour-long sessions every Thursday, and at first I was excited to be seeing that many people in one day. The hours were too long for me, though, and I ended up compromising what was best for me and getting hurt. The chiropractor also forced every patient to get a massage from me whether they wanted one or not, just so he could collect money from the insurance. Some patients lay down on the table and burst into tears because they didn't want to be there. I knew this wasn't right for me, so I began searching for something better."

Julia's search eventually led her to Dr. Teresa Brennan, who had been interviewing massage therapists for five months, seeking a good match of her own.

Though she always wanted to work with a chiropractor, Julia says it was a challenge finding one with the right belief system of how to treat people. There is such stiff competition that many have developed a "get 'em in, get 'em out" mentality.

"I was very fortunate to meet Teresa. A friend of mine told me about her, and when I went to interview with her, we clicked right away. She offered me the job that same day. She was moving into a new office space, so I ended up moving in with her, and I stayed for eight years.

"I went to work with her because of her approach. She listened to her patients first before treating them. She was also a trained psychologist, and she had a very holistic manner. It was important that I respect the way she worked with people, especially after my initial experience."

(continues)

Julia Cowanh (continued)

The working arrangement they conceived was atypical of chiropractor/ therapist setups. Julia had a quiet room of her own off to one side of the reception area, where she could control the music, lighting, and other environmental factors. At first Julia split the income from her sessions with Teresa, but then she began renting the space out as her own, becoming almost completely independent.

"Ninety-nine percent of the massages I gave were an hour long," Julia states. "Teresa understood the power of what I could do in an hour session, and she didn't try to push patients on me. Typically, I gave patients massage after their adjustments, which was also different than most chiropractic offices. I recommended they try it both before and after their adjustments to see what worked best, and Teresa recommended that, too. People had choice about their own treatment.

"We developed a rhythm of consulting about clients. I reviewed charts, took good notes, and looked over Teresa's notes. Patients saw Teresa first, and although they were not required to go to her for adjustments, they would if necessary. We kept our practices separate but complementary, and I always felt like my treatment room was my own space—calm and soothing like a massage room should be.

"Teresa allowed me to figure out what schedule worked for me, which included 30-minute breaks between each session for stretching and review—a very sane and civilized way to approach massage within the chiropractic setting, but one which you hardly ever see.

"During the eight years I worked with her, my respect grew every day. Her patients raved about her. This brings up the one point I'd like to highlight. It is extremely important for a therapist to be *proud* of who they're affiliated with and where they're working. A lot of therapists are *not* proud, and that colors their work. When you go on a job interview at a chiropractor's office or anywhere else, remember that you're interviewing them as much as they're interviewing you."

You will need at least one of the following ingredients to make a go of it in your own office, and a little bit of each ingredient would be even better.

1. An incredible location

2. Some substantial financial backing

3. Overwhelming, unstoppable enthusiasm and persistence

4. A good business background

When you buy or lease your own office, you will become as responsible for it as if you had bought a house. Plumbing, wiring, and appliances, not to mention taxes, will all be yours to worry about. Of course, just like when you buy your own house, you'll be free to upgrade, too, adding such niceties as a sauna, shower, or new carpet.

The most appropriate time to take a realistic look at your financial situation is *before* you put any money down on a particular place. Do what business people do: Write a proposal and figure out assets versus expenses. Massage therapists, as opposed to business people, tend to be exceptionally optimistic about finances until they have to actually start spending money. It's better to be realistic and postpone a few cherished dreams than it is to be idealistic and lose everything.

As a very general guideline, I'll give you an imaginary budget to use in the opening of a clinic. The first is for a one-room, no-frills office, where you not only do massage but everything else, from the painting to the bookkeeping to answering the phones. The second example is for a multiple-room suite, where you do massage and are also in charge of other therapists who work for you and an office person, as well.

Remember, these are make-believe costs. You will find things to be more expensive, or perhaps less, depending on the neighborhood and the part of the country you're in. Use these examples to get an idea of the proportional outlays you should make on certain necessary items.

Example 1, a One-Room Massage Office for Yourself

So you have found the perfect little niche, perhaps a room in a medical services building (Figure 7-4). This budget is for just that room, with perhaps a small antechamber, plus a phone line. You'll take your linens home every other night to wash yourself, and you'll keep your own books. Someone on a shoestring budget, economizing wherever possible, will find this option appealing. Remember, any advertising or outreach will cost extra, and you'll have to do something to let people know you're there. See chapter 9, "Creating a Professional Image."

Figure 7-4 | A minimum-sized massage room. You can perform massage in a room smaller than 12 × 9—by placing the table diagonally and squeezing yourself in some slightly tighter spaces—but it's not recommended.

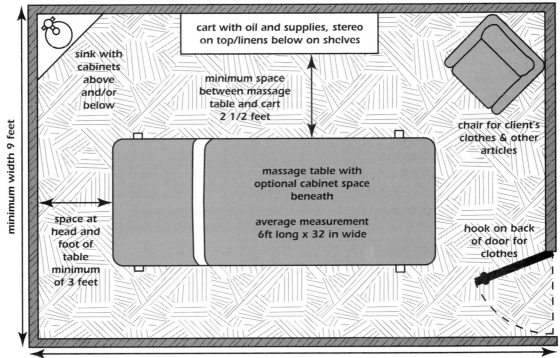

Startup costs

Down payments, closing costs, or deposits and initial fees	$2,000
One portable massage table	600
Misc. furniture, chair, cart, hamper, filing cabinet, wastebasket	250
Oils/linens/other massage supplies	175
Utilities hookup and deposits	350
Phone plus deposit and hookup	200
Portable CD player for massage room	150
Printed materials, printing	290
Total	4,015

Ongoing costs (monthly)

Lease/mortgage	$800
Utilities	120
Phone	60
Supplies	40
Insurance	60
Total	1,080

Next, figure out what your approximate income will be for the first month, the next, and so on, remembering that you don't really know what that figure is until you actually get there. If you had just two customers a day, five days a week, for example, at $50 apiece, your income would be $2,000 a month—plenty to cover business expenses; but remember that you have living expenses, as well. You have to determine how many paying customers per day you'll need to break even. And you may have to struggle to keep that minimal number of people coming through your door, at least in the beginning. On the other hand, your initial enthusiasm may attract more clients than you had anticipated, and your problem will end up being, as it has for many beginning therapists, how to avoid burnout (more about this in the next chapter).

You will be able to find ways to bring your costs down farther, I'm sure. In fact, the price will probably drop as an inverse ratio of your growing persistence and ingenuity. You can try to find someone to bankroll you at this early stage to take some of the pressure off, but be aware that the very best collateral you have will be your own positive energy and enthusiasm. If you have to make it happen, you will. If you fail, you will try again until you succeed. The people who never try are the ones who are really missing out.

Please be aware, though, that if you attempt to create a scenario similar to the one I have outlined, it will be easier to stay positive and enthusiastic if you have approximately $8,000 dollars in the bank to begin with.

Example 2, a Two-Room Massage Office for Yourself and Other Therapists

In this scenario, you have more money saved and more to spend. You envision an office where you are working as a therapist, and you also have other therapists working for you, either renting space from you or sharing the profits (see Figure 7-5). This space could be in a conventional office setting, or you could follow the example of many therapists before you and convert a more exotic setting like a garage, gas station, or bank. Your income potential is obviously greater in this situation, but you have more expenses, too. Here are some potential numbers:

Startup costs

Down payments, closing costs, or deposits and initial fees	$4,000
Two stationary massage tables	3,600
Desk, chairs, coffee table, sofa, filing cabinets	2,800
Washer/dryer	460
Oils/linens/other massage supplies	200
Phone plus deposit & hookup	180
Utilities hookup and deposits	400
Printed materials, printing	500
Stereo system	600
Total	12,740*

Does not include rebuilding or remodeling or buying a place to convert

Ongoing costs (monthly)

Lease/mortgage	$1,200
Receptionist's salary (part-time)	700
Utilities	240
Phone	100
Supplies	100
Insurance	180
Total	2,520

In this case, with ongoing monthly expenses in excess of $2,500, you'll need some deeper pockets to start out with. You'll be generating income from other people's work in that second massage room, though, which will help out. If you do four massages a day at $60 and receive 40 percent of four done by an employee for the same rate, that's $336 per day or $6,720 per month. Not

Figure 7-5 | Floor plan for massage office with two treatment rooms.

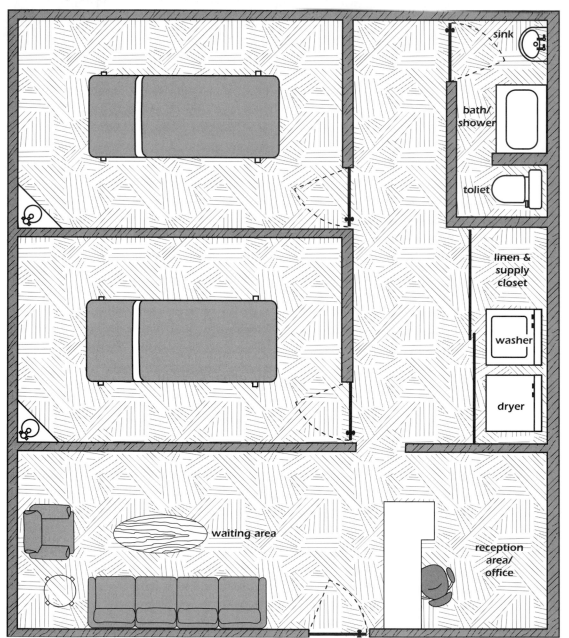

bad! Before you rush out to lease your first storefront, however, remember that you're getting yourself into a supervisory situation and tying yourself securely to the success of this particular establishment. Before you sign any papers, determine whether or not your personality is suited for that type of responsibility. In addition to your love of massage, you'll need to really focus on your people skills and business knowledge. Of course, having $26,000 dollars to start out with will help smooth the rough edges of your startup pains, if necessary.

To Summarize

The permutations of the preceding two examples are endless, and the details will vary tremendously from one city to the next. Once you get your business set up, you will soon notice that it will change right before your eyes on a somewhat consistent basis. In business, as in life, nothing is static or fixed. The course of your career and progress will be as fluid as the bodies beneath your fingers. Be ready for transformation.

ELEMENTS COMMON TO ALL MASSAGE ENVIRONMENTS

Whether you move into a 1,000-square-foot professional office suite or shuffle some furniture around at home, you're going to deal with some of the same basic questions when you're setting up your massage space:

- ❋ What type of lighting is appropriate?
- ❋ How about sounds and music?
- ❋ What equipment will I need? Where do I get it, and how much will it cost?

Lighting

When you adjust the lighting in your room at the beginning of a massage, you will almost always adjust it *down*. In general, people like to feel sheltered from the bright, outside world when they enter your massage sanctum. Therefore, it is of great benefit to you and your clients if you install adjustable lighting in your massage area. Rheostats are not terribly expensive. Candles are fine for those of you who enjoy the flickering natural glow they produce, and many clients love them. Be aware, though, that some clients do *not* love them, finding the aroma or the dimness daunting, and they'd prefer other forms of lighting. Also, some therapists have the tendency to overdo it when it comes to candles, creating a tableau that looks more like a séance than a massage session.

Some therapists prefer to leave the lighting at normal levels to avoid any New Age, nonclinical implications about their work. This is understandable. However, you don't want your clients to suffer as a consequence of your professional intentions. In my opinion, the lighting in your massage room, as with the music, should be left up to the discretion of the person who's presently paying for the experience they are having—the client on your table.

Tips: If you are budget conscious or working in a temporary room where you don't have control over the permanent lighting situation, use a colorful piece of fabric or scarf to drape over a lamp, as mentioned earlier, thus creating a completely different mood in a matter of seconds. In your home, try to arrange the draperies so that you can control how much light enters the room at any time of the day.

Music

The mixture of music and massage is not for everyone. Some clinical practitioners feel that music lessens the seriousness of their work. "Massage music" is probably not appropriate in a doctor's office or the training room of the local major league baseball team, although in either situation you may indeed find it playing. Many therapists, however, probably the majority, feel that music not only makes their work more enjoyable for both themselves and their clients but actually makes their work better. How does this happen?

Music can take the therapist and the recipient on a shared journey that expands the experience of a massage because it introduces a third consciousness into the picture, that of the musician. This third consciousness can act as a kind of guide, mentor, teacher, or friend, depending on the mood you're in and how focused you are while giving a particular treatment.

Think of it: When you're giving a good massage, both you and your client are focusing inward, blocking out the million distractions that can steal your mind away at any given moment. You're trying over and over to bring your mind down to that one point where your hands are contacting his body and to make that contact the center of attention. This is usually difficult. The natural tendency of your mind, as any Zen master will tell you, is to wander.

A therapist's internal dialogue while in the middle of a massage may typically sound like this (especially at the end of the day when she's tired):

> *Boy, his rhomboids sure seem to be tight here. Maybe if I bend the elbow to open up the scapula a little . . . That's better. I wonder what Tony's cooking for dinner tonight, because if it's that same tuna casserole he made the last time I came over, I don't think I'll be able to stomach it. Tony's such an excellent sculptor, but a chef he is not. Why didn't he call me this morning, anyway? My phone bill's late this month. Better stop by and pay it in person, and I hate that. The traffic's so bad in that part of town. Oops, there goes that rhomboid, releasing a little bit now. I'd better tell him to breathe.*

When you introduce the right music into this type of picture, it is easier for you to bring your mind back to your hands on a more consistent basis throughout the massage. Music offers a mental lifeline to grab on to so that you don't drift off onto the sea of random thoughts your mind is prone to produce.

I have given approximately 1,200 massages to the accompaniment of George Winston's *December* CD, and I feel like I know George as well or better than I know most of my clients—or at least I know the George who was playing the piano while he recorded that CD. I know by heart every moment of rapturous pause, every humble diminuendo and crashingly bold crescendo. I know the moments when he cared more for the notes and the moments when he could just let go and watch his fingers play, as if he had set them loose from his mind, just like I can do with my fingers in the massage. He cared and cared and cared about that music while he created it, and if I focus enough on the sound, timing my rhythm and movements to that caring, I begin to care just as deeply about the keyboard of human tissue I am playing upon. It doesn't matter whether my client is focusing on the music or my hands at first or not. The power of my focused mind is much stronger than the wandering, unfocused mind of a person in "normal" consciousness, and he will soon be brought into a focused state, too. It is automatic.

Every time, as you use the power of your mind to bring your client with you into that space of concentration, you will recognize that you are really listening to both the music *and* your own bodies as they do the dance of massage. The two are inseparable. Perhaps that is the best analogy—massage as a dance. Without music, where would the dancer be?

For a special approach, try doing your massage accompanied by *live* music. If you have a musician friend, have him sit in the same room and play some extemporaneous tunes based on the mood and movements you create through your therapy. This can be a truly deep experience for everyone involved because the consciousness of the third person is physically in the room with you. You will often come away with three people who all feel as though they've received a great massage. Make sure to record the session so that your client can take the music home with him. Of course, certain instruments are more conducive to this type of experience than others, and it will help if your friend plays keyboards, flute, violin, vibraphone, or guitar rather than tuba, which is more of a challenge.

If, indeed, you are a therapist who uses the power of music in your work, you will find no lack of choices when you head to the music store. The New Age section alone contains hundreds of titles, and you shouldn't let your search be confined to just that one area. Classical music, jazz, contemporary flamenco, light reggae, Native American, and some popular music are also good accompaniments.

I've given great massages to Bob Marley, the Cowboy Junkies, Beethoven, the Gypsy Kings, and Ella Fitzgerald, as well as the standards like George Winston, Yanni, Kitaro, Shadowfax, and Enya. Stephen Halpern's music is a favorite of many therapists, and he's composed music especially for us. Paul Horn has taken his flute into such sacred chambers as the Taj Mahal and the Great Pyramid in Egypt to create music that seems to flow directly from heaven. Several artists specialize in interweaving music with the sounds of nature. Paul Winter has done this on some of his titles, and others have created entire lines of nature CDs, such as Dan Gibson's *Solitudes*. Other titles traditionally favored by therapists include *Music to Disappear Into, Deep Breakfast* by Ray Lynch, *For God Alone* by Mark Kelso, *Chant* by the Benedictine Monks of Santo Domingo de Silos, and Johann Pachelbel's *Canon*.

Certain record labels like Narada and Windham Hill specialize in music most suitable for massage, but don't be limited or categorized in any way when it comes to selecting the music you'll use. Your massage is *your* massage. It is your dance. Ultimately, you should be your own choreographer and choose your own musicians. After all, it is your own special audience of one at a time for whom the dance is performed. They are counting on you for inspiration. Make musical choices from your heart, just like you did when you chose massage in the first place.

Equipment

When you enter the massage profession, you will find an entire industry waiting for you with open arms, ready to welcome you in and ready to sell you as much equipment as you care to buy. Massage therapy may indeed be a low-overhead business when compared to doctors with their operating suites and dentists with their x-ray machines, but you'll have no trouble spending thousands of dollars on equipment you didn't even know existed before you received your massage training. A few of these items include:

* Stationary heating units called hydrocollators

* Pneumatic stools to sit on while working

* Paraffin baths into which clients dip hands, feet, elbows, and more

* A special lighting unit that sends beams of colored light toward various chakras

* A tent that arches over your massage table and fills with steam to warm your clients

* Computer software for billing and scheduling

* Special support cushions for your massage table that sometimes cost almost as much as the table itself

* Carved stone and wooden massage tools

As you go through school and when you begin to network with other therapists, you'll hear recommendations and be able to try some of these products firsthand to see how you like them. In a few cities, you'll even find entire stores, such as the Massage Company and Bodywork Emporium devoted to the sale of massage-related products. Several mail-order sources are available, as well. See the appendix for a complete listing.

Your First Massage Table

Buying your first massage table is similar to buying your first car. Should you get a new one or a used one? Should you invest in an expensive top-of-the-line model or an economy version? What's important? Weight? Size? Material? Brand name? Of course, quality is always a concern, and luckily, most massage table manufacturers are quite reliable (see Figure 7-6). In almost every case, the people who became manufacturers were therapists first. Their

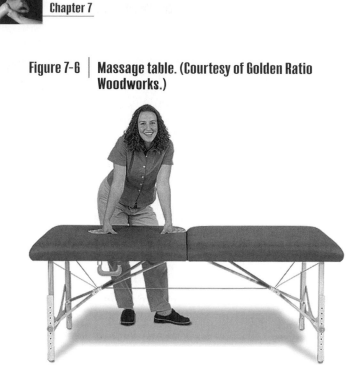

Figure 7-6 | **Massage table. (Courtesy of Golden Ratio Woodworks.)**

desire to build tables and other equipment grew naturally from their own experience.

If you attend one of the massage conventions, you'll find a much larger variety of tables and equipment available than you ever thought possible. You can spend thousands of dollars on a silent electric-lift table, for example. You'll see people selling tables that split into sections, arching up and stretching clients into better positions for massage. The number of people manufacturing standard massage tables has also grown significantly in recent years. The choices can seem overwhelming at first, and many beginning therapists end up feeling more frustrated than fulfilled by the bewildering selection. How should you choose?

Chances are, if you attend a well-known massage school, you'll find several makes and models of tables available for purchase there. Some manufacturers have a special arrangement with certain schools, and their tables receive preference when the staff are asked for recommendations. Don't feel that you have to buy under these circumstances or that your choices are limited because of what is offered at your school. The truth is that every manufacturer is capable of shipping a table right to your doorstep. You can find in-depth information about all of them by calling the numbers listed in the appendix.

Although it is still very much a specialty market, massage retailing has become a bona fide business opportunity of its own in recent years. Stores where you can buy a variety of massage products from several manufacturers have been part of massage schools for years; but now several have become freestanding entities, and they are doing a good business.

"The sheer volume of people is difficult to handle sometimes," reports Noel Martin, manager of the Massage Company in San Francisco. "We're busy on the phone all day long with mail order, and people are coming in and out a lot, too."

Noel tempers a busy retailing career with her own private practice, a balance that she finds optimal. "I wanted to do something in addition to hands-on massage," she says, "and I happen to love business, so this was the perfect match."

Noel became interested in massage after receiving several sessions and having some profoundly positive experiences. She wanted to help people in the same way and so signed up for massage school right after she left college. Her first job was at the La Costa Spa in southern California, where she found herself belonging to the Teamster's Union along with the rest of the spa's employees. "I never thought I'd be a union worker as a massage therapist," she says. "I imagined a more personalized career. The job didn't pay very well, either, and the atmosphere wasn't fulfilling to me because there were no repeat clients. Everybody was gone by the end of the week. And even though the spa was a great place to start out, and I learned from working on a lot of different clients, I was already getting burned out.

"I wanted another job, and since my major in college was economics, I naturally thought of the business world, but I couldn't see myself with a typical corporate position. That's when I started with the Bodywork Emporium in San Diego, doing massage in their clinic at first and then moving more and more into the retail end of the business. They have a chain of stores in southern California. Working there was much more supportive of who I was and what I wanted to do."

At the Whole Life Expo, Noel talked with the owner of one of the massage table companies, who explained he was thinking about opening a retail store of his own. He was impressed with the way Noel handled sales of his products at the Bodywork Emporium. "There aren't a whole bunch of other people involved in selling these products in a retail environment," she says. "I guess my skills were pretty unique."

(continues)

Noel Martin (continued)

Noel's job is certainly different than the average sales position, but it has many of the same challenges found at a GAP or Banana Republic. "Retail is retail," she states. "The store is so busy, I don't get to pace my own day because I have to deal with people when they come in. But the customers on the whole are wonderful . . . they are mostly people who are interested in healing and bodywork, which tends to draw nurturing folks.

"My favorite part of the job is the interactivity. When people are shopping for massage equipment, it's not like they're going to the supermarket and already know exactly what they want; there's a lot of explaining and demonstrating to do, which I love. Probably the most common question I hear is, 'What is *this*?' because there are so many tools that people can learn about . . . I get to make good connections with customers because they need my help."

Noel has witnessed the massage business up close from both perspectives—the seller's and the buyer's—and she has some counsel for each. "If you're thinking about manufacturing and selling something for massage therapists, give it to some therapists to try first. Take it to trade shows and get some feedback. A lot of times I see people who are not doing massage day-to-day who invent things they think will work, but it's not right.

They should test it first before they put a lot of money into packaging and marketing.

"On the buyer's end, I used to think I should temper the students who wanted to spend money on equipment when they were just out of school and didn't even have a job yet. I'd say to them, 'Have you thought about how you're going to make money to pay for all this?' But lately I've been thinking it's appropriate for them to make that first major step in their careers. Paying for massage school is an investment in their lives and their personal development, but when they buy that first table, it really brings it home to people that this is an investment in their *business*. It's a way for them to say '*Yes,* I'm doing it, and I'm a professional now.' A lot of people go to school and then don't make that next level of commitment by purchasing the equipment. If you don't have the right equipment today, you can't be charging professional rates. I feel good about encouraging people to buy the high-end products we sell here because in many cases they'll be good for a lifetime."

Noel's encouraging attitude about massage retailing extends to the career itself. "I think the whole concept of what you can do with massage is really opening up today," she says. "People are finding many positions within the field that are outside the traditional

(continues)

role of massage therapist. The opportunity of doing a great variety of things with massage is growing, and *now's* the time to do it.

"If people really want to do something like I'm doing, they can.

More and more therapists are able to blend some kind of business with their actual hands-on work. It's a way to stay in love with what you do, not burn yourself out, and keep helping lots of people."

Seek the opinion of somebody who is not tied either economically or emotionally to one particular brand of table. An older, more experienced therapist who has used various brands of tables over the years will be able to give you a better perspective from which to choose wisely.

When you try out a few tables to see how they work for you, spend 99 percent of your time lifting the table, carrying it up stairs, opening it, setting it up, checking for ease of adjustability, closing it, stowing it in your car, and leaning it up against a wall. These are the areas where you'll experience the most frustration if you purchase the table that's not right for you. Once it's set up and your client is lying on it, there isn't a great difference between various tables, except for their strength and comfort. Check for bracing beneath the table. Are the corners solid? Do the legs wobble? Is the table height easily adjustable? How thick is the foam padding on top? (Most companies offer a choice of thickness.) Does that padding extend over the sides? Is the table wide enough for comfort? Is the face cradle adjustable, and can it be positioned at either end of the table? Is the fabric on top in good condition and attached smoothly to the wooden frame, or are there exposed staples?

The table you choose is going to be a big part of your life for several years. You want it to look good and work well. Consider your table to be a huge business card that you carry with you whenever you're on assignment. People will notice the table and, if you're fortunate, ask you about what you do. Your table doesn't have to be brand new, and it doesn't have to be expensive, but it should be clean and presentable.

As you upgrade your skills (and your income level) over the years, you'll be able to upgrade your massage table, as well. They get better every year—more comfortable, stronger, and lighter. A good, solidly built, older table can be compared to a vintage automobile. It builds more character as it ages if you

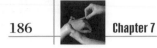
take care of it. Some therapists become attached to their original tables, and they work perfectly well for years and years. You may have to do a little patching up now and then because no material is immune to wear and tear; but, with a little TLC, a good table can last the better part of a career.

Massage Chairs

Massage chairs can be as expensive as massage tables. Good ones are light, easily opened, fully adjustable, and very comfortable. Besides all that, they look really cool (Figure 7-7). Some therapists give in to temptation and buy one of these pieces of artistic massage furniture before they are completely sure how they are going to go about making a living actually using it. It's a good idea to scout out the possibilities in your area before you plunk down your money.

Every major massage table manufacturer also makes a version of a massage chair (they are listed in the appendix). It's a good idea to comparison shop. Be aware that people who try to sell you a chair at the massage chair seminars they teach will usually offer just one brand—from the company that sponsors the workshop or pays them the most commission. They'll offer discounts to

Figure 7-7 | **Massage chair. (Courtesy of Golden Ratio Woodworks.)**

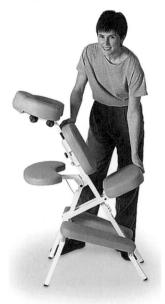

PROFILE: John Fanuzzi
Golden Ratio Woodworks, Inc.

In the late 1970s, John Fanuzzi was working construction in New Jersey when he visited Florida and received his first massage. "I finished that session with Clarity with a capital C, and it changed my life," says John. "It was energy work, which was completely foreign to me. When I returned to Jersey, I got totally hooked when another therapist worked on me. My fingers felt like they were three feet long and I was seeing visions through my third eye—whoa! I decided I needed to know how to do that.

"I signed up for Polarity training in New York; then a deep-tissue bodywork course in Florida; and I studied with Dr. Vasant Lad, the famous ayurvedic healer. I traveled around from Santa Fe to California and back to Jersey, and I was thinking it was going to be the end of my construction career, but fellow students started asking me to build them massage tables. I started in a basement, with a $100 deposit from someone who wanted me to build them a table. I went to a lumber yard, bought two pieces of oak and some foam, and that's how it all started."

Then came advice from a spiritual messenger, which further changed John's life. "A while later, this guy named Swami Virato suggested I put an ad for tables in his Philadelphia magazine called *New Frontiers*. He asked me if I would like to make $100,000 a year. A hundred thousand! That was a huge number for me back then. I was only thinking in small terms, living hand-to-mouth. But the ad paid off. More and more people started asking me to build tables.

"In November of 1982, I went to my first trade show, the Whole Life Expo in New York. I sold 17 tables and picked up my first distributor. At the time, I was still doing some construction work as an assistant project manager. It's a good idea to keep your full-time job until you're really ready to break into the massage industry.

"After a year and a half, I was just too busy. The curve of the massage-table construction business was going up, and I saw more potential there, whereas my salary in construction was just flat. I started thinking maybe there was a career here. I had driven through Montana in 1981 and loved it, and I said to myself, 'If I can save up enough money, I'm going to move.' I was 35 years old.

"I had $10,000 in the bank by June, so I rented a Montana property sight unseen, packed up my five-year-old and my two-year-old and my entire table-making shop on an old gutted school bus, towed my car behind me, and headed to Montana. I established Golden Ratio Woodworks in Emigrant, and folks in the area were happy to have new job options. I quickly put

(continues)

John Fanuzzi (continued)

people to work, paying them $10 to assemble a table, $10 to upholster one, etc. It was piecework and people appreciated it. At first we had to ship most of our tables on Greyhound buses, but I contacted a regional manager for UPS and got them to start accepting larger parcels. That was the start of a nationwide trend."

Along the way, John's flair for design and his close ear to the needs of therapists helped him implement several milestones in the industry. John created the first lightweight wet-treatment table with a built-in drain, a four-panel upholstered top so clients could recline in various positions, and a table with a built-in pedicure foot spa. He also brought his QuickLite™ massage chair to trade shows to drum up business. His extensive array of spa equipment is the mainstay of Golden Ratio's business today, with massage therapists representing 30 percent of sales and spas 70 percent.

John's 50,000-square-foot manufacturing facility in Emigrant has expanded to include a showroom and mini-conference center and Wellspring Healing Hearts Center with a full-service spa and guest rooms. "The first five or six years, we doubled sales every year," says John, "and now we're doing millions of dollars a year. It would be well over 10 million if we hadn't lost part of our business to cheaper imports from China. Pretty amazing when you

consider it all started with that $100 deposit for a table I put together in a basement!"

John's personal list of qualities to look for when buying your own massage table follows:

- ✻ Wide variety. It's important to be able to choose from an assortment of styles, weights, and designs.

- ✻ Structural design. Golden Ratio's CenterLock™ leg design, for example, has no cables around the sides to trip on or rub against.

- ✻ Easy opening. You'll be opening and closing your table thousands of times, so it should be quick and simple.

- ✻ Sturdiness. Your table should be able to withstand prolonged use and heavy clients.

- ✻ Customization. It's great to be able to add your own logo, options, and accessories, and to choose your wood and colors.

- ✻ Upholstery. UltraLeather™ is often the preference on massage chairs because the clients feel the fabric more. But even if your massage table is covered most of the time, color and texture are still important for most people, and it's a good idea not to skimp in this area.

entice you, and you'll be excited about getting this tool so that you can use your newfound skills right away. That makes you vulnerable. You have to make sure that you're really going to pursue chair massage as a business or else you may be making an impulsive purchase you'll later regret.

If you don't have enough money to invest in a massage chair right away, or you're not sure if on-site work is right for you, consider working for a time at one of the companies that offer this service to the public through storefront businesses or kiosk setups in malls and airports. It's a great way to gain experience while saving up for a chair of your own, and some therapists enjoy not having to worry about finding clients. At these establishments, which are gaining quickly in popularity, the clients will come to you.

Linens

Although the purchase of your first massage table will probably be a momentous occasion and you'll put a lot of thought into choosing the perfect one, most of your clients may never even see your table directly. Every time they get a massage, the table will be covered by sheets or towels. Your clients will feel the table, but they will look at the linens. It behooves you to put a little thought into what kind of linens you use.

Of course, your clients will also touch the linens, so you'll want to have a fabric that feels as good as it looks. Flannel is a favorite fabric of many therapists because it's so soft and comforting to the touch. It feels especially good on cold days. Consider the following tips:

✻ For an added touch that many clients appreciate, warm the linens before giving a massage by either placing them in the drier and taking them out right before beginning the treatment or placing a Thermophore heating element (see the sidebar, "The Temperature Dilemma") on top of your prepared table.

✻ Shop for some expensive designer sheets that have been deeply discounted because they are "irregular" in some way. Usually this means that they have imperfect seams, an uneven edge, or some other minor flaw that your clients will never see while on the table. The high-quality texture far outweighs any tiny imperfections.

✻ Darker solid-color sheets work well. Regular white sheets are great for clinical settings especially, but they can end up looking a little shabby after multiple washings and oil exposure; make sure to use an oil remover (see "Oil Removers" later in this chapter). Flowery patterns may appeal to your aesthetic sense, but some clients may find them unprofessional.

✳ Fitted sheets are fine but only if they're the right size. Many massage manufacturers and suppliers have fitted sheets designed for tables (see appendix).

✳ Have a separate little cover for your face cradle or face hole. It makes a big difference in client comfort. These are available from the same suppliers.

You can personalize your linens *and* save money if you buy fabric by the yard and sew sheets yourself. I've been practicing for 20 years now, and my mom still personally sews all of my sheets for me. Your clients will appreciate it when they find out about the special efforts you've made for their comfort.

Some therapists cover their clients with another sheet, and some use towels. If you use towels, you'll want to make sure they are thickly woven and large, at least bath size. Smaller-size towels may save you money, but when it comes time for your client to turn over and your towel is not big enough to cover them modestly, you'll wish you'd made the extra investment.

Oils and Lotions

Therapists are known by the oils they keep. The oil or lotion you use in your massage is more than a simple lubricant. It is an organic substance that literally penetrates the pores of your clients, being absorbed through their skin into their bodies. The product you choose to work with says a lot about your commitment to those clients. You'll be amazed at how strongly they will respond to the different types of oils you use—but only if you choose ones with character and depth. Simply spreading a palmful of safflower oil onto somebody's back will probably not elicit odes of appreciation. If, however, you use Edgar Cayce's special almond-scented Aura Glow oil made with a blend of cold-pressed peanut oil, olive oil, lanolin oil, and vitamin E—the formula that came to the famous healer while he was in trance—you're quite likely to have clients request that particular oil again and again. Many therapists have learned how to blend their own oils, and some have even started their own line of essential oil products (see the profile on Doug Rasmusson). Some people have allergies or sensitivities to certain oils, and you'll have to be aware of this when applying your own lubricants or aromatherapy products. Be sure to ask clients beforehand if they have any allergies or sensitivities.

Doug Rasmusson's father owned a bakery, and from age five to seventeen Doug helped out in the business, kneading dough and growing up amidst the deliciously pungent aromas every day.

"I suppose that's what drew me to massage and aromatherapy later in life," remembers Doug. "I must have been looking for a way to recreate all that kneading and all those good smells from my childhood.

"I was somewhat interested in aromatherapy oils during massage school, so when we had to pick a topic for our term paper, that's the one I chose. I took a two-day class from a woman named Sylla Shepard-Hanger, director of the Atlantic Institute of Aromatherapy in Tampa, and after that I was hooked."

Doug picked up *The Art of Aromatherapy* by Robert Tisserand and began experimenting on his own, using the knowledge he'd gained to mix and blend oils and incorporate them in massage. After graduation from massage school, he took several more classes by well-known teachers and then found a job with a company called Whole Spectrum Oils.

"After that, I realized that I could put together my own oils," Doug says. "I started bottling them with my own labels, dealing with a superior grade of oils, not the type you'd find on the shelf of the local health food store."

With his wife Kim, Doug has taught aromatherapy workshops around the country, offering both a beginners class in blending oils that stresses safety issues and basic knowledge (phase one) and a more advanced three-day class (phase two) that deals with oil chemistry, the botanical families of different types of oils, and some more esoteric uses.

Doug also set up a mail-order oil business in his home, which has done well. "We get a lot of our business through going to the massage trade conventions and through advertising in the trade magazines like *Aromatic Thymes*," Doug states. "I've been a district director of the National Association of Holistic Aromatherapy for a while now, too, and those contacts help us get the word out. Besides that, it's mostly word of mouth. Kim does most of the development of new oil blends, and I deal with sales. Plus we both see massage clients. It's a great way to 'blend' different ends of the business together."

My own personal favorite, which I've used for years, is called Bindi Body Oil. It contains a special blend of healing herbs that are actually cooked into the oil and then strained out, leaving an incredibly aromatic scent evocative of India and the Far East. The recipe is based on the principles of ayurveda, the ancient natural healing system. I've seldom massaged a new client with Bindi Body Oil without her asking me where she can buy some for herself.

The Bindi Body Oil and several other popular massage blends are not cheap. I've been paying $70 per gallon for mine. Some therapists may think this is an extravagance; but, as I said, the oil is one of the crucial components of your massage practice. If it's at all possible, make an investment in the best oils; that will make it all the easier for clients to respond favorably to you and your business. If you're careful, you'll be surprised how far one gallon of massage oil can go, stretching for hundreds of clients. Make sure you use a control-flow cap, and apply only the amount necessary, no more. Some therapists have a tendency to be heavy-handed with their oil, ending up with stains on their linens and soggy clients on their tables. Investing in a top-quality oil will help you avoid this because you won't want to waste any.

As far as creams go, one product seems to have taken over the massage therapy market and is by far the most popular. Biotone Dual Purpose Massage Creme is used by many therapists, a number of whom have come to prefer it to oil because it is absorbed more readily by the skin and therefore leaves no stains on sheets and towels. It takes a little more product to create a lubricating layer, but it works as well as oil. Some therapists like the slightly less slippery feel; they say it allows them more control in their work. When you visit any massage convention, you'll find Biotone represented, and you can get free samples.

Whether or not to place your bottle of oil or cream on the massage table while giving a massage is a controversial point that has been discussed endlessly by a surprisingly large number of therapists. Each person, it seems, feels strongly about one point of view or the other. Certain massage schools make special policies regarding this issue, turning out class after class of students who then claim to "know" whether it's right or wrong to place their bottle on the table. The reason for the furor will soon become obvious after you've given a few massages. The most convenient place to put the bottle is on the table, and yet it is also the most unstable place. Clients are always shifting their bodies, sending bottles clattering to the floor. Your client will invariably say, "I'm sorry," but then you have someone who feels bad about something that was actually your fault. With time, you may become adept at placing the bottle in the exact position where it won't get knocked over; you may even come to know the shifting and leg-twitching habits of each of your clients, allowing you to deftly swipe your bottle away moments before disaster strikes. However, you are probably better off using the floor or a nearby steady area to place your bottle until you become extremely fluid and dexterous around your table. The real point here is, don't be lazy. Don't leave your bottle on the table just because it's easier to reach there. Put it where it will help you give the best massage for your client.

Some therapists wear oil holsters (Figure 7-8) around their hips like six-gun holsters, ready to unsling their bottle and apply some lubricant at any moment, without the need to bend over and lift the bottle off the ground or balance it precariously on the massage table. Regardless of the method you choose, the most important thing is to provide your clients with an experience that feels seamless. You don't want them to notice those staccato breaks when you're searching for your bottle or picking it up off the floor when it falls. Put yourself in your client's position, and practice fluidity. With a little practice, you'll get there.

Following are some sources for the oils I have mentioned (see the appendix for more sources):

✳ The Edgar Cayce Aura Glow oil can be ordered from Heritage Products, Box 444, Virginia Beach, VA 23458; phone (757) 428-0100; http://www.heritagestore.com.

✳ Bindi Body Oil can be ordered from Tara Spa Therapy at PO Box 222639, Carmel, CA 93922; phone (800) 552-0779; http://www.taraspa.com.

✳ Biotone products can be ordered from Biotone at 4757 Old Cliffs Road, San Diego, CA 92120; phone (800) 445-6457; http://www.biotone.com.

Figure 7-8 | **Oil holster. (Photo reprinted with permission from Living Earth Crafts.)**

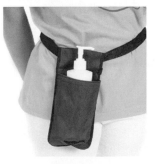

THE TEMPERATURE DILEMMA

When you start practicing massage on a consistent basis, you will quickly become aware of a particular problem that all therapists run into and has to do with the very nature of the practice of massage. You, the therapist, are clothed and standing up and moving and working, while your client is lying down, unclothed, and for the most part completely still. So while you're working up a sweat, your client is getting chilled. Of course, you should always set the temperature in your room for your client's comfort, but sometimes this makes it almost unbearable for you, especially if you are prone to sweat a lot.

I dealt with this problem constantly when I was the supervisor at a large spa. We had 26 massage rooms controlled by four separate thermostats, and all day long therapists were running out of their rooms in the middle of treatments saying their clients wanted the rooms warmer. Dutifully, I would adjust the thermostats of the appropriate areas, and then at the end of the hour the therapists would emerge from the rooms pink-faced, moist, and bedraggled.

What to do? One solution is to bury the client under a mountain of blankets. While this may make some people feel warm and protected, it certainly doesn't make it easy for you to massage them. A better alternative is to provide warmth precisely where it's needed. I learned this lesson from the client's perspective when I went to receive a massage in Maine one time. Although the air outside was frigid, and the temperature even inside was quite crisp, I was comfortable the entire time. The therapist used an electric moist-heat device called a Thermophore to keep me warm. The unit worked so well that I immediately bought three of them, one for me and two as gifts for clients. They have an automatic release switch that the client controls. After the first time they use one, people seem to find them indispensable.

Ways you can beat the temperature dilemma: Dress lightly so that a warm room isn't uncomfortable for you, use thick towels and/or flannel sheets to cover your clients, invest in an oil-warming unit (a baby bottle warmer works for this), and buy a Thermophore. Battlecreek Equipment makes this product, and they are still available where I originally encountered them, at the Downeast School of Massage Bookstore, PO Box 24, 99 Moose Meadow Lane, Waldoboro, Maine 04572. The phone number there is (207) 832-5531.

Oil Removers

A good share of the oil that therapists put on their clients inevitably ends up on sheets and towels and tables and even clothes. If you try washing it with regular detergent, you will discover what so many therapists have discovered before you: It takes more than soap and water to get rid of oil stains. Before you spend money needlessly on new linens or drive yourself crazy washing the same sheets a dozen times in a row, purchase one of the special products on the market to help you with this massage-specific problem. Clean Again has been formulated with the massage professional in mind—and it works. Clean Again is available from Biotone (see "Oils and Lotions"). You can also order a special water dispersible massage oil that does not stain sheets or towels. It washes out in normal laundry and also rinses easily off your skin. Living Earth Crafts carries Oasis Water Dispersible Massage Oil. Call (800) 358-8292 to order.

COMPUTERIZING YOUR MASSAGE BUSINESS

Because massage is high touch rather than high tech, some new therapists assume that computers wouldn't find a place in their new business. They never even give computers a thought. The impersonal nature of the keyboard and screen turns them off before they have a chance to discover what they're missing. I mention computers in chapter 9 in regard to advertising and promotion. But there are several other good reasons for incorporating them in your business:

- Scheduling and client records
- Bookkeeping
- Education
- Communication
- Internet use

When you open your own office and find yourself in the position of accountant, bookkeeper, and manager, as well as therapist, you will be thankful that you've invested in a modestly priced computer and added some useful software. If you visit your local computer store, you'll find a multitude of business software options, some of which are probably much more powerful than you need. If you're looking to simply get yourself organized, try Microsoft® Outlook. If you need to keep track of who's paid and who hasn't, with a running total, any spreadsheet program will suffice. Quick Books is a more advanced bookkeeping program.

Of course, if you are a part-time therapist who sees only a handful of clients each week, and you have no plans to expand, a computer is probably not necessary for your everyday business. You can schedule clients in your Daytimer and keep track of billing on a ledger. But that doesn't mean you still don't have a lot to gain from computerizing your business—and your life.

The computer has become an incredible learning tool. As each month goes by, it is increasingly indispensable as a communications tool, as well. For example, there are some informative (and fun) multimedia CDs on the market that will take you on an in-depth voyage of discovery within the human body. This is a great way to help you learn the minutiae of anatomy. One such CD is called BodyWorks by SoftKey, available in most computer stores. On it, you'll see anatomy professors talking to you from the screen, describing each bodily system. ADAM Software offers a range of CDs, from less expensive ones aimed at high-school students to their flagship product, ADAM Interactive Anatomy. This program is for people seriously interested in learning anatomy on the computer. Log onto http://www.adam.com or call (770) 980-0888. As technology progresses over the next few years, your potential for learning through this medium will increase rapidly. It would be a shame not to take advantage of the opportunity.

All throughout this book, I've mentioned how to use the Internet to get in touch with successful therapists, business advisers, and other people who can help you. You can even join an E-mail list especially for therapists (see the appendix for details). This electronic forum will grow rapidly in the coming years. As in most realms of the business world today, the massage business is becoming connected to the whole world through computerization. Would you like to find out how your counterparts in Australia or Europe are faring? The information is just seconds away.

If you don't want to deal with computers in your massage business, you probably have one of three main objections:

1. Computers are too expensive.

2. Computers confuse you.

3. Computers are high-tech impersonal machines, the opposite of your reasons for being in business in the first place, which is the interpersonal warmth of a high-touch environment.

Let me address those (valid) points. First, a computer needn't be terribly expensive. The models you see advertised in the catalogs and newspapers are the latest, most powerful versions that high-end users are searching for. These tend to start around the $2,000 mark. But you can buy a used, reconditioned, or less-powerful machine for under $600, with some software already installed. It will still have everything you need, which includes the basic operating system and a way to connect to the Internet (including a modem).

Second, if computers seem too confusing, try getting one of your friends who understands them to help you out. How can you entice him to offer assistance? How about trading massage?

Third, every business you can think of has benefited greatly by adding computers. The massage business is no exception. The fact that massage involves the least high-tech and the most high-touch learning about the technological side of the business will provide you with much-needed balance. Besides, everybody's going digital, and you don't want to be left behind. If worse comes to worst, you can put off learning that new software program for a rainy day and use your computer to play music CDs, just like all the other technical whizzes out there.

Island Software offers several programs to help therapists with everything from booking to client tracking to insurance forms and soap notes. Massage Office 2.2 is their premier product. Contact them at http://www.islandsoftwareco.com or (877) 384-0295. There is also an on-line massage therapy appointment booking service, which can be found at http://www.appointmentquest.com. This program allows your customers to book directly with a professional service, freeing you up to do the work you love best and saving you the cost of hiring a receptionist.

More sources are listed in the appendix.

Figure 7-9 | The massage universe. Page numbers for relevant passages are noted after each subject.

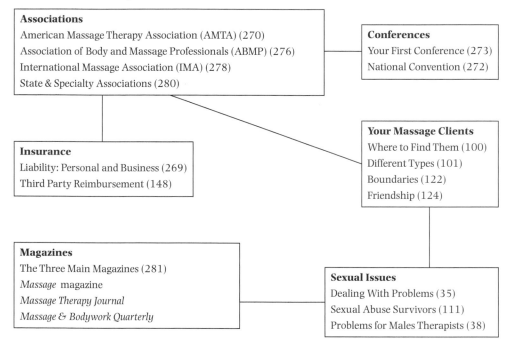

Associations
American Massage Therapy Association (AMTA) (270)
Association of Body and Massage Professionals (ABMP) (276)
International Massage Association (IMA) (278)
State & Specialty Associations (280)

Conferences
Your First Conference (273)
National Convention (272)

Your Massage Clients
Where to Find Them (100)
Different Types (101)
Boundaries (122)
Friendship (124)

Insurance
Liability: Personal and Business (269)
Third Party Reimbursement (148)

Magazines
The Three Main Magazines (281)
Massage magazine
Massage Therapy Journal
Massage & Bodywork Quarterly

Sexual Issues
Dealing With Problems (35)
Sexual Abuse Survivors (111)
Problems for Males Therapists (38)

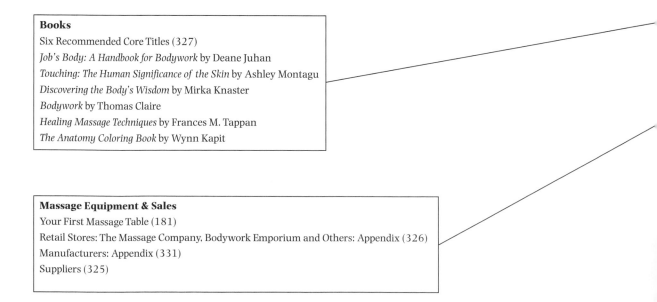

Books
Six Recommended Core Titles (327)
Job's Body: A Handbook for Bodywork by Deane Juhan
Touching: The Human Significance of the Skin by Ashley Montagu
Discovering the Body's Wisdom by Mirka Knaster
Bodywork by Thomas Claire
Healing Massage Techniques by Frances M. Tappan
The Anatomy Coloring Book by Wynn Kapit

Massage Equipment & Sales
Your First Massage Table (181)
Retail Stores: The Massage Company, Bodywork Emporium and Others: Appendix (326)
Manufacturers: Appendix (331)
Suppliers (325)

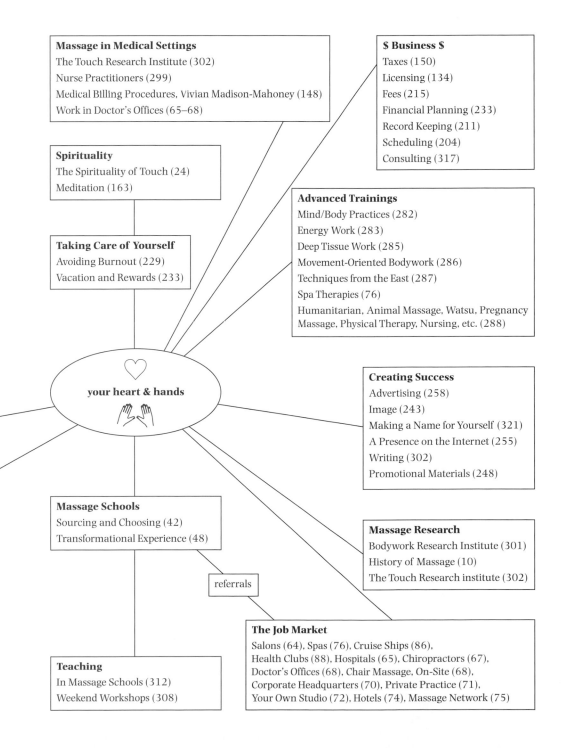

Massage in Medical Settings
The Touch Research Institute (302)
Nurse Practitioners (299)
Medical Billing Procedures, Vivian Madison-Mahoney (148)
Work in Doctor's Offices (65–68)

$ Business $
Taxes (150)
Licensing (134)
Fees (215)
Financial Planning (233)
Record Keeping (211)
Scheduling (204)
Consulting (317)

Spirituality
The Spirituality of Touch (24)
Meditation (163)

Advanced Trainings
Mind/Body Practices (282)
Energy Work (283)
Deep Tissue Work (285)
Movement-Oriented Bodywork (286)
Techniques from the East (287)
Spa Therapies (76)
Humanitarian, Animal Massage, Watsu, Pregnancy Massage, Physical Therapy, Nursing, etc. (288)

Taking Care of Yourself
Avoiding Burnout (229)
Vacation and Rewards (233)

your heart & hands

Creating Success
Advertising (258)
Image (243)
Making a Name for Yourself (321)
A Presence on the Internet (255)
Writing (302)
Promotional Materials (248)

Massage Schools
Sourcing and Choosing (42)
Transformational Experience (48)

Massage Research
Bodywork Research Institute (301)
History of Massage (10)
The Touch Research institute (302)

referrals

The Job Market
Salons (64), Spas (76), Cruise Ships (86),
Health Clubs (88), Hospitals (65), Chiropractors (67),
Doctor's Offices (68), Chair Massage, On-Site (68),
Corporate Headquarters (70), Private Practice (71),
Your Own Studio (72), Hotels (74), Massage Network (75)

Teaching
In Massage Schools (312)
Weekend Workshops (308)

8

Day-to-Day Realities: Dealing with the Details of a Thriving Massage Practice

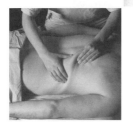

As the months and years go by and you work at your new career, you will gradually realize that the massage lifestyle you had so eagerly anticipated is actually the one that you are leading every day—with all of its ups and downs and all of its quiet joys, surprises, and ordinariness. The day-to-day realities of the massage business, like any business, will at times crowd your mind, and you may occasionally have trouble recalling exactly what inspired you to head off on this path in the first place. It is especially important, then, to have developed certain skills that will help you survive and prosper as new challenges arise. In this chapter, I will give you some specific instructions on how to deal with the day-to-day realities you'll face, especially when you begin experiencing some of the burdens of success. These are burdens many of you may be devoutly wishing for, but they are burdens nonetheless, and you'll be a better therapist if you know how to deal with them.

First of all, just to give you an idea about some of the challenges you may face while leading the therapist's life, I'm going to offer you a "nightmare" scenario that is composed of actual events in my experience and those of other therapists, condensed and combined for impact and entertainment. Do you remember having one of those days when nothing you did could pull you out of your negative spiral? The following description is "one of those days" exaggerated to an unrealistic degree. It's not meant to alarm you but rather to emphasize some of the challenges you'll likely run into as you travel the healing path. Remember, when you have "one of those days," the next day is often one of your best—as you'll read about in the last section of this chapter, "A 'Dream' Day in the Life of a Massage Therapist."

A NIGHTMARE DAY IN THE LIFE OF A MASSAGE THERAPIST

You wake up to the sound of the phone ringing at 7:00 A.M. It's your first client saying she has to cancel her 9:00 appointment. She's the client who called last night around midnight to plead for the 9:00 appointment, and so you've rearranged another appointment to accommodate her. Now she's not coming, and it's too late to call your other client. You can't get back to sleep, so you head to your home office to do a little bookkeeping and file updating, only to find on the way there that your washing machine stopped working sometime last night in the middle of the rinse cycle, and now it's filled to the brim with soggy sheets and towels. You ignore this debacle for half an hour while you make coffee and toast, but then you come back to face the inevitable. Armed with a flashlight, you crawl behind the washing machine to see if there is any hope for a quick do-it-yourself repair job. When you are thoroughly wedged behind the appliance, the phone rings. Fearing it's one of your clients, you extricate yourself laboriously and grab the phone only to hear the voice of the receptionist at the local massage school calling to tell you that the weekend workshop in Thai massage you've registered for was canceled due to lack of interest. You'd been looking forward to the experience for over two months.

The washing machine turns out to be irreparable, and the rest of your linens are dirty. You don't know if you can get them to the laundromat and back in time for your first client, who is now coming at 11:00 A.M. Deciding to risk it, you stuff everything, soggy sheets and all, into two pillow cases and head out the door.

Things at the laundromat go amazingly smoothly, and you're back at 10:59, but your client is there on your front steps waiting, and she swears you had rescheduled the appointment for 10:30, not 11:00. The massage she gets is the worst you've ever given, and she politely declines to sign up for another 10-massage package.

Over a lunch of peanut butter and jelly sandwiches, you read the morning's mail, which includes the dues statement from your massage organization plus the license reinstatement bill. Also, there's an envelope from the editor of *Massage Today* magazine, passing along a letter sent in by a reader in response to a article you'd written several months ago about a massage experience in Jamaica. The reader claims that you made racist remarks in your article. This chills you, and you dig through your pile of magazines to reread the article yourself. You can see where she might have read something into the article that wasn't there, and you remind yourself, reluctantly, that you have to be more circumspect the next time you write for the magazine.

After lunch, you head out for a house call at the home of a new client, who has been referred by a therapist who's on vacation. As you place your precious massage table gingerly into the backseat of your two-door Toyota, you hear the horrible slashing sound that means the creamy Ultra-Leather cover has ripped against the sharp little lever on the back of the seat. It was a brand-new table, and you haven't ordered the protective cover for it yet.

Negotiating through snarls of midday traffic, you finally reach the correct address, press the buzzer, and the Hulk comes to greet you at the door. He's a solid-as-rock ex-football player, and no matter how hard you try, you can't seem to make any progress on his frozen trapezius muscles. As you leave, he crushes your hand in a death grip, grimaces, and asks when his regular therapist is coming back from vacation.

Time for your three-hour stint at the local day spa. The management still hasn't insulated the massage room as they've promised you, and you give three treatments in hair-dryer hell, sniffing the fumes from the coloring station right outside the door.

At 8:00 P.M., you're scheduled to make a presentation about massage at the local health club where you work occasionally, leaving you no time to eat a proper dinner. Wiping the grease from the Chicken McNuggets from your fingers, you enter the club, where only two people are waiting to hear your speech. You give it anyway, all the way through, even though half of your audience leaves before you're five minutes into it.

As you're leaving the club, you approach the owner and ask if he has the money he owes you for the four clients you worked on there last month. "Sorry, a little tight right now," he says with a smile, slapping you on the back.

When you pull into your driveway, you find that your massage oil bottle has accidentally flipped open and spilled on the backseat of the car, all over the cloth seats of the Toyota.

You have two messages waiting for you on the machine. An angry-sounding official from the Department of Professional Regulation has called to say you've been subpoenaed to testify against a former employer who is operating without a massage establishment license. This means a day's revenue lost while sitting in court, in addition to possible implications about your own professional standing. The other call is from a friend you went to college with. He's a physician now, living across town in a large new house. In a robust voice, he asks how the "rub biz" is going, and then he invites you to a barbecue at the country club where you were turned down just last week for a therapist's position.

You head directly to bed, too tired to even raid the refrigerator. Falling onto the covers with your clothes still on, you succumb to a moment of doubt. Was massage the right path to choose after all? Blankness and depression inch around the edges of your eyeballs, until suddenly you see the spine of a book you've left by the bedside with the intriguing title *Job's Body: A Handbook for Bodywork.* You've been meaning to read it for months. With the last ounce of positivity left in your spirit, you reach for the book. Opening it to a page at random, your eyes fall on a certain phrase, and you keep reading. . . .

(continued in the last section of this chapter)

SCHEDULING AND MANAGING YOUR TIME EFFECTIVELY

One of the best parts about working in the massage business is that, during a typical work day, you'll often be "in the flow" when you're actually giving a massage, and time will seem to stop for both you and your client. Your problems will disappear, and you'll know you've made the right career choice by the way you feel and how you're helping your client to feel, as well. However, you're going to have to pull yourself out of that luxurious space on a consistent, cyclical basis as each massage comes to a gradual end and stops and then another one looms ahead. To get the most out of your time, you'll be smart to learn the basics of structuring your schedule just like any other busy professional.

Some therapists blur the lines between their professional lives and their personal lives when they first start out, and it seems like they never have enough time to do everything they need to. The massage business has a way of ballooning into every nook and cranny of your existence, expanding into your private life and choking off your free time. Busy therapists sometimes get overwhelmed. You'll benefit by learning a few basic rules concerning effective scheduling.

Here, then, are **seven keys** to time management for massage therapists:

1. Perhaps more important than the time you schedule for each massage is the time you schedule *between* massages. Be generous with this buffer zone, especially in the beginning of your career when you may be overanxious to achieve. It's better to allow yourself an extra 15 minutes to get from one appointment to the next, even if that means telling a client she'll have to wait a little bit.

2. Make sure you have some type of late policy that your clients are aware of. When a client is late for her appointment and another client is scheduled immediately afterward, you can proceed with the first massage but explain that you may have to cut her time short. If she arrives too late (about halfway into her scheduled time), you'll have to postpone the massage.

3. Determine which clients are perpetually 10 to 20 minutes late, and schedule around them. If necessary, tell them that their appointment is earlier, just to make sure they get there on time. This type of client is very difficult to reform because the habit of tardiness usually carries over into all areas of life. It's better to adjust your schedule accordingly rather than get upset by their actions, which you can't control.

4. When you're on the road, give yourself some extra time in case of unforeseeable difficulties like traffic or bad weather. If you arrive early to your client's home or your place of employment, you can spend a couple minutes in the car, calmly breathing and centering yourself for the work you're about to do. It's difficult to soothe others when you're a nervous wreck yourself.

5. Try to schedule appointments as far in advance as possible. That way you can begin to visualize your workload and plan accordingly.

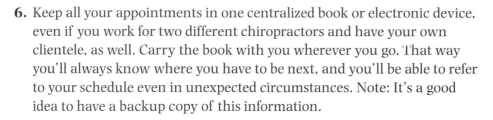

6. Keep all your appointments in one centralized book or electronic device, even if you work for two different chiropractors and have your own clientele, as well. Carry the book with you wherever you go. That way you'll always know where you have to be next, and you'll be able to refer to your schedule even in unexpected circumstances. Note: It's a good idea to have a backup copy of this information.

7. When you're scheduling work, don't forget to schedule relaxation, too. Even if it's just 10 minutes to meditate before the start of a busy day (see the sidebar "Meditation and Your Massage Space" in chapter 7), your psyche will benefit by knowing it has some "space" amidst all the activities you have planned.

As massage therapists, we don't have the same luxury as physicians, whose patients expect to be kept waiting even when they arrive on time for their appointments. Most people, in most circumstances, will expect you to be ready for them at or near the agreed-on time, whether you're seeing them in your own office or at their vacation rental cabin an hour's drive from your house. Therefore, we need to become consummate schedulers and yet maintain a great deal of flexibility for those inevitable occasions when the schedule must be adjusted.

Therapists, like people in general, fall into one of three basic categories when it comes to the levels of detail they work best with. Some like looking at the *big picture* and will be happy using a monthly planner to schedule their days. Others need a *closer focus* and prefer to use a weekly planner. Still others need to see the *minute details* of each and every day, using a daily planner to get their time scheduled right.

I've taken a sample page from the appointment book of each type of therapist in order to show you how the mind of each works. Perhaps you'll recognize yourself in one of the categories, and you'll know how to proceed when it comes time to create your own scheduling system.

The Monthly Planner

This person who chooses a monthly planner (Figure 8-1) enjoys seeing an overview of what is going on. She would rather fill in the squares with cramped handwriting than flip through a series of pages to see where her

Figure 8-1 | **Monthly planner page.**

June
2007

Sun	Mon	Tue	Wed	Thu	Fri	Sat
					1 Bill W. 4:00 PM	2 Lisa R. 9 AM Angela R. 10:30 AM
3	4 Mr & Mrs Rubenstein 2 & 3:00 PM Dave S. 5:00 PM	5 Karen 2:00 PM	6 Liz R. 5:30 PM	7 Dr Sal. 10:00 AM Angel S. 12:00 PM Beth K. 4:00 PM	8 Bill W. 4:00 PM	9
10	11 Lawrence 10:00 PM	12 Katie 11:00 AM Angel S. 7:00 PM	13 Liz R. 5:30 PM	14 Julia S. 3:00 PM NEW CLIENT!	15 Bill W. 4:00 PM	16 Enrique 11:00 AM
17	18 Christina 10:30 AM	19 Tom V. 9:00 PM Jill 11:00 PM Angel 5:00 PM	20 Lisa R. 10:30 PM	21 Dr Sal. 10:00 AM Julia S. 3:00 PM	22 Bill W. 4:00 PM	23
24	25	26 Fred B. 4:00 PM Alice B. 5:00 PM	27 Lisa R. 5:30 PM Christina 9:00 PM	28 Dr Sal. 10:00 AM Julia S. 3:00 PM	29 Bill W. 4:00 PM	30 Wedding Party 5 massages

next appointment with Client X falls. The advantage to this system, of course, lies in its ease of use. It's perfect for part-time therapists who schedule occasional appointments and seldom see more than three clients on any given day. On the downside, monthly planning pages tend to get messy and unreadable if the therapist isn't neat when inputting appointments and other information.

The Weekly Planner

The therapist who chooses the weekly planner (Figure 8-2) is a little more concerned with the details of each week's schedule. She likes to open her book on Monday morning and see immediately who is coming when, but she doesn't need to know in one glance how her entire month is shaping up. This type of planner allows more room for scheduling. It is good for therapists with a medium to medium-heavy work load.

Figure 8-2 | Weekly planner page.

the week of the 4th–10th • June 2007

Monday, June 4		Thursday, June 7	
Dr. Harvey	**9:00 AM**	**Kathleen**	**9:00 AM**
Frederick	**10:30 AM**	**Heather**	**10:30 AM**
		Garth	**12:00 PM**
Theresa	**2:00 PM**		
Rosa	**3:45 PM**	**Bert (2 hours)**	**7:00 PM**
	(1 1/2 hour mass)		

Tuesday, June 5		Friday, June 8	
Salomé	**10:30 AM**	**Paula**	**12:00 PM**
Roderick	**4:00 PM**	**Francine**	**2:00 PM**
Sandy	**5:30 PM**	**Mr & Mrs Silver (1 1/2 hr each)**	**5:00-8:00 PM**
Rhonda	**7:00 PM**		

Wednesday, June 6		Saturday, June 9	
		Yuhio	**10:00 AM**
Scuba Diving 8:00 AM !			**2 hour massage**
Deborah	**2:30 PM**	Sunday, June 10	
Bill	**4:00 PM**		
Suzanne	**5:30 PM**		

The Daily Planner

The therapist who chooses the daily planner (Figure 8-3) needs to see every detail of the day's events. She likes to be able to peer inside each hour and see how it's broken up. Is a client coming at 9:45 and staying until 11:15? She needs to see it graphically. Is lunch from 12:10 to 12:55? She wants to see the minutes blocked out. This system is only for those people who actually *like* to spend time scheduling because they have to commit to constantly updating their information. Of course, if therapists have somebody else to do this for them, such as a secretary or receptionist, that can be a big help, but many therapists find that they need to both speak to clients personally and fill in the appointment book themselves in order to have a handle on their own schedules. This is extra true for the daily planner, who often has a very full plate of appointments.

Figure 8-3 | **Daily planner page.**

the week of the 4th–10th • June 2007

Monday, June 4	Tuesday, June 5
8:00 AM _____	*8:00 AM* **Breakfast Presentation - Rotary Club**
8:30 **Dr. Hofstra (45 min)**	*8:30* _____
9:00 _____	*9:00* _____
9:30 **Suzanne (1 1/2 hrs)**	*9:30* **Community Center 1 hr sessions**
10:00 _____	*10:00* _____
10:30 _____	*10:30* **c.c.**
11:00 **Frank**	*11:00* _____
11:30 _____	*11:30* **c.c.**
12:00 **12:15 - 12:55 Lunch w/Sally**	*12:00* _____
12:30 _____	*12:30* **Lunch at Community Center**
1:00 **Work for Dr. H, 1/2 hr sessions**	*1:00* _____
1:30 **- session**	*1:30* **Mr & Mrs Foxworth (1 1/2 hr each)**
2:00 **- session**	*2:00* _____
2:30 **- session**	*2:30* _____
3:00 **- session**	*3:00* _____
3:30 **- session**	*3:30* _____
4:00 **Drive to gym**	*4:00* _____
4:30 **Work out**	*4:30* **Drive home**
5:00 _____	*5:00* **Snack, WATER PLANTS**
5:30 _____	*5:30* **Joel (REMEMBER TO**
6:00 **Dinner w/Steve**	*6:00* **SAY HAPPY ANNIVERSARY)**
6:30 _____	*6:30* _____
7:00 **Donald (first time client)**	*7:00* _____
7:30 **DO SOAP CHART**	*7:30* **Do laundry**
8:00 _____	*8:00* _____
8:30 **Tape Football game**	*8:30* _____
9:00 _____	*9:00* _____

To Summarize

Of course, you may find that a common computer program such as Microsoft® Outlook or perhaps one of the more therapist-specific programs will work best for you when it comes time to schedule your clients. For a discussion of computer programs that will help you in scheduling your massage appointments, see "Computerizing Your Massage Business" in chapter 7.

As mentioned in chapter 4, therapists are a special breed of employee, and one of the issues that they are most particular about is that of scheduling. When you're in charge of a group of massage people, it can seem like they all have a long list of constantly fluctuating needs as far as their schedules go. The following are some words of advice from Valerie Sasso, an enterprising young therapist who became the manager in charge of a group of therapists at Capellini's Day Spa in Woodmere, Long Island.

"We massage people definitely all have our own pet peeves," she says. "For example, one of the therapists at the spa is a male who does not like working on men; plus, he won't do more than three massages in a row. It can get frustrating, working around specific conditions like that.

"Still, I've found that therapists in spas really can't be blamed for their idiosyncrasies. After all, they're inside a dimly lit room all day, with the same slow music playing over and over again. Working more than three hours in a row in that environment can make them feel like they need to escape sometimes."

Valerie worked as a therapist in the spa for several months before an injury prompted her to move into management. Sometimes she wishes she had the chance to do it all over

again, and there are definitely a few lessons that she's learned along the way. Her fiery dark eyes flash as she talks about self-care for her fellow practitioners, one of her favorite subjects. "The most important thing for therapists who work in a spa," she counsels, "is to not hurt themselves. Some new therapists would come in to the spa fresh out of school and do seven or eight treatments a day, then quit after a couple months because of injuries (see "Keeping Yourself in Shape Mentally and Physically: Combating Burnout Syndrome" later in this chapter). That's the same thing that happened to me. On Thursdays I used to work the nine-to-nine shift. If you work a 12-hour day as a massage therapist in a darkened room, you'll go crazy.

"Spas are great for the customers, who come and go. They're very relaxing for the first four hours, but after that you sometimes feel like you're going to slip into a coma. It's rough on the employees, and you have to take that into account when you're making their schedules.

"Therapists appreciate the security and convenience of having all their appointments booked for them. Even so, in the beginning they try to do private massages at night after getting off from the spa. I tried not to overwork those people, even when they were

(continues)

Valerie Sasso (continued)

requesting it. That kind of behavior usually ends after a little while anyway because it's just too tiring."

As a manager, Valerie also lobbied the owner of the spa for better schedules for the therapists. "I constantly had to convince the boss that he couldn't overwork these people and expect them to make his customers happy at the same time. If they work too many hours in a row, therapists end up praying for cancellations, which is counterproductive. It's the long-term therapists who are actually gaining clients for the business and keeping them there. Because of that, they've got leverage, and they can request better schedules."

Scheduling is always about balance, and it's the same in a private practice as it is at a day spa. No matter what your situation is, when it comes time to schedule your appointments or have them scheduled for you, you'll be OK if you follow Valerie's Golden Rule: "Take care of your body," she states simply.

Enough said.

RECORD KEEPING: CLIENT RECORDS AND FINANCIAL RECORDS

Let's face it; you probably didn't enter the field of massage therapy so that you could spend an hour a day filling out paperwork. Chances are, if you've become a therapist, you are a people person who would rather interact with the hamstrings of a distance runner than a form or chart. This is as it should be. However, as with any job or avocation, a lot of groundwork must be laid and a lot of background information must be assembled before you can successfully pursue the path that you love.

Your clients only expect you to be great when they are actually with you, and a large part of your energy will be spent fulfilling this expectation. But it takes preparation beforehand to be great in the moment. Consider the actress who wows an audience with a gripping performance on stage, for example. The audience doesn't see the years of schooling and training, the months of rehearsal, the detailed attention to every last step, gesture, and expression that seem so effortless and natural. This is what you will be striving for, too, and the "effortless" performance of your great massage has to be built upon a foundation of understanding and detailed attention to each particular client's needs and conditions. This is where record keeping comes in handy. Client intake forms (Figure 8-4) and session notes (Figure 8-5) are not Broadway on opening night, but they're what make you professional and successful.

Figure 8-4 │ **Client information form.**

Client Information

Date:_____

Client ID:_____

Referred by:_____

Client Information

Name:_____

Address:_____

_____

City:_____

State:_____Zip:_____

Phone:_____Fax:_____

Emergency contact number:_____

E-mail address:_____

Birthday:_____

Occupation:_____

Employer:_____

Employer address:_____

Employer phone:_____

Massage Background

Approximate number of
massages received before:_____

Local therapists seen:_____

_____

_____

Type of work preferred:_____

Depth of pressure preferred:_____

Reasons for seeking massage therapy:_____

_____

_____

Problem areas (eg. sensitive
lower back, ticklish feet, etc):_____

_____

_____

Medical History

Are you under medical care now?_____If so, for what condition(s):_____

Past accidents or operations:_____

List any medications being taken:_____

Please describe any physical problems or conditions which you are currently experiencing:_____

_____

Physician's name:_____

Address:_____

City:_____State:_____Zip:_____

Phone:_____

Figure 8-5 | **Client record.**

Client Record

Name:_____

Client ID:_____

Date	Time	Session #	Description of Session	Fee	Balance

Comments:_____

_____

_____

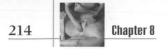

You may be surprised how well clients react to filling out forms and how quickly you'll get used to it yourself. There is something comforting about answering the same questions you've answered a thousand times before in doctors' offices and dentists' offices and insurance offices and hospitals and schools and everywhere else.

Also, you'll want to have a form that keeps track of your existing clients, charting them treatment by treatment. The information you gather on these forms will serve you in a number of ways:

1. You'll be able to chart the progress of every client over the course of their treatments, making it easier to serve them better.

2. You'll be able to send out birthday and other special-occasion cards on the appropriate dates.

3. You'll have extensive background data for tax purposes (see "Taxes" in chapter 6).

4. You'll have a way to chart your own progress as a professional because you can go back over your files to see how your techniques and insights have improved over time.

5. In case of any liability problems, you'll have the records to show exactly what you did and what you hoped to accomplish.

One very specialized type of form used by many massage therapists is called the SOAP form. *SOAP* is an acronym that stands for *subjective, objective, assessment,* and *plan.* These forms are very useful for massage therapists, just as they are for other professionals in the health care field. However, some therapists find them difficult to work with at first.

I had a firsthand experience with the SOAP form problem when I was put in charge of the student clinic at Educating Hands Massage School in Miami. The owner of the school and I decided that both the students and the public who came in for massages would benefit by the use of SOAP-form record keeping, and we implemented its use at the beginning of one semester. The clients didn't mind answering a few extra questions, but the students were honestly confused. What is SOAP supposed to mean anyway? Did it have something to do with cleaning the massage linens? Mutiny was in the air at first, but within a matter of two or three weeks, the students were comfortable with the new forms, and they ended up taking pride in the thoroughness of their new methods.

A few words about each category on a SOAP form follow:

- ✹ **Subjective:** In this space, write what you *hear.* Your client will tell you what she thinks her problem is or simply what she's feeling, and you write down what her condition is from her *subjective* point of view. This point of view may also be that of another health care practitioner or massage therapist who is passing the information along through your client to you in the form of written charts or spoken opinions.

- ✹ **Objective:** In this space, write what you *see.* In your *objective* opinion, what is going on with this client? What you observe may coincide with the subjectively reported experience of the client, or it may be something entirely different.

- ✹ **Assessment:** Here you'll write down what you *think.* This will include your observations of your client's response to past treatment. You'll analyze all available information and, using your experience and knowledge, come up with a treatment plan.

- ✹ **Plan:** Finally, you'll write down exactly how you expect to *act* as regards to this client. You'll map out your treatment strategy as well as specific modalities or maneuvers to be used.

One good book that can help you learn the details of SOAP charting is Diana L. Thompson's *Hands Heal.* See the appendix for details.

When you keep records of your massage business, you will in essence be creating a written history of your interaction with your clients, your profession, and your "self" as you grow through the years. If you value watching old home movies or videos and if you treasure an occasional glance back through your personal diaries and memorabilia, you'll be grateful that you've taken the time to create a history of your massage journey, as well. In addition to being professional, record keeping is also gratifying on a personal level. Of course, keep in mind that all SOAP notes, intake forms, and other records you may keep regarding your clients should remain strictly confidential.

FEES: SETTING THEM, BARTERING, KEEPING THE BOOKS

When you first decide on the amount you'll charge for your massage services, you will probably learn some interesting facts about yourself. In a sense, you'll be telling yourself (and the rest of the world) how much you and your time are worth. This can be a tricky business because there are two basic, opposing perspectives you can take:

1. On the one hand, you, as a human being, are inestimably worthy and no amount of money could ever come close to equaling your true value— especially when you are talking about the value of your touch. Your touch, in a sense, *is* you, and you certainly don't want to undervalue that.

2. On the other hand, as a massage therapist, you are basically an hourly employee of whoever is contracting your services at the moment. You are a skilled manual laborer who is competing against other skilled manual laborers in the marketplace.

When most people are formulating their fees, they look at the situation from perspective number two. They ask themselves the question: What's the right amount to charge to earn a decent living and still offer my customers a good value? This is an entirely appropriate and realistic method and one that I will elaborate on at the end of this section. However, you may benefit from taking a look at your value as a therapist (and as a human being) from another point of view for just a few moments.

Ask yourself this, and answer honestly: Have you ever heard that Therapist X charges an outlandish sum (say $350) for a massage and then thought to yourself, "That guy is just ripping people off. His massage can't be worth that much. I'm sure I'm as good as he is." Conversely, have you thought, "Wow, that guy's way out of my league. He must know some secrets I'll never understand."

I confess to feeling both of those sentiments when I came across a listing of "top" therapists in a trendy magazine recently. One of the featured therapists who worked on movie stars in Los Angeles did in fact charge $350. My mind went through the contortions just described for several minutes until I finally stopped myself and thought, "Hey, wait a minute. Money, after all, is relative. It only has as much value as we give it. If this therapist was able to convince people that his massage was worth $350, why should that bother me?" And it was then that I understood why it did bother me. It bothered me because *it was outside of the value system I had constructed for myself.*

How much you can charge for a massage has nothing to do with value. It has everything to do with *perceived* value. You can receive an excellent, two-hour massage from a highly skilled veteran therapist and pay only $8 for it in one of the temples of Thailand. Is that therapist's work worth less simply because he's the citizen of another country? Would you insist on paying him $75 instead of the normal fee because you thought he was worth it? Or would you do what almost every other human being would do, which is pay whoever massages you the appropriate *perceived* value of that massage in whatever culture, country, city, or neighborhood you happen to be in?

Do you understand what I'm getting at? On a certain level, *we are making all of this up.* Personally, I believe in offering people a valuable service at a price that they can afford; yet at the same time, I desperately want to break out of the constraints I have created for myself, with a little help from society, religion, and family.

Why not challenge yourself? Why not experiment with shifting the *perceived* value of the services you render under certain circumstances? Try an experiment: make up a flier or simply use word of mouth to spread the news that you have a new service to offer. Call it Mega-Massage or Ultra-Massage or something along those lines. Tell people that you've discovered a new level of giving; that this special massage lasts longer than your normal massage; that the techniques are applied with exquisite care; and that you schedule only one or two clients on that particular day because you focus all of your attention on them, holding nothing back. Charge double your normal rate for this massage, and see if anyone takes you up on it. If they do, you may well be amazed to find that the massage actually *is* a Mega-Ultra-Massage. Both you and your client will be utterly focused on the event, and the simple power of your conscious attention will make the massage better than most. The *perceived* value of what you have created in your mind and your client's will usually be fulfilled.

I now receive over three and a half times as much for a massage from some clients than I did when I first started. I have personal goals to receive much more, not because I'm worth more than somebody else or because I want to overcharge people but because I want to continually broaden my own perceptions of what's possible.

The value of your massage, and of you, is what you *create* it to be. Assuming, however, that you won't be charging an infinite amount for your massages, a few basic rules may come in handy when you begin creating your own particular set of perceptions. The following five *conscious fee principles* may help you when it comes time to translate your thoughts, dreams, training, and goals into a simple business transaction in the "real world."

※ When someone asks you what your fees are, have them figured out beforehand, even if they vary according to circumstances. Calmly and clearly state the fees without mumbling. It helps if you have a flier or brochure outlining your rates. Decide in advance if you're going to offer discounts or not so you won't be caught off guard if you're asked to lower your rates.

※ Be aware of what others are charging for similar services in your area. If someone asks why you charge more, be ready to explain why you're worth it—and be ready to believe it!

※ When your client physically hands you the money or the check to pay for a massage, look him or her in the eye and say, "Thank you" so that it's obvious to both of you that you are thankful for the payment itself rather than thankful for their "business" or "support" or any other word that is really just camouflage for money.

※ When you raise your rates, tell all of your clients what you've decided to charge, even those who have been with you for a long time. You may decide to keep a lower rate for long-standing clients, but it's good business for everyone to stay updated about your increasing worth.

※ Start off on the lower end of the fee scale and work your way up rather than struggling to find clients because you're charging prime rates when you're fresh out of massage school.

The following worksheet could as easily be used for any type of massage situation—in a chiropractor's clinic, a spa, a health club, or your own office. I've chosen the out-call massage at a client's home as an example because it involves little overhead and is often used as an indicator of the going rate for massage in any particular area.

First, fill in these figures about massage fees in your community.

1. What is the lowest any therapist charges in your area, even if you feel this therapist *under* charges and the price is unrealistic?　　　　　$ _____

2. What is the going rate in your community for an $ _____
average hour out-call Swedish massage session?

3. What is the highest a customer will pay for the same $ _____
service in your area, even if you feel this therapist
*over*charges and the price is unrealistic?

Then, ask yourself the following questions. Be completely honest with
yourself. Spend a few minutes of introspection to come up with accurate
numbers here.

4. How much do you feel totally comfortable asking $ _____
for right now in return for one massage, even if
the number is a little low on your scale of
expectations?

5. How much would you be willing to ask for, even $ _____
though the thought of asking for that much makes
you a little uncomfortable?

6. What is the most fantastically high price you think $ _____
you are worth right now and would ask for if you
did not think you would be laughed out of town
for doing so?

Now, take the figures from columns 1, 2, and 3 and compare them to 4, 5, and 6.

1.	4.
2.	5.
3.	6.

Notice that what you've placed in the first column are figures perceived to be
out there in the world and the second column holds the numbers that only
you can see, the ones in your mind. How closely do the two compare? While
the first column may be more realistic, the second, in my opinion, is more
important.

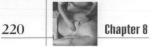
Somebody once said, "You don't get what you deserve, you get what you negotiate." With massage, this is especially true. You may be a tremendous, highly skilled, and extensively trained therapist, but if you don't negotiate the fee you deserve, nobody else is going to do it for you. In fact, you may run into people who willingly take advantage of your youth or your newness to the profession. You have to become worth more in your own mind—and be ready to ask for it—before others will pay you what you really want.

Are you just starting out in your career and want some specific advice about how much you should charge? Here's a little technique that may help you. Referring to numbers 4, 5, and 6, ask yourself those questions again. Now choose the lower number, the one you feel absolutely confident about asking for because you know you can get it and the potential clients in your area are willing to pay it.

Now add $5 to that amount.

That's how much you should charge. If you know you can comfortably get $40, charge $45. If you know you can get $65, charge $70. Just that little extra push will give your subconscious mind the message that you can *grow*.

Income Expectation Chart

Even while you are in the midst of creating prosperity for yourself, you will have to deal with the current reality of your situation. In fact, you can most quickly move on to the economic levels you desire if you first fully admit to yourself the level you're on right now. One pitfall many therapists tumble into is a sort of dreamy, unexamined lifestyle in which they make just enough money to pay the bills but can never seem to get ahead. This can last for years as they continue to dream of great windfalls and expanding profits while in the meantime they can't figure out why their checking account is constantly teetering toward zero. I know; that was my lifestyle for years.

The table on the next page is a simple way to determine if your expectations are likely to keep pace with reality. It is meant to reflect the first year of your massage practice, while you are still getting it off the ground. You'll be wise to look at the reality of your situation early on, thus avoiding some of the economic growing pains many therapists have gone through. Of course, these numbers will vary widely from case to case, but there is a predominant tendency for new therapists to heavily overestimate their cash flow during the first few months of business. This can tend to create an unpleasant *slap in the face* when they actually sit down and do the numbers.

All figures in the following table are based on monthly estimates.

Type of practice	Typical expectation	Typical reality	Slap-in-the face factor
Private (out-call visits only)	$2,000/month	$1,000	$1,000
Private office (yours)	2,500/month	780	1,720
Chiropractor's office	2,000/month	720*	1,280
Doctor's office	1,800/month	800*	1,000
Health club	1,800/month	600*	1,200
Destination spa	2,500/month	1,500	1,000
Day spa/salon	2,000/month	1,200*	800

*At times you may have to pay rent for the space where you do massage when you work at one of these facilities, in the same manner that many stylists rent space in a salon.

Keep in mind that these are *generalizations* and *estimations*. Some people do incredibly well their very first year, becoming completely booked in a private practice and earning over $50,000. Some find jobs in health clubs that just happen to offer an excellent pay scale and have a complete clientele waiting for them. But many put their first ad in the paper only to hear a deafening silence in response. People take jobs at health clubs and find themselves sitting around trying to think up ways to get someone to buy a massage. You may find that you can barely make ends meet and decide that you have to seek other employment while building up your practice. In fact, this is a typical occurrence and you shouldn't feel defeated if you find yourself flipping burgers or selling clothes at the GAP while getting yourself on your feet. In fact, most people end up only practicing massage part time. As a result, the median income for massage therapists in the United States is under $20,000.[1]

One typical path that beginning therapists follow is to find part-time employment at a health club, spa, or clinic that gives them a base salary to live off of while putting in place the promotional and marketing pieces that will eventually get them the private clientele they desire. The owners of such

1. Associated Massage & Bodywork Professionals booklet, *Thinking About Career Options* (2002).

businesses know that beginning therapists are willing to work for peanuts while they gather experience, and, accordingly, the pay scale at many of these places is low ($12 to $25 per hour). My advice to you on this point is *SA*: smile anyway. Regardless of how low the pay is, continuing to work someplace when your attitude is negative will get you nowhere.

Figure 8-6 shows one therapist's income during the first year of massage practice, doing out calls in clients' homes. The price per massage was $40, and the total income for the year was $13,000. Notice the slow beginning in January, the slow steady climb, then the unexpected slump in the summer, which often happens. Massage is seasonal in many areas. People with the discretionary income to spend on massage often go spend a good deal of time away during prime season.

Now, even though I've warned you about getting your economic hopes up too high when you first start out, we're going to look at some graphs of what will happen to your income if, after this first year of gradually increasing your business, you are able create a steady flow of 18 massage clients per week, not an astronomical goal at all. In Figures 8-7 through 8-11, the first thing you'll notice is the great difference in the annual income of a therapist who charges a mere $10 per session more. Ask for $20 more, and you'll jump from $37,440 to $56,160 per year. So, is it worth it for you to raise your rates gradually as your reputation, skills, and confidence grow? You better believe it.

Figure 8-6 | **Monthly income during first year.**

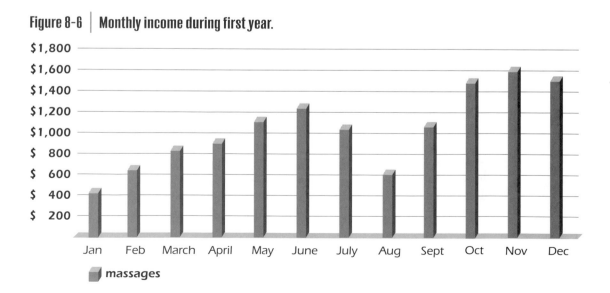

massages

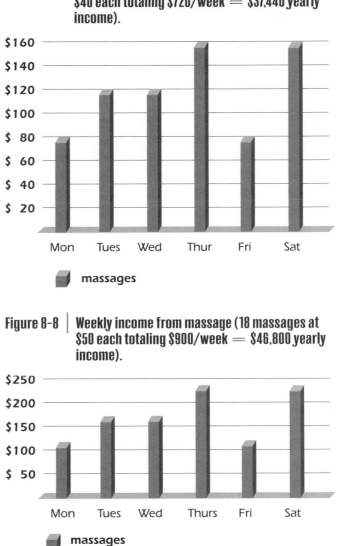

Figure 8-7 | Weekly income from massage (18 massages at $40 each totaling $720/week = $37,440 yearly income).

Figure 8-8 | Weekly income from massage (18 massages at $50 each totaling $900/week = $46,800 yearly income).

Bartering

Imagine walking around with a new, potentially unlimited supply of self-replenishing dollar bills in your pockets, bills that you could pull out at any moment and exchange for the things you want and need. This is essentially what you have in the form of your newfound massage skills. Your skills are liquid assets that can be traded at a moment's notice for a wide variety of

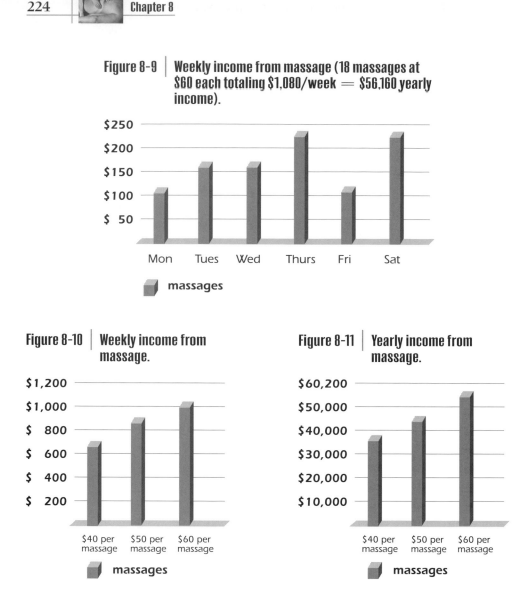

Figure 8-9 | Weekly income from massage (18 massages at $60 each totaling $1,080/week = $56,160 yearly income).

massages

Figure 8-10 | Weekly income from massage.

massages

Figure 8-11 | Yearly income from massage.

massages

goods and services; and when you make such a trade, you will be engaging in an ancient system of commerce known as *bartering.*

I personally haven't "paid" for a haircut in over 20 years. I've been offered Caribbean cruises, world-class meals, professional graphic design services, and much more in exchange for massage. This type of trading is something I highly recommend as your reputation grows.

The word *bartering* itself may not have a completely positive connotation for you because it is sometimes used—incorrectly—in place of *haggling* to describe arguing over price. Also, some people may associate the word with a communal lifestyle in which everything is shared with everybody.

In fact, today bartering has become a sophisticated system of economic exchange, and it's becoming more popular all the time. People are setting up bartering networks in communities across the country, and exchanges are made totaling billions of dollars a year, with the current participation of over 300,000 small companies as well as some larger ones.

How can you as an individual therapist benefit from the world of bartering opportunities? It may be to your advantage to join one of the bartering networks; or you may, like many therapists, choose to exchange just a massage or two at a time with people you already know. You'll be amazed at how many people will be willing to trade an hour of what they do for an hour of what you do.

As a member of a bartering network, the value of your services will be predetermined and you exchange with other people using vouchers or credits. If you make private exchanges, you'll have to agree on a fair exchange rate with each individual. This may prove a little tricky, especially when you're trading such disparate items as massage and television repair; but bartering seems to bring out the instinct of fair play in most people, making most exchanges a pleasure and a bargain for both parties. To give you some idea of what you may ask for in return for your massage, the following page lists some sample exchanges that can be made. Of course, the relative value of each commodity may differ depending on where you live, availability, relative experience levels of the people concerned, seasonal considerations, and so on. When in doubt, simply compare your hourly rate with the normal value of what you're trading for.

There are assuredly many more items you could successfully barter for massage therapy. The only limitation is your imagination. Also, don't forget to give Uncle Sam his due, even in this seemingly personal exchange of favors. The Internal Revenue Service (IRS), by law, is entitled to receive its share of the proceeds even though the transaction involved no exchange of cash. Here's what the IRS has to say about bartering on a page of its official Web site:

> Bartering occurs when you exchange goods or services without exchanging money. An example of bartering is a plumber doing repair work for a dentist in exchange for dental services. The fair market value of goods and services exchanged must be included in the income of both parties.

What to Barter For

What to barter for	Recommended trade	In exchange for
Haircuts	2 haircuts	1 massage
Local moving	1 full day's moving, including truck	10 massages
Auto repair	1 hour of labor (parts extra)	1 massage
Musical instrument lessons	2 lessons	1 massage
Voice lessons	2 lessons	1 massage
Lawn mowing/yard service	Monthly maintenance	2 massages
Plumbing	1 hour of labor	1 massage
Electrical work	1 hour of labor	1 massage
House painting	Small house, including paint	15 massages
Carpentry	2 hours work (supplies extra)	1 massage
Artwork	1 painting or sculpture	1 to 100,000 massages depending upon artist
Marketing/publicity	1 month's retainer fee	20 massages
Videography/photography	1 hour (tape or film extra)	5 massages
Advertising space	1 small ad in local paper	4 massages
Other massages	1 massage	1 massage
Computer training	2 classes	1 massage
Tax preparation	1 return	3 massages
Accounting	1 hour	1 massage
Dental work/orthodontics	1 child's braces	Weekly massage for a year
Chartered cruises	1 week-long island cruise	20 massages
Language or academic tutoring	3 tutoring sessions	1 massage
Meals	1 gourmet meal or 3 regular	1 massage

Income from bartering is taxable in the year in which you receive the goods or services. Generally, you report this income on Schedule C, Profit or Loss From Business, Form 1040. If you failed to report bartering income on returns you have already filed, you should correct this by filing an amended return, Form 1040X (PDF), for each year involved.

The home page for the IRS is http://www.irs.ustreas.gov, and the page concerning bartering can be found at http://www.irs.gov/taxtopics/tc420.html.

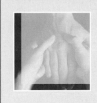

TRADING MASSAGES

How are you, as a therapist, going to receive the massages you need to keep functioning at optimal levels? One traditional method that many of your colleagues use is the massage trade—one session for one session. This is a great way for you to experience the techniques of others while simultaneously keeping yourself in top form. If you're like a lot of therapists, you'll probably become friends with your massage exchange partners and use the opportunity to deepen relationships with other people in your field. However, along with the advantages of this system, there are some disadvantages, as well.

It's fairly easy to find someone to exchange a single massage with; you'll meet them at trade shows, workshops, in school, on the job, and through networking. The challenge is to find someone with whom you're compatible; who likes your work as much as you like theirs; and who, above all, can be depended on to honor the exchange in a timely manner on an ongoing basis.

Once you've found someone and established a good rapport, certain issues may arise that put a kink in your mutual plans to go on blissfully trading session per session for years on end. Here are a few of the points that many therapists get stuck on:

Should you trade on the same day or different days? Same-day massages are probably better because they take care of the entire process in a finite, controllable amount of time. Even with the best of intentions and a solid commitment to complete the trade at a later date, difficulties often arise that make it more difficult than expected to complete the process.

Who should go first on a same-day trade? The partner who is willing to do the massaging first ends up on the table last, which can make the other partner jealous. In general, the partner who is feeling strongest, most awake, and positive should *receive* first because she is more likely to get off the table after her massage with enough energy and enthusiasm to complete the trade, especially when it's later at night.

What do you do when one partner isn't holding up her end of the bargain? Camille Hewton, an Australian therapist who constantly ran into the problem of massage-trade partners who failed to pay her back, had this idea: each pair of massage partners should reserve a $50 bill that they can trade back and forth over and over again, in essence "paying" each other for the massage but never really spending the money. If one partner isn't in the mood to return a massage, she forfeits the cash.

You can find a lot of interesting information about bartering on the World Wide Web. Try typing in http//barter.net, the home page for BarterNet, a service that can put you in touch with many of the networks.

Another good source for help and knowledge about bartering is the *Bartering News Magazine.* Copies can be requested from: Bartering News, PO Box 3024, Mission Viejo, CA 92690. Call (949) 831-0607 or subscribe on line at http://www.barternews.com.

KEEPING YOURSELF IN SHAPE MENTALLY AND PHYSICALLY: COMBATING THE BURNOUT SYNDROME

Giving six or seven full massage sessions every day for weeks on end is comparable to any other form of manual labor, but most of us don't think of it that way because massage therapists work in peaceful, low-stress environments and often seem to be not moving much at all. "How could *that* be so hard?" people ask—until, that is, they try it themselves.

In a workshop I took at a massage association conference recently, one of the attendees—a burly, well-muscled man in his early 50s who looked like he could hold his own among a company of longshoremen—spoke with tears in his eyes as he confessed to the group that he had "just plain broken down and burned out" from doing too many massages. He couldn't take it any more.

It was not this man's physical capacity that had reached the breaking point, although even the strongest therapists have to be aware of certain limits, especially as they mature. What broke down was not tendon, muscle, or bone; it was his will.

As melodramatic as it may sound, the daily repetition of multiple therapeutic massages can be compared to the work that nurses and doctors go through in triage during times of war. Session after session, client after client, day after day, massage therapists are always spending hands-on, in-depth, focused attention on the needs and feelings of others while their own bodies and spirits may be suffering from neglect and overwork.

For a successful massage professional, the flow of clients through the door can seem unceasing, like a river of bodies; and the demands of each client can at times seem childish, selfish, and strange. Nobody is paying attention to the therapist because the therapist is the giver, the strong one, the rock.

Unfortunately, that perception is not the entire truth, and therapists end up paying a price for it in the end.

The number of therapists who complain of burnout is quite large, so much so that entire seminars are devoted to the prevention of it. Before you find yourself signing up for one of these classes yourself, try observing these few basic steps that have helped other therapists avoid—or at least diminish—the impact of this problem.

Fourteen Techniques to Combat Burnout

1. Get sufficient exercise, fresh air, and water. Unless you are one of those fortunate therapists who has created an outdoor work environment, you will quite likely be spending a large amount of time cooped up in a small indoor space, sometimes without windows as in many spas and medical offices. Artificial air and lighting take their toll. Try to spend at least a little time out in the natural elements each day. Try to make some kind of aerobic movement a part of your day, as well. Although massage is hard work, you won't be using your cardiovascular system while doing it. A separate effort is required to exercise, one that may seem difficult at the end of a day spent working hard. You'll find, though, that exercise refreshes and energizes you. Instead of adding to your fatigue, it helps you overcome it. Remember to consume a large amount of pure drinking water, at least two quarts throughout the day. If you spend all day inside a room giving massages, you may easily become dehydrated and not even know it.

2. Let other therapists help you. With the network of massage friends you've built up (see Commandment 9, chapter 6), you'll have a great natural resource to help you avoid the stress of overwork. For example, you may be handling your responsibilities just fine and then one last-minute call from a client tips the scale toward overload. You don't want to turn this client away and force him to look elsewhere for therapy, but you just can't do the session yourself without putting your well-being at risk. What can you do? The wise therapist will call on one of her colleagues to step in for her. In that way, you're the one who fulfilled the requirement for the client, even though you don't directly perform the massage. It takes a confident therapist to do this, someone who isn't afraid to let her clients experience someone else's work. It's no coincidence that these confident therapists are the ones with more clients than they can handle.

3. Receive massage as well as give. This is another commandment from chapter 6. It bears repeating that besides all the physical benefits you'll receive, getting massages will remind you about how good you're helping your clients to feel. This is something that's easy to forget. Remembering it can make your job seem more worthwhile and give you a much-needed boost of enthusiasm when you need it most.

4. Don't give more sessions than you can handle, and allow sufficient time between sessions. Everyone will have a different cutoff point, and you will quickly learn where yours is. For some therapists, two or three massages a day is completely draining. For others, seven or eight is possible, at least for limited periods of time. Know your own limits and when to say No.

5. Have clients come to you instead of going to them. Sometimes the biggest stress in the massage business comes from driving from client to client. If they come to you instead, you'll be a little calmer and cooler when you work on them and you may give a better massage. The downside of this, of course, is that the clients have to do the driving and perhaps get stressed out themselves. Try alternating your options—having clients come to you once a month, for example. They may like the change of venue and enjoy getting out of the house occasionally, too.

6. Use proper body mechanics, from your toes right up through your fingertips. You'll learn about body mechanics in massage school, but you may forget about them in the course of your busy career. That's one sure way to develop some new aches and pains and perhaps even do yourself some serious harm. Remember: Don't place undo stress on the joints of the hand (being especially careful with the thumbs); use your body weight to your advantage; keep the knees bent; don't hunch over at the shoulder; place the feet solidly on the floor; and be aware of your own breathing. If you forget body mechanics over time, you can take a refresher course at the local massage school. Weekend workshops are occasionally offered on the subject; one therapist teaches an entire course on how to give treatments without the use of your thumbs! That may sound extreme right now, but it sounds perfectly reasonable to an overworked therapist with sore, swollen thumb joints.

7. When possible, choose which clients you will work on and which clients you won't work on. Many therapists don't realize that this is a choice left

distinctly up to them. They feel that it's compulsory for them to take everyone who calls and that they'd be losing a valuable customer if they turn anyone away. Not everyone is valuable as a customer, however, and some are downright worthless. When you run into somebody who degrades you or tries to force you to perform sexual favors or in some other way just gives you the creeps, resolve never to see that person again. If you've already worked on him or her and you're left feeling sick or nauseous, use some cleansing or protective rituals to rid yourself of the negativity. Burn a candle. Light a sage stick. Make shaking movements and say, "Ha!" very loudly over and over. These may seem like silly suggestions, and I really can't explain exactly what somebody's negative energy feels like, but it is a very real experience. I've felt it myself, as have countless other massage people, medical practitioners, members of the clergy, and anyone else who comes into regular intimate contact with people they don't personally know. Sometimes it's best to admit that some kind of negative force really is there, although you can't see it, and use the power of your mind along with some abrupt, focused actions to get rid of it.

8. When you go away, *really* go away. Don't touch a body therapeutically even once while on vacation. Don't bring any books about massage. Don't even talk about massage. Sometimes taking a complete breather like this is a way for you to regenerate quickly and come back with fresh excitement for your job. This drastic step isn't always necessary, but it often helps if you feel yourself on the verge of burning out and want to avoid it.

9. Reconnect with the earth. Much of our healing energy comes from our connection to nature. It's a good idea to physically touch elements of nature (trees, rocks, dirt, sand, water) on a consistent basis to stay in contact with the foundation of our energy. When you make contact, close your eyes, breathe deeply, and concentrate on the replenishing of your reserves. (See the profile of Ellen Porr later in this chapter.)

10. Pursue a favorite pastime that has nothing to do with massage. If you develop a hobby, skill, or pursuit that isn't related to bodywork, it may be easier for you to find balance in your life. For instance, one therapist friend is an avid cyclist. Every weekend, she heads out with a group to pedal dozens, and sometimes even hundreds, of miles. This certainly

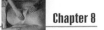

fulfills her quota of fresh air, *and* it gives her the opportunity to spend time among people who have other careers and other interests.

11. Vary your technique. If you always start a massage with your clients facedown, change and start with them faceup. Change the height of your massage table so that you are forced to use different muscles to do the same work. Sit on a chair while working at the head and foot of the table; or, if you already sit in a chair, try working without one.

12. Take classes in new forms of therapy, some of which may be completely different from what you practice now—Different movements, different effects, different needs for strength and balance. This type of diversity will keep your interest alive.

13. Play varied music while you work. Instead of classical guitars, try light jazz. As an experiment, put on some dance music and see how your routine changes along with the rhythm.

14. Get new customers. One thing that can burn you out is repeating the same moves on the same customers over an extended period of time. New bodies inspire new work. Your personality will have to stretch a little, too, as you accommodate new people into your life.

If you are experiencing hand or wrist pain, in particular, you may want to consult a book written specifically about the problem, *Save Your Hands: Injury Prevention for Massage Therapists* by Laurienne Greene. Another choice is *Conquering Carpal Tunnel Syndrome and Other Repetitive Strain Injuries* by Sharon J. Butler.

REWARDS: VACATION TIME AND THERAPY FOR THE THERAPIST

Once therapists start to experience some success, being the givers they are, they sometimes get into a mode in which they do little else but work. This situation is compounded by all the money coming in, which makes continued working seem like a very good idea indeed. The ladder-of-success syndrome can develop, leading the well-intentioned and humanitarian therapist into an escalating series of needs and acquisitions, not unlike any other person in the capitalistic system. Massage therapists are every bit as susceptible to these problems as their corporate counterparts; and even though they've set themselves out on a trajectory that is meant to encompass health, rejuvenation, and well-being, they can end up with a duodenal ulcer or facial tic just as easily as an account executive or the vice president of a start-up company. Just because your work consists primarily of sitting quietly with one person at a time in peaceful surroundings, that doesn't mean you don't have to get away from it once in a while.

Many therapists find a way to incorporate some aspect of their professional lives into their vacations, thereby providing a way for them to both feel productive (a need common to many crusading therapists) and supply an excellent tax write-off. Some examples of this type of vacation include:

- Trips to other countries to study the indigenous forms of massage found there

- Trips to conferences, workshops, and seminars that just happen to be held in beautiful resort areas

- Trips to provide research material for magazine articles and books

- Trips on which you provide lecture services to guests at a hotel, passengers on a cruise ship, attendees at a special event, and the like

Of course, you can also schedule trips to spas, healing centers, and other massage meccas to experience other types of bodywork for your own benefit and understanding. Unfortunately, this type of vacation is nondeductible.

Let there be no mistake; if you're doing what you truly want to be doing, performing work you love, and helping people directly through your touch, there may be no vacation that seems like it could compare to the fun and enthusiasm you're experiencing already. If you enter a phase of your career in which a vacation sounds like torture, by all means continue what you're doing with spirit and enthusiasm. However, it may help you to be aware that there are other therapists who have gone before you and have been burned. Finding the middle road between devotion and relaxation is probably the best choice.

REWARDS: FROM FINANCIAL PLANNING TO FINANCIAL FREEDOM

One appealing aspect of the massage business is that you can make a very tidy sum of money through your work. This is a good thing, of course, but it can also present some challenges. Unless you perform all of your massage work as

PROFILE: Ellen Porr
Vacation Time for Massage Therapists

The lifestyle of Ellen Porr typifies exactly what many people dream about when they first get into the massage business. Each year, for up to two months at a time, Ellen leaves on an extended trip to Greece where she cavorts with friends at a holistic retreat and communes with nature in the semi-inhabited wilderness of some of the more remote Greek islands.

"I'm so blessed," Ellen says. "It really is a great way of life. But I don't think my lifestyle should be the exception. All massage therapists deserve to treat themselves this way. Most therapists are unconventional people . . . types who don't want their lives to become boring. Massage gives you an inner freedom to do what you want to do and go where you want to go.

"The way I look at it, our touch is a gift that we have to take care of so we can keep helping other people. You give and you give and you give, and what happens is you eventually get dried up inside if you don't take time for yourself. People are amazed when I go scuba diving on a Wednesday, for example, but it's one of the things I do for myself to maintain the quality of my work. I work 10 months a year, and I don't get two full days off like most people. Near the end of those 10 months, I start to feel in my heart that I can't give as much anymore. There's a well inside me, and when it gets dry,

the only way to replenish it is to completely *stop* putting my hands on people for an extended period of time.

"At those times, I need to reconnect with nature, too, to physically lie down on the earth, and I do a lot of that while I'm camping in the Greek islands. It replenishes me. Here in the city we're surrounded by this scratchy music in the background of everything we do, even while we're sleeping. Nature is silent and regenerating. To help me reconnect while I'm still here in the city, I go visit my favorite tree every day. I just sit in her and breathe for a while between working on clients."

Ellen claims that her connection to nature is what makes her work come alive for her clients. "I think that when we're connected to Mother Earth, there's a part of us that is silent inside and paying attention, which is exactly the quality a good therapist needs to tune in to her clients as well.

"I think all therapists should do this for themselves if at all possible. Most of us are such givers, we're in danger of giving too much and not receiving enough back for ourselves. The way to receive is to take time for yourself.

"Younger people I talk to are sometimes afraid for me when I tell them about my lifestyle. They say, "What, are you crazy? What if all your clients find another therapist while you're away? What if you can't afford to

(continues)

Ellen Porr (continued)

pay the rent when you get back? What if, what if, what if?" My older clients, on the other hand, think it's great that I take this time for myself because they know what's important in life. They say, "That's great, honey. You go to Greece, and have a **great** time." They hate it when I leave, but they love it when I come back and have all these stories to tell them. When I ask anybody who's older what they wish they could change about their lives, they say they wish they'd spent more time with their families or doing the things they loved like traveling, *not* worrying about money!"

Ellen has settled on a money management system that works perfectly for her. She started as a therapist five years ago, charging $60 per massage, and now she only accepts 10 clients per week who will pay $100 for an hour and a half treatment. She saves a minimum of a $100 a week, and by the end of her 10-month work year, she has between five and seven thousand dollars for her trip.

"It helps knowing that money's growing and I'm going to have that

extended time off each year," she says. "I have one client who lives in a beautiful mansion and drives fancy cars, but when he sees me, he often says, 'I wish I had your life. You know, I think I'm jealous.'"

Ellen's Tips to Make the Massage Life Easier

1. Take minivacations in your hometown by reconnecting with nature, even if it's just by sitting in a tree for a few minutes. As an alternative, try taking a moon bath on a full-moon night.

2. Leave massage sheets at your clients' houses and have them put them in the wash for you. It's no problem at all for them to clean one extra sheet and towel, and it will save you a load of laundry every day or two.

3. When you're on your vacation, send a postcard to each one of your clients. It will help solidify your relationship, and it will be a conversation starter when you get back.

an employee, you will have to manage your own income, your own taxes, your own social security payments, your own insurance, and so on. This is on top of the fact that you're going to have to find your own clients. While this can be a blessing, it also strikes fear into the hearts of many massage therapists who are uncertain about starting out on their own. This fear has several components, including the fear of failure, the fear of embarrassment, and the fear of abandonment.

Even though we U.S. rugged individualists don't like to admit it, many of us would rather feel protected by a "parent" company that we work for and that takes care of many of our needs. To be independent is to be, by definition, all alone, and that can be difficult, both emotionally and financially. What if we fail? What will others think of us? Who'll be there to help?

Many therapists have made the switch to that independence, however, and they couldn't imagine ever going back. In this section, I'll introduce you to the basic information you'll need to strike out on your own, manage your income wisely, and plan for a secure future. You may even find yourself better off than you ever thought possible. Some of the information also applies to those therapists who choose to work for somebody else. Regardless of where your money comes from, you're going to have to learn how to use it wisely or it will magically disappear.

The number one rule that will help you with your finances is: **Pay yourself first.** If you consistently set aside a certain percentage of your income, you'll be accomplishing two important goals. One, of course, is the saving of money. The other, and probably more important, is that you'll be telling your subconscious mind that you are a person who can *have* money. A huge majority of us *make* money throughout our lives, but we never end up having any because we spend it and it's gone.

As a massage therapist and independent contractor for over 20 years, I've made an extensive study into the sometimes confusing role that money plays in our lives. I've found that while some of us definitely do very well financially, a much greater number of therapists find themselves struggling through much of their careers, constantly on the edge, it seems, of poverty. They are truly living hand-to-mouth.

During one particularly penurious stage of my early career, I had to keep putting change together each morning and deciding whether I could afford the six-inch or the twelve-inch sandwich from Subway for lunch, my main meal of the day. This was during the heat of a Florida summer, and I had no air conditioner nor the money to buy one. With no savings to fall back on and not much clientele built up yet, I had no shield from the heat or the hunger; but, strangely enough, not for one moment did I yearn for a job in a big cool glass office building downtown. I did know, however, like so many therapists before me, that I needed to gain some insight and mastery over the whole issue of money.

Thus began the quest, one familiar to many therapists, in which we reach out for the wisdom that others have to offer on the subject of finances. A good place to begin on this quest is in the pages of an aptly titled book that succinctly states the nature of our problem: *The Trick to Money Is Having Some* by Stuart Wilde, published by Hay House. As mentioned earlier, so many of us in the massage business experience money coming and going but not staying. It's an extremely simple concept that somehow eludes us. The trick is . . . *having* some!

Most of us, as we progress through our massage careers and our lives, eventually decide that, yes, we do want to have some money. This happens at different stages and different ages for each therapist. Indeed, some may start out feeling this way. Regardless of when we make this decision, we are then immediately faced with the challenge of carrying it out; and this is when we run head-on into the next set of barriers.

At this stage, after we've decided that we'd like to have some money, we discover that money is still somehow the enemy. This is when we need the simple yet profound wisdom of another book, *Money Is My Friend* by Phil Laut. In it, Mr. Laut puts the emotions we have about money under scrutiny, until we can see why, up until now, money has *not* been our friend at all. Is it any wonder that we've had a hard time holding onto it? You can find this book in many bookstores or order it on line from Amazon.com and other Web booksellers.

The granddaddy of all works on the psychology of money is *Think and Grow Rich* by Napoleon Hill. At a young age, Mr. Hill was given a mission by the wealthy industrialist Andrew Carnegie, who asked him to spend several years studying the lives of wealthy and successful people. The resulting insights have helped thousands of other people prosper, as well—not just financially but in the riches of the heart and spirit, too. Indeed, as all of these authors point out, success and spirituality go hand in hand—which brings us to the final barrier.

To make the final leap to the lifestyle we want, there is one more step. We have to believe that it can be so. Do you truly believe that as a massage therapist you can lead a fulfilling life in which you not only help many people but remain healthy and happy yourself, experience both spiritual and emotional growth, *and* become financially successful? You'd better believe it because if you don't, it won't happen.

Three basic concepts that hold many therapists back at this point include:

1. Money is not spiritual, and therefore if I have money I am not spiritual.

2. People who have a lot of money are selfish and spoiled.

3. If I focus on money, I can't focus on what really matters, which is the quality of my work and my interactions with other people.

Now, let's shoot these concepts down before they shoot you down:

1. Money is inert. It is neither spiritual nor unspiritual. It is what you do with money that creates value and spirituality, or emptiness and materialism. Search yourself for traits of the philanthropist type of therapist (see "The Parameters of the Profession" in chapter 6). Does a part of you still feel that you can't be good and well off at the same time? If that's true, then nothing outside of you is holding you back from attaining your dreams. It's an inside job.

2. There are many very nice, very spiritual, very giving rich people, some of whom would be happy to share their insights and inspiration with you were you wise enough to listen to them. Rich people give money to charities, start crusades to aid the needy, establish scholarship funds, and donate to worthy causes. Sure, there are some miserable, selfish rich people, but there are many miserable selfish poor people, as well.

3. If you don't *have* money, you'll be worried about *getting* money all the time, and you won't be able to focus on what really matters, which is the quality of your work and your interactions with other people.

So, now that you've decided that the trick to money is having some, that money is actually your friend, and that you're ready to use your thoughts to grow rich, what are you actually going to do about it? The books I've cited and many other similar volumes are filled with practical advice in this arena, and I hope you take it to heart. The best guidance I can offer is to say, once again, **pay yourself first.** Set up a plan of savings, investing, and growth. Take advantage of the tax-deferment options offered to you, either as a self-employed therapist or as an employee of a larger company.

Absolutely the smartest thing you can do is to go out *today*, if you haven't already, and start your tax-deferred retirement fund, either an Individual Retirement Account (IRA), a Simplified Employee Pension (SEP), or a Keogh.

You gain a tremendous advantage by starting early on this. For example, if you start at 18 years old instead of 30, it could mean the difference between having $300,000 at retirement age or $1,200,000. Do you think saving $2,000 a year from the age of 18 to 30 is worth $900,000? Even if it means you have to settle for the six-inch sandwich instead of the twelve-inch for lunch today, do it anyway, and **do it now.** Go to your bank. Ask your employer. Call an investment firm. Act.

If you think you can skip the part about paying yourself first and simply live off Social Security when you retire, think again. The entire Social Security system is undergoing rapid change, and it definitely will not be able to support the U.S. population very far into the future. Even today, Social Security benefits afford a very meager living for those people forced to rely upon them. In the future, there may be no benefits at all. Keep in mind, however, that you still have to pay Social Security taxes today. If you are a self-employed therapist, you are responsible for your own self-employment taxes, which go to support the Social Security fund (see "Taxes" in chapter 6).

Many eager and idealistic people start out thinking massage will provide them with a direct route to riches. Others feel that massage will provide just enough money so that they can shelter themselves from the commercialism of the modern world and live at peace. At either extreme and everywhere in between, as a therapist you'll have to deal with money and pay attention to it in one way or another.

Money is simply one of the ways humans decide what to concentrate on. Whether you're deciding between a six-inch or a twelve-inch sandwich or between a 40-foot or a 50-foot yacht, the same powers are at play. Why not upgrade?

A "DREAM" DAY IN THE LIFE OF A MASSAGE THERAPIST

To finish this chapter, I'll leave you with some of the brighter moments that can happen in the daily life of a massage therapist. Once again, this is a conglomeration of actual events from my experience and those of other therapists.

(Continued from the "Nightmare Day" section at the beginning of this chapter.)

You were up reading until 1:30 a.m., yet you still feel refreshed this morning. You were inspired and found solace in the words of Deane Juhan in his book *Job's Body: A Handbook for Bodywork.* "Touching hands are not like pharmaceuticals or scalpels," you read. "They are like flashlights in a darkened room. The medicine they administer is self-awareness. And for many of our painful conditions, this is the aid that is most urgently needed."[2]

Yes! This is exactly why you chose this path as a massage therapist in the first place. You wanted to administer self-awareness and relief to many people through your touch. Your old friend the physician may be helping people, too, with his scalpel and his drugs, but you knew you had a different kind of mission to fulfill. His house near the country club may be bigger than yours, but you are following your heart; and who knows what kind of successes await you?

Your first appointment this morning is with a new client, recommended to you by a dentist friend. After arriving punctually, she tells you that she has been suffering chronic pain in her head, neck, and shoulders for several years now and her dentist thought it might have something to do with her temporomandibular joints. You've had experience with TMJ problems because you are a trained craniosacral therapist, and your dentist friend has referred several cases that you've treated successfully. This woman, however, reacts more positively than anyone you've seen before. Within 20 minutes, she is having an emotionally charged resurgence of a long-lost memory in which she recalls exactly what caused this pain of hers in the first place. It was a blow to the head she suffered as a teenager and had long since forgotten. This is what all of your training is about, to be able to help someone on profound levels through your skills. The woman on your table has tears of gratitude and relief streaming down her face.

Another punctual client arrives at 10:00 for a great, playful session in which you both laugh a lot. You attended the birth of her daughter several months earlier, and you realize that she has become a lifelong friend.

After she leaves, you put on your shorts and head out for a brisk jog in the nearby park. With a smile on your face and a glow deep inside that still lingers from your interactions of the morning, you breathe in the scent of freshly mown grass and enjoy the sensation of sun on your face. On the other side of the street is a row of glass and concrete office buildings, where hundreds of people are working away, probably gazing out the window at that very

---

2. Deane Juhan, *Job's Body: A Handbook for Bodywork* (Barrytown, NY: Station Hill Press, 1987).

moment, wishing they could be in the park, too. This is one of the most precious gifts your lifestyle as a therapist has provided—the freedom to make your own schedule and your own rules.

After stretching out and cooling down, you drop in for a smoothie and a healthy sandwich at the little shop you love down on Main Street, beating the noontime rush.

Back home, you meet the mail delivery woman at your doorstep, and this time it's great news. The American Massage Therapy Association has accepted your proposal for a presentation at their upcoming educational conference in San Francisco! That means you get to present your latest ideas and techniques to a roomful of colleagues and receive national-level recognition for it. Plus, San Francisco is your favorite city in the world!

Another letter is from the owner of the massage school you attended, asking if you'd like to offer the new weekend workshop you've created as a part of its very popular continuing education program.

Your last piece of mail is a letter from a reader of the booklet you wrote about the art of giving and receiving massage. In heartfelt words, he explains how you helped him find new focus and improve his relationship with his wife, how the two of them now exchange massages on a regular basis following the guidelines and inspiration you provided. He wrote, "Thanks to you, we learned how to care about each other all over again, using the magic of touch."

While you're still holding the letter, the phone rings. It's the man from the Department of Professional Regulation. Sure enough, he wants you to testify in court against the employer without a massage establishment license. The date is set for next week. You have no choice in the matter, but instead of feeling depressed about it, you begin to think that this employer deserves to be testified against and you look forward to doing your duty. The conversation you're having becomes amicable, even pleasant, and you feel good to be part of a profession that takes itself seriously enough to deal out court time and penalties to those who don't follow proper guidelines.

In the afternoon, you pay visits to two regular clients, and each of them decides that it's time to take advantage of the special offer you've announced recently, giving a sizable discount for 10 sessions paid in advance. So you stop at your bank to deposit two hefty checks and still make it home in time to avoid rush-hour traffic.

To celebrate your good fortune, you decide to take your favorite yoga class. The teacher is a friend of yours; when she sees you, she asks yet again if you'll join her in signing up for a training course in Rubenfeld Synergy, the advanced technique you've wanted to study for years. The training commitment includes making several trips a year to New York City, however, and you've never had the extra money necessary. You begin to tell your friend this one more time when you remember the new funds in your account and the promise of the upcoming workshops at the massage school, which normally bring in between $1,000 and $2,000 per weekend—and you realize that you can sign up for the training after all. You're going! A whole new chapter in the book of your massage career is about to begin.

Your muscles and joints seem especially loose, and you go home after the class feeling buoyant and fulfilled. Too excited to sleep, you turn on your computer and begin composing the opening comments of your presentation for the educational conference. Before you know it, three hours have gone by and you have the entire format of your half-day seminar completely filled in. You read back over it with satisfaction. Suddenly, it seems, you've turned a corner. Perhaps tomorrow will bring with it another set of challenges; but you're a professional now, and you'll know how to face them. By never giving up and by following what your heart told you was right all along, you've reached heights of fulfillment that many people only dream about. The view from your new vantage point, at least on this particular day, is breathtaking.

9 Creating a Professional Image

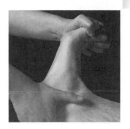

Massage therapy is one of the most "internal" professions you can choose. Your clients will experience the benefits of your work *inside* their own bodies, often with their eyes closed. In massage school, you learn about the *inside* of the human body, not just the surface. When you are doing your best work, you may likely have your own eyes closed as well; you'll be working from that quiet screne space *inside* your self from where all healing flows. Yes, massage is definitely an *inside* job, and yet . . .

For you to enjoy the most success as a therapist, you'll want to learn the best way to present yourself on the *outside* as well. The general public, as well as prospective employers, future business partners, and your fellow therapists, all perceive your external image before they have a chance to get to know the quality of your work. That external image is the door that they must pass through before getting to know how good you are. If the door is shabby or hidden down a dark alley or plain and unadorned, few people will take the time to come inside and find out what it is you have to give.

IMAGE ENHANCERS

Creating a professional image for yourself is extremely important. In this section I'd like to share with you some simple, effective ways that you can put together a dynamic, successful image without spending a lot of money. The image enhancers I'll discuss include:

1. Your attire

2. Résumés

3. Business cards/letterhead/logos

4. Brochures/fliers

5. Photographs of yourself

6. A presence on the Internet

7. Press kits

Your Attire

As I've mentioned, a lot of people choose the career of massage because they have an artistic, independent nature, and they don't want other people telling them how they should look or what they should wear. I respect this attitude, and yet I also feel that therapists should always be aware of the image they are presenting to the public through their appearance. Massage therapists should look good; they should look clean; they should look bright and neat and approachable.

Depending on where you live and what time of year it is, different types of dress are appropriate. In California, for instance, if you are driving to a client's house for an out-call massage in one of the small redwood communities of Humboldt County, chances are that you're already friends with your client and he or she is expecting you to show up in simple, neat attire, perhaps something with a personal accent like a bright rainbow shirt or a loose-flowing cotton dress. If, on the other hand, you are arriving for work at a chic day spa in the trendy Buckhead section of Atlanta, Georgia, you'll want to be wearing a crisp white outfit that bespeaks professionalism and elegance.

PROFILE: Michael McGillicuddy
Leadership and Service

Often, massage therapists are not completely comfortable with the idea of marketing themselves. They would rather focus on the *inside* rather than the *outside,* on giving rather than getting. They believe in service and true leadership, not just creating a superficial image, no matter how professional that image may be. Well, sometimes these disparate elements can come together. There are therapists who have dedicated themselves to the profession, and through that dedication they have achieved new levels of recognition. Michael McGillicuddy is one such therapist.

You may have a vision of yourself heading toward a rosy future in the industry, following a smooth trajectory toward ultimate success. But as any one who has reached high levels of leadership in this field can tell you, the road is often winding and the path at times unclear. Michael, like many therapists, has had to deal with setbacks and even tragedy on his way to becoming a person who is looked up to and admired by all who know him and work with him. This, in his own words, is how he got started and then developed his career to its present peaks.

"The very first time I was exposed to bodywork was at a community college," says Michael. "A therapist was there giving a demonstration of Rolfing®, and

as I watched, my first thought was that Rolfing® looked mighty painful! I got over my fear within a few short weeks, though, as I watched my roommates at the time come back from their own Rolfing® sessions. They seemed to be changing and they seemed to be happy about it. I became curious.

"I signed up for the 10 sessions of Rolfing® and experienced firsthand how powerful bodywork really is. After I went through my initial Rolfing® series, it took another nine years for my life circumstances to get to a place where I could enter massage school. When I finally did attend, I knew almost from the beginning that I would be specializing in sports massage.

"The very first month the school offered a weekend sports massage workshop. I signed up and have been practicing sports massage ever since. Once I graduated from massage school I took every sports massage workshop I could find. I also volunteered to provide massage at every sporting event I could. It did not take long for my reputation as a sports massage therapist to build in the community.

"Soon the owner of the local massage school asked me to teach sports massage to her students. She liked what I did so well that at the next faculty meeting she announced to my amazement that I was now part of her core faculty and tripled the hours I was

(continues)

Michael McGillicuddy (continued)

teaching! The school then developed an advanced sports massage internship program in connection with a local state university. My job then required me to supervise students massaging in the athletic training room on all teams at the university.

"After 10 years of teaching experience, I developed my own series of sports massage workshops and became a continuing education provider. I now write sports massage articles and continue to teach sports massage workshops."

Michael says he then began to think about the possibilities of increasing the reach of his teaching. "I had been teaching sports massage for a number of years at different massage schools and would often think about the possibility of opening a school of my own," he says. "One day I got a call from someone who was starting a school and wanted me to consider being a partner. When we started, the school was just an empty building. Our first day-class had four students in it. It has definitely grown in popularity since then, and today we graduate about 60 students a year."

After a time, owning a thriving school and offering his services as a sports massage therapist did not fulfill Michael's need to give back to the industry, and so he became involved with his state massage association. "I have served the Florida State Massage Therapy Association (FSMTA) in numerous positions for 17 years and eventually became the executive president," says Michael. "I believe that when you volunteer, especially for positions you have never done before, it allows you to grow as a person. I had been involved in promoting the profession for so long that I felt I was the best person to serve in that position at the time. I was recently re-elected to a second term so I believe the membership had faith in my abilities also.

"My biggest challenge as president is trying to stay on top of everything that is happening to a profession that is growing so quickly. When I started my career, there were about five massage schools in the state, and there are now over 120. There are over 22,000 licensed massage therapists in the state of Florida at this time.

"My greatest fulfillment is watching the reputation of massage therapy grow in professional stature. Through hard work by many volunteers, the citizens of Florida now have some of the best trained massage therapists in the country."

Then, Michael experienced a tragedy in his personal life and professional life as well when his wife was killed. Cheryn had been a big part of the massage school. "From the day I found out about Cheryn's death," says Michael, "everyone—students, teachers, staff,

(continues)

Michael McGillicuddy (continued)

FSMTA members, and massage therapist friends—have all been extremely supportive. Cheryn was a human being who was a true servant to humanity as well as my wife. There has not been a day since her death that I have not wished to see her smile and hear her voice. She was the heart and soul of the Central Florida School of Massage Therapy. The hardest thing I had to do was to walk into the school every day without her being here. It was only through the support of the staff, teachers, and students that I could do it. I also knew that she gave so much of her life to growing our school that if I did not continue she would have been very disappointed in me. It is my intent to make the Central Florida School of Massage Therapy the best massage school in the country and dedicate it to Cheryn McGillicuddy."

Through all of the ups and downs, the triumphs and the tragedies, the constants in Michael McGillicuddy's life have been leadership and service. This has tempered his philosophy about life and about his profession. "I really believe that the practice of massage allows the therapist to develop his or her own interpersonal communication skills in a very loving way," says Michael. "No matter what type of massage you perform, it always involves another human being. I believe that good therapists are always trying to communicate through touch a better way for their clients to experience their lives. I study now more than I ever have before, and after 21 years I still feel I am only beginning to learn. Practice with constant childlike curiosity and amazing openness and you will never tire of the massage therapy profession."

You'll have to use your own judgment to adjust the image you portray through your clothes. To help you, here are a few general guidelines to keep in mind when you're building your wardrobe or getting dressed for a day of work as a therapist:

1. White is the color of choice of many therapists. White is the color associated with healing and care, like a nurse's uniform. It looks good on therapists and is often the most appropriate choice for many work situations. White jeans, white polo shirts, and, in warmer climates, white Bermuda shorts are acceptable. Make sure to wash your outfits often; massage oil can easily spot the material.

2. Other color clothes are fine. Bright, positive colors are appealing, as well as darker earth tones. All garments should be in good repair.

3. Avoid belts with big buckles because they can scrape against clients' skin during the massage.

4. If you have long hair, keep it pulled back from your face when you're working. This is more sanitary and it also looks neater.

5. If you tend to perspire a lot when you work, wear an undershirt beneath your clothes. Sweat-absorbing headbands and wristbands can help with this, too.

6. Therapists should be aware that revealing outfits may give the wrong impression. Even in warm weather, a shirt with some sort of sleeve is best. Midthigh-length shorts are fine.

7. Keep nails trimmed and smooth.

8. Remove any jewelry, rings, and so on that may interfere with the massage.

Résumés

The résumé is an important tool for you to use in the beginning and into the intermediate stages of your massage career, until you've acquired enough material and experience to create your press kit. The objective of a résumé is to attain employment at a specific facility. Therefore, my recommendation is that you tailor your résumé separately for each prospective employer, inserting the name of the company and what you intend to do specifically for them. You should also get the name of the person you have to deal with at each place— either the office manager, personnel director, or owner—and address a personal, one-of-a-kind cover letter to that person, submitting it with your résumé.

A sample cover letter is provided in Figure 9-1, and a sample résumé is provided in Figure 9-2. The résumé is for a beginning therapist fresh out of school with only a few private clients. She still doesn't have enough "meat" to put together a press kit, but she can make herself attractive to employers nonetheless with the skillful construction of words on paper.

Business Cards/Letterheads/Logos

A logo is a symbol that tells others who you are with one brief, impacting image. Choose your logo wisely, use it in a creative way on your printed materials, and you're bound to attract positive attention.

Figure 9-1 | Sample cover letter.

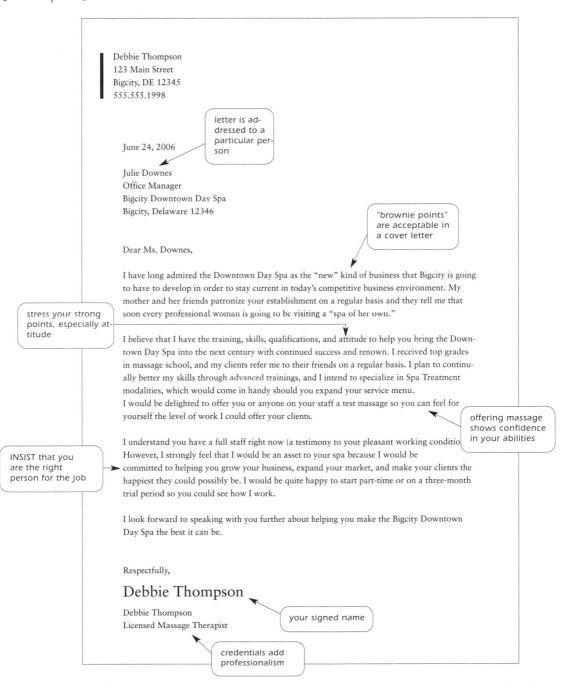

Debbie Thompson
123 Main Street
Bigcity, DE 12345
555.555.1998

letter is addressed to a particular person

June 24, 2006

Julie Downes
Office Manager
Bigcity Downtown Day Spa
Bigcity, Delaware 12346

"brownie points" are acceptable in a cover letter

Dear Ms. Downes,

I have long admired the Downtown Day Spa as the "new" kind of business that Bigcity is going to have to develop in order to stay current in today's competitive business environment. My mother and her friends patronize your establishment on a regular basis and they tell me that soon every professional woman is going to be visiting a "spa of her own."

stress your strong points, especially attitude

I believe that I have the training, skills, qualifications, and attitude to help you bring the Downtown Day Spa into the next century with continued success and renown. I received top grades in massage school, and my clients refer me to their friends on a regular basis. I plan to continually better my skills through advanced trainings, and I intend to specialize in Spa Treatment modalities, which would come in handy should you expand your service menu.
I would be delighted to offer you or anyone on your staff a test massage so you can feel for yourself the level of work I could offer your clients.

offering massage shows confidence in your abilities

I understand you have a full staff right now (a testimony to your pleasant working conditio). However, I strongly feel that I would be an asset to your spa because I would be committed to helping you grow your business, expand your market, and make your clients the happiest they could possibly be. I would be quite happy to start part-time or on a three-month trial period so you could see how I work.

INSIST that you are the right person for the job

I look forward to speaking with you further about helping you make the Bigcity Downtown Day Spa the best it can be.

Respectfully,

Debbie Thompson

Debbie Thompson
Licensed Massage Therapist

your signed name

credentials add professionalism

249

Figure 9-2 | Sample résumé.

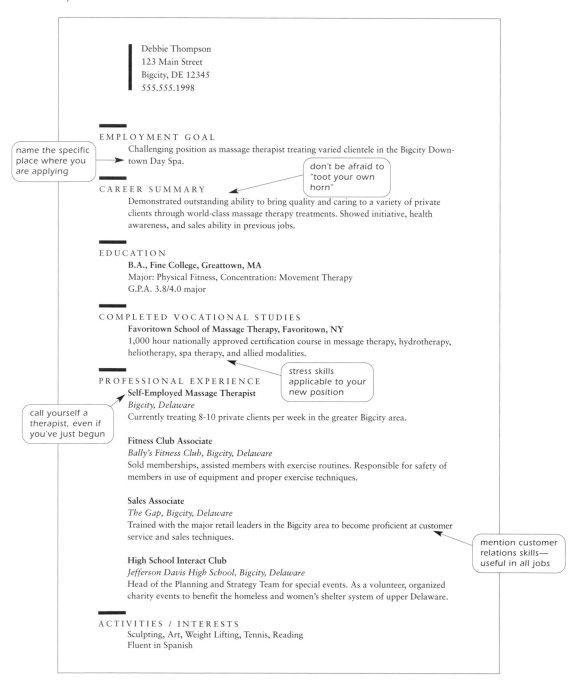

Debbie Thompson
123 Main Street
Bigcity, DE 12345
555.555.1998

EMPLOYMENT GOAL
Challenging position as massage therapist treating varied clientele in the Bigcity Downtown Day Spa.

name the specific place where you are applying

CAREER SUMMARY
Demonstrated outstanding ability to bring quality and caring to a variety of private clients through world-class massage therapy treatments. Showed initiative, health awareness, and sales ability in previous jobs.

don't be afraid to "toot your own horn"

EDUCATION
B.A., Fine College, Greattown, MA
Major: Physical Fitness, Concentration: Movement Therapy
G.P.A. 3.8/4.0 major

COMPLETED VOCATIONAL STUDIES
Favoritown School of Massage Therapy, Favoritown, NY
1,000 hour nationally approved certification course in message therapy, hydrotherapy, heliotherapy, spa therapy, and allied modalities.

PROFESSIONAL EXPERIENCE
Self-Employed Massage Therapist
Bigcity, Delaware
Currently treating 8-10 private clients per week in the greater Bigcity area.

stress skills applicable to your new position

call yourself a therapist, even if you've just begun

Fitness Club Associate
Bally's Fitness Club, Bigcity, Delaware
Sold memberships, assisted members with exercise routines. Responsible for safety of members in use of equipment and proper exercise techniques.

Sales Associate
The Gap, Bigcity, Delaware
Trained with the major retail leaders in the Bigcity area to become proficient at customer service and sales techniques.

mention customer relations skills— useful in all jobs

High School Interact Club
Jefferson Davis High School, Bigcity, Delaware
Head of the Planning and Strategy Team for special events. As a volunteer, organized charity events to benefit the homeless and women's shelter system of upper Delaware.

ACTIVITIES / INTERESTS
Sculpting, Art, Weight Lifting, Tennis, Reading
Fluent in Spanish

How you design your logo will depend upon your circumstances. Many beginning therapists don't have enough money saved up to hire the services of a graphic designer, which can be quite expensive. If this is the case, you can try the following scenario: Locate the designer you want through friends or by word of mouth or ask who did the design work for printed materials that you find attractive. Next, approach this person and offer to trade massage services for help in the creation of your logo. You can make things easy for the designer by coming up with some creative ideas of your own as suggestions. Work out an equitable trade for the designer's time. He or she will provide you with "camera-ready copy" that you can then take to a printer to be made into business materials.

I personally think this is a good way to get started if you don't have much money; it's the method I used myself. When I was just getting by as a therapist, I had an inspiration for a logo. The company name I had in mind was Massage Adventures, and the logo was a backpacker "hiking" over the terrain of somebody's back (see Figure 9-3). I had no idea how to get this idea on paper, and so I approached an acquaintance who had his own design business. He provided the design in exchange for several massages for both him and his assistant.

You want your logo to tell the world who you are. Many therapists choose an image of hands or an anatomical design like Leonardo da Vinci's drawing of the human body. If you can think of something unique that grabs people's attention, you may help your business get off the ground in a big way. Within a year of creating my Massage Adventures logo, I was approached by a massage industry leader and asked to help create and then teach massage workshops all across the country. When I asked later why they had chosen me for the job, I was told it was in large part due to the unique, professional look of my logo and materials.

In addition to your printed materials, other simple objects can be turned into effective massage therapy marketing tools, as well. Coffee mugs, windshield blinds, calendars, license plate holders, pens and pencils, water bottles, and many more items can all be emblazoned with your logo, name, and number. This will help people keep you and your business in mind.

The time, effort, and investment you put into your image will create rewards that you can't presently foresee. Don't neglect this important aspect of your new career.

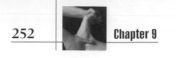
Figure 9-3 | Sample logo on letterhead.

Once you've created your logo, take it to the printer to make business stationery (letterhead) and business cards. There are many ways you can use your printed material to promote yourself:

1. Pass out your cards at all social functions and to any prospective clients.

2. Give your cards to clients so that they can give them to friends who will then become clients, too.

3. Write letters on your letterhead to the media and include them in your press kit.

4. Send out all your correspondence on your massage business letterhead. In that way, everyone you communicate with will start to think of you primarily as a massage therapist.

Brochures/Fliers

You can inexpensively produce your own business brochures and fliers using a computer. If writing is not your forte, try exchanging massages with a friend who has a gift for language. Between the two of you, you'll be able to come up with some interesting copy to include in the brochures. Another alternative is to take advantage of preprinted massage newsletters, brochures, and fliers from experts who prepare them for a living. For a fee, they will provide you with these materials and your name will be strategically inserted in the blank spaces so that the feeling of a personal promotional piece is conveyed.

For all your printed materials, use good quality paper. The look and feel of the paper will reflect on your business. If you have access to a computer, you can order specialized papers that are already precut and prefolded as brochures, letterhead, fliers, business cards, and more. One company that has great products and quick service is Paper Direct. It also offers computer software with templates so that you can design your own materials right on the screen. You can call Paper Direct at (800) APAPERS for a free catalog, or visit http://www.paperdirect.com.

Photographs

Get at least one high-quality photograph of yourself from the chest up (known as a "head shot") to use in your promotional materials. Most head

PREPRINTED NEWSLETTERS

Would you like to offer your clients pertinent information about massage therapy, wellness, and your business in the form of a slick, professionally produced newsletter? Would you also like to avoid much of the cost usually associated with this type of endeavor? Then you may consider membership in Associated Bodywork and Massage Professionals (more information about ABMP can be found in chapter 10). As an added perk to joining, members receive access to a special section of the Web site where they can plug in their own information and within minutes print out a beautiful, informational newsletter. Alternatively, they can send this newsletter via e-mail as a PDF attachment to all of their clients and associates. What could be easier? Visit http://www.abmp.com, send an e-mail to expectmore@abmp.com, or call (800) 458-2267 to get more information about this newsletter and how it can boost your practice.

shots are in black and white because it is more expensive to reproduce color photographs in volume. As an alternative, some therapists choose an "action" shot of themselves giving a massage. You can have a friend take the photographs, but a professional will know how to greatly enhance your image with the right lighting, backdrop, and so on. This is another instance in which you can profitably trade massage services; offer a photographer massages in exchange for your promotional shots.

Once you've chosen the very best photograph, reproduce it in 8×10 or 5×7 size, at least 50 copies. You can choose to have your name and the words "licensed massage therapist" superimposed over the photograph if you want, and you can also have your contact information printed on the back.

The old saying that a picture is worth a thousand words is doubly true when the subject is a massage therapist. Many people want to be recommended by a personal friend before they will accept the services of a therapist they don't know. A photograph may help them feel they know you a little better.

You can miniaturize your photo and include it in your brochure or even on your business card. It can also be printed on gift certificates. And make sure to include one with every press kit you send out.

A Presence on the Internet

If you haven't visited the massage section of the World Wide Web, you may have a surprise in store for you. Enterprising therapists and marketers have turned the Internet into a forum for a rich and interesting exchange where manufacturers promote products, therapists promote services, clinics promote facilities, spas promote vacation packages, doctors promote alternative healing practices, and everyone promotes the benefits of massage therapy.

As each year passes, a proper understanding of the Internet and how it can serve you and your business is becoming increasingly important. Don't let the high-tech nature of computers scare you away; access to the Web is so simple that almost anybody can learn the basics of using it in a few short minutes.

You can help promote your massage business by computer in a number of different ways. By creating your own home page, you'll have a distinctive presence on the Internet where people can look you up when they are browsing through various directories. Home pages can be as simple as a photograph of your business card, or they can be complex multimedia entertainment experiences, depending on your needs and your budget. You can design your own simple home page using popular programs like America Online. Or you can find people in your area who specialize in professional home page creation; ask your local computer store staff or look up computer specialists in the yellow pages.

Another way to get your message out there is to subscribe to a service that lists therapists in different parts of the country with their contact numbers. People interested in massage can browse the list and look you up.

There are literally thousands of sites on the Internet that have something to do with massage. Instead of burdening you with a long list, I'll give you the address of just two sites. From there, you'll be able to point and click your way to many other sites on the Web that have something to do with massage.

❋ http://www.aboutmassage.com

❋ http://www.royaltreatment.com (my Web site)

Check the appendix for more Internet addresses. Happy surfing!

Press Kits

When you have assembled enough material to promote yourself as an "entity," you'll want to put it together into a package that can be easily distributed and easily understood. The package has to look as good as the contents. Find a high-quality laminated folder in a color that matches your business design. Buy labels or print them on your computer to advertise your name on the outside of the folders. If you spend a little money on this outer shell, you'll let those you come in contact with know that what awaits them inside is going to be equally as beautiful.

With your press kit, you can contact local media and tell them what you do. Many smaller publications will be happy to feature a local person who has an interesting business. When the community paper runs an article about you, clip it, make copies, and add it to your press kit. In that way your kit will constantly keep growing. Another way you can use your press kit is to approach community and business clubs and offer to give a free speech at their meetings. After the speech, hand out business cards and brochures.

Your press kit will come in handy whenever you are trying something new with your business. If, for instance, you decided to start teaching massage workshops, the materials in your press kit can be rearranged to create a promotional brochure about you for future workshop attendees.

Promotion with Heart

If all of this talk about the *outside* of things has made you start to feel that we're abandoning the *inside*, please stop for a moment and take stock of what really matters to you. If you're like me, you feel as though you are on a mission of sorts and you'd like to make as many people as possible wake up to their bodies, receive massage, and know that there is a deeper level of relaxation and health that they could be experiencing. How are you going to reach these people? There is only one way: You have to show them who you are. You have to create an image and let them know that you are available and that they can come to you.

You can achieve this level of communication through the creation of an image, *your* image, and it can serve you as you go forth and serve others. When you become a massage therapist, whatever you do to make yourself more successful benefits others as a matter of course. Get successful, do a good

HOW TO BE A SUCCESSFUL THERAPIST

Whatever choice you make regarding your work situation, and even if you haven't been able to decide yet, *you will benefit by making as many concrete goals as possible.* The following seven rules will help you get to where you want to be as a therapist faster and with fewer side trips. These basic concepts were inspired by the work of Napoleon Hill in his classic motivational text *Think and Grow Rich,* which, by the way, is highly recommended reading for all therapists.

1. Decide exactly how much you want monetarily from your massage income—for the first year, then five years, and into the future. Even if you don't really know the amount at this time, pick a specific, reasonable number. Write this number down someplace where you can look at it every day but where no one else will see it.

2. Look at this number each day when you wake up and each day before you go to sleep. Concentrate on the amount. Feel what it would be like to be a therapist making that much money.

3. Decide where you want to work as a therapist, and then proactively approach the people there with the power to give you that job. Don't wait for the right opening to come up in the papers. Businesses are always looking for the right people who will increase their profits and reputation. If you present yourself as that person, in a persistent and yet respectful manner, chances are you'll eventually get in.

4. Whatever position you find yourself in now as a therapist, even if you're making much less than your ultimate goal (**especially** if you're making less than your goal), *be grateful* for the work you are getting as a therapist, no matter how scant or poorly paid the jobs may be. Strive to be the best therapist during each and every massage you give.

5. While you are on the road to accomplishing your goals and meeting your financial and professional dreams as a therapist, you will encounter obstacles. That is a definite, not a maybe. As each of these circumstances arise, instead of complaining about them or retreating into your shell, go forth *immediately* and *ask* for what you really want. And when you are turned down, *ask* again. Keep on asking and never stop until the answer is **Yes.**

6. Do at least a few hours of volunteer massage work per month. This will not only help other people; it will also send your subconscious mind the message that you have plenty to give—and more where that came from! Act the part of the successful humanitarian and you will eventually be it.

7. When you begin to achieve success as a therapist, help others to do the same by inspiring them to look into massage as a career, too.

job, become well known and well paid, and you will then be able to touch others with the message of healing and wholeness that you believe in.

One of the greatest things about massage therapy is that it offers those who follow it as a career a way to re-create themselves, and that re-creation is *always* in a more positive light than was available before. That is the reward for helping others. While you are in the act of this re-creation, my advice to you is to **have fun!!** It's exciting and challenging to forge a new image for yourself. If you approach your new career in a lighthearted, upbeat way, people will respond to your enthusiasm; you'll get lots of clients; and everyone will profit by your success.

ADVERTISING OPTIONS

A few basic guidelines apply to advertising your services as a massage therapist. If you follow them, you won't have to spend much money at the beginning of your career. If your practice begins to flourish, you can then think about investing more in other options.

In general, taking out expensive magazine and newspaper ads will not be cost-effective in the long run. There are therapists who have proven to be exceptions to this rule, of course. Unfortunately, in some areas, many calls that come in from advertisements end up being for sexually oriented massage; and sometimes people find ads too impersonal as a criterion to buy something so personal as massage services. The exception to this is the massage-business owner. Strategically placed ads promoting your day spa or massage clinic or referral out-call service can bring in good clients.

By far the best advertisement is word of mouth. If you can find ways to get your clients to tell their friends about you, you will be well on your way to building a solid clientele. One way to begin this process is to make 100 special business cards with your name and logo on them, plus these extra words: FIRST MASSAGE HALF PRICE WITH THIS CARD. Give a few to your current clients and ask them to give them to anybody they run into who is interested in getting a massage. If people are amenable and your client gives you their numbers, it's OK for you to call them and inquire about their interest in massage. Make sure to follow through if they express interest.

Instead of posting your card or brochure on a bulletin board at the local market with 100 other cards, try approaching nearby business owners on a one-to-one basis and ask if they would mind prominently displaying your material. Before even asking, offer to give each owner a free massage. Then if they like it (which they surely will), they will feel that it was their decision to place your information in their establishments. In this way, you will be the only one who is promoted in those businesses and you will have excellent allies to help drum up new business.

MARKETING

As you hone your new therapist self-image and seek to expand your client base, low- or no-cost "guerilla marketing" is one of the best tools you can use. It is often a better option than paying for advertising. *Marketing,* in this definition, is everything you do (besides pay for advertising) to get people through your door, whether they are repeat customers or new ones. The following are some ideas you may use to get the word out about yourself and your massage offerings.

You Are a Writer!

That is correct. You are a writer. All of us are, but we limit ourselves by thinking that only "other people" write. You have all the talent necessary to pen a simple article for the local section of your community paper that is always looking for new material about new businesses. You can also write press releases that can go out to media outlets. This is not difficult. You can also put together a small booklet and "publish" it yourself at Kinko's, thus instantly becoming an expert about, for example, stress reduction, how to relax at home with partner massage, what to look for in a therapist, and so on.

Give Away Free Services

It is tactically wise to give free treatments away to people who can help you promote your practice. These include travel agents, hair dressers, waitresses, media personalities, journalists, car mechanics, shop owners, and other similarly well-placed people. Give them a full taste of what it is you do and let them do the rest. Also, you can choose a particular local charity to associate yourself with and create a special event, with all proceeds going to benefit the organization.

PROFILE: Lynda Solien-Wolfe
LMT, NCBTMB

Lynda Solien-Wolfe is a massage therapist who has taken the concept of marketing to a whole new level. While always staying within the boundaries of the industry that she loves, she has expanded her horizons and now helps promote not only herself and her own practice but also other individuals and companies in the massage, spa, and health care markets. She sees herself as a resource for everybody involved, bringing together many participants for the mutual benefit of all.

Her business development company, Solwolfe Resource Group, has been in operation since 1994, helping untold numbers of therapists expand into greater realms of success. I can personally vouch for her effectiveness because Lynda has touched my life and brought me increased wealth and happiness.

Happiness? Yes. When Lynda brings people together, she *really* brings them together, and the result is usually a fun event of some kind that leads to major bonding among the participants. For instance, she invited me once to take a four-day cruise in the Bahamas aboard the Dolphin Star, the research vessel for the Upledger Institute. We 12 participants swam with the dolphins, practiced Ocean Therapy (a kind of Watsu in the waves on the sandy, palm-fringed Bahamian beaches), ate conch together, shared our stories, and then

went back to our various homes to write about the experience for massage publications. So, you see? It benefited the Upledger Institute by spreading the word across the land about its new boat, and at the same time it afforded an opportunity for us to form long-lasting friendships. Those of us lucky enough to be on that trip refer to ourselves now as the "POD," as in dolphin pod, and we've been able to help each other further our careers, as well as have a great time whenever we meet at conventions and industry events. Lynda also connected me with a company that now promotes my workshops nationwide and paid me to help develop their training program.

For Lynda, massage is all about relationships and strategic alliances. First, she sees a need, then she puts people together who can help each other fulfill it. And while her main focus in the past few years has been to promote companies like Biofreeze, Golden Ratio Woodworks, and Scrip Massage & Spa Supply, the way she got started in this industry was as an individual therapist struggling to get her name out there—just like the rest of us. So, her first love has always been helping therapists help themselves, and it was with this passion in mind that she created one of the most exciting educational events ever offered for therapists to promote and market

(continues)

Lynda Solien-Wolfe (continued)

themselves. The event was offered at the largest massage convention in the United States, the Florida State Massage Therapy Association annual convention. Over 200 people packed a standing-room-only hall in Orlando for her Successful Start program, which brought together nine leaders in the profession who freely shared their insights and advice on topics such as leadership, compliance, setting up an office, ethical retailing, insurance billing, public relations, and more. Lynda got the idea for the program while presenting at the Florida Chiropractic Association convention and experiencing their Right Start program. She wrote the massage component for that program to highlight the benefits of massage therapy for chiropractors, and she thought it would be a good idea for therapists to start thinking in terms of a "successful start" also. Thus, her program, "Tips to Kick Start a Successful Massage Practice," was born. I asked Lynda if she would share her own personal top 10 tips for marketing yourself as a beginning therapist; and, blessing me with one of her distinctive laughs, she readily agreed.

Lynda's Top 10 Marketing Tips for Beginning Therapists

1. First, make sure you have the passion and the drive to really be a part of the industry. Build up that fire in the belly and focus it on the goals you want to achieve.

2. Next: network, network, network. Networking is one of the most important tools for LMTs to promote their business. It's important to master the art of bringing people together, because if you're helping others, you're going to be helping your own business, too. Be a part of your community. Go to chamber events and city events and local get-togethers. Get yourself known.

3. Use the power of your touch. Get out there and volunteer your skills. "I got started volunteering at the March of Dimes," says Lynda. "I'd massage anybody and everybody at any one of their events anywhere. You've got to be willing to go the extra mile."

4. Never stop learning. It's very important to be the best massage therapist you can be and always be sharpening your skills. Plan on continually racking up CEUs (continuing education units) as you go through your career.

5. The number one item therapists must have is business cards. "I've known many massage therapists who have built their practice on word of mouth, networking, and business cards," says Lynda. "Of course, it always helps if you give a great massage, too."

(continues)

Lynda Solien-Wolfe (continued)

6. Take advantage of co-op advertising and marketing opportunities with other small businesses.

7. The newest marketing is Web-based marketing, using e-mail lists, your own Web sites and others' Web sites. Do not neglect this important area.

8. Reach out to other professionals in your community. Form bonds with doctors, physical therapists, dentists, and others. Work together to raise the level of awareness for all professionals. "I made up press kits for chiropractors and doctors in my area," says Lynda. "I still bring each of them a press kit during massage therapy awareness week every year. I even wrote the Florida Massage Therapy Awareness Proclamation and had the governor of Florida declare it!

9. Do research and know what's going on in your industry, making sure you're offering up-to-date information and treatments to your clients.

10. Become the expert. "I was the in-house massage expert at my local Barnes & Noble early in my career, fresh out of school," says Lynda. "I would write articles on massage for their newsletter, and then it expanded to other publications, growing from there. I also did talks on massage therapy and chair massage at the store every month. It really helped me get known."

You can contact Lynda at the Solwolfe Resource Group, (321) 459-0133 or SOLWOLFE@aol.com.

Co-Op Yourself

Take advantage of the power of like-minded businesses in your community to work together toward mutual success. You can cross-promote with health food stores, health food restaurants, fitness studios, counselors, nutritionists, beauty salons, and similar establishments. Have your collateral available at their places of businesses, and you can display their information for your clients. You may even take out an ad together in a local magazine, splitting the otherwise prohibitive cost. This is one of the few instances in which it would be appropriate for a new small massage business to advertise.

Open House

When you open your doors or when you add new services to your practice, use the opportunity to throw a party and invite the local media. Give away free treatments and small retail items.

Discount Card

Offer clients a special card good for 10 percent off of your services for a specific period of time. This will drive business to you during what may otherwise be a lull. You can specify "blackout dates" such as weekends or peak hours. Alternatively, you can offer a card that is marked each time a service is bought and after 10 the next one is free.

Seasonal Promotions

Always keep current with the calendar, offering weekly or monthly specials, discounts, and themes to go with holidays such as Mother's Day, Valentine's Day, and so on.

Off-Menu Service Items

A great way to have a trial period on new services prior to putting them on your menu is to offer them as a special. For example, give a free mini face massage with herbs and lotions or a salt scrub with every full-body massage. You can create new services as an offering, especially for established clientele who may not have tried anything new in a while.

Educational Events

Use your space as a teaching venue. If you have the room, invite experts, authors, and teachers to give classes on topics you are enthused about. This will drive in new potential customers while offering a valuable service.

Massage Dollars

Massage dollars are a kind of mini gift certificate that can be given or sold in any amount. Gift certificates in general are very important and account for a good percentage of some massage practitioner's sales, especially around the holidays. Be aware of laws concerning gift certificates in your area.

Keep in Touch

Keep yourself in clients' minds by sending out periodic messages for anniversaries and birthdays. Thank-you cards after a referral are a nice touch, too. You can also send out a quarterly or semi-annual newsletter to keep clients up-to-date with your practice; include coupons and special offers. See the sidebar, "Preprinted Newsletters," earlier in this chapter.

Join a Group

Men's groups and women's groups are very popular, and they're excellent places to network with people about your business. You can also start your own support group or "healing circle," offering your home as a meeting place for people who wish to discuss such issues as emotional growth, overcoming trauma, stress relief, and interpersonal relationships. Many of the people who come for discussion will end up as massage customers, as well.

Discount for Series Massages

For already existing clients, offer a discount for massages bought in a series. For example, if you charge $50 for a normal massage, offer to sell 10 massages for $400 *if the client pays up-front.* Don't make the mistake of agreeing to take $40 per massage and ending up with a client who gets a 20 percent discount for nothing. It benefits you to receive the money up-front to cover expenses, and it benefits the client to pay less. Tell clients you will give refunds in case of emergency or if they have to move out of town. Otherwise, you keep the payment. When people have paid up-front, they tend to come more frequently. This is a good way to keep your practice busy and give you the feeling of success, especially if you're at the beginning of your career and still actively seeking clients.

BUSINESS PLANS

If you're serious about branching out from private practice, hiring other people, and putting your own massage business on the road to big-time success, you're going to need a plan. This is especially true if you're going to need financing from a bank or venture capitalist to start you in your business. A business plan should be a document filled with facts and figures, but it should also contain the personalities and the "fire" that you feel is going to turn your business into a winner. Be sure to describe everything about your business team, along with realistic estimates of earnings and expenses. Many business plan templates can be found on the Internet, some of them at no charge. Try looking at http://www.planware.org, or searching under "business plans" on the Web.

10 | The Path Ahead: How to Advance Your Career in Massage

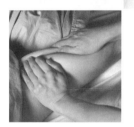

As time goes by and you spend months and years working hard to mold a new career for yourself in the massage business, you'll notice something peculiar happening. The further you advance in your skills, learning, and experience, the more you realize that you're just beginning. The human body has a way of humbling us with its majesty, like a great cathedral; it has a way of frustrating us with its capricious forces, like a massive hurricane; and it has a way of silencing us, like a single perfect rose or a child's wide-eyed innocence. We will never know an end to our study of and fascination with the body and the mind, and you'll eventually understand that this big step, this fundamental change you made by choosing to become a therapist in the first place, can be looked on as merely the first step in a long journey that lasts throughout your life.

Yet, at the same time, it all goes by very quickly. Each person is available to be touched only briefly. We are born, flourish, then fade, even while the impressions of our hands and fingers linger in each others' memories. Every day, countless people slip out of the embrace of the body, and we can no longer do what matters most: touch them. And every day countless others appear for the first

267

time on this planet, each one of them craving touch as if it were oxygen, sunlight, or love itself. Use your time wisely. Profit by the opportunity you've created for yourself to be with others in this profound manner, to interact with them in ways that count, to touch not only their tissues but the ephemeral living heart within them—and perhaps their very soul.

As you grow in your own unique way, you may add your own legacy to the long list of therapists who have shared their insights, creativity, knowledge, and caring in this profession. In this chapter, I'd like to introduce you to some of the ways that people have moved forward along the path of massage, propelled by their own quest to do more, help more, and express more fully their growing need and capacity to successfully, effectively reach others. As you'll see, this quest has inspired therapists to form professional associations, to create new methods of therapy, to offer therapy in innovative ways, to write about it, teach it, and even share it with their families. In the end, massage becomes much more than a business. It will be your life's adventure.

RESOURCES

Professional Associations

One of the unique aspects of the massage business is that you will be spending 90 percent of your professional life in a room with just one other person at a time. This can be a great boon for meaningful exchanges with people, and it is an ideal environment to nurture the growth of inner tranquillity and peace; but, after a while, it can leave you craving more interactions. Just like everyone else, massage therapists are social creatures and we need to relate to our peers in meaningful, exciting ways. It's helpful to form relationships with other therapists in your area, building a support group and network of friends. When you're ready to reach out and join a nationwide network of therapists, you'll have several options to choose from. Big families of therapists are out there, ready to welcome you in and help you on your way. Massage associations are booming and bursting at the seams with new members, new services, and exciting new opportunities for you to make connections and contributions to your newfound profession.

For those of you who already appreciate the benefits of professional associations, I don't have to convince you of their worth; but you may not think of yourself as the joining type. Perhaps you've never joined a professional association before and the idea is intimidating. Or, maybe the reason you entered the massage profession was to maintain total independence. That's fine, and nobody is going to come knocking on your door with a summons to sign up. You can stand to the side of the association scene throughout your entire career. However, if fear or aversion or a habitual loner tendency is keeping you from making the first move, let me offer a few words of encouragement.

First and foremost among the reasons to join, in my opinion, is the fact that a large number of very cool people are already members and, by joining, you'll get to meet them, hang out with them, and become friends with them. When massage people get together outside of their work environments, they can sometimes turn into party animals and be a really fun bunch to be around. At an association convention, for example, it's almost as if someone has opened all the closed doors to all those separate therapy rooms at once and the therapists come swarming down to the meeting place, eager to be with each other after hours and days and months of focused work in their separate cocoons.

You'll enjoy a certain amount of protection as a member of these massage families as well, just like you do as a member of your biological family. They'll take care of you, offer you insurance in case you are sick or disabled or sued, keep you informed about issues that affect your career, help promote massage to the public, uphold educational and ethical standards in the profession, and give you the opportunity to help in return.

One of the biggest benefits of membership in all of the associations is the **liability insurance** coverage you'll automatically receive. Knowing that you have millions of dollars worth of protection behind you can help put your mind at ease when you contemplate the litigious atmosphere of today's marketplace. (This point was covered in some detail in chapter 6.) Associations also offer group rates on disability, business, health, and dental insurance, which comes in extremely handy—especially if you're self-employed.

Some therapists think that they'll wait until they become more established and then join one of the organizations, not realizing that joining is precisely the step that would help them become more established in the first place. The cost may seem prohibitive when you are first starting out; but when you break it down, you'll realize that the cost of membership for an entire year is the equivalent of just two to five massages. Instead of waiting to be convinced of the benefits before joining, why not join while still a student and get the student-level discount or give yourself a membership as a massage-school graduation present? Then decide whether or not the expenditure is worth the benefit. Memberships only last a year, and you can change organizations or drop out completely whenever you like.

The main national professional organizations for massage therapists are the American Massage Therapy Association®, Associated Bodywork & Massage Professionals, and the International Massage Association. Each organization has its own proponents and detractors, but they are all focused on the same fundamental goals: the growth of the profession and the success of its practitioners.

When you join one of the associations, you'll receive more than you expected in terms of networking, education, insurance, information, and many other factors vital to your success. At the same time, however, nobody will force you to play an active role and you may feel slightly on the fringe of the group at first. Over time, though, you will forge alliances and friendships that will eventually lead you to become more involved. If you stay with massage therapy for several years, you'll probably be able to look around one day and realize that most of your closest friends are members of the same organization. You share the same commitments, fulfillments, frustrations, and vision; and membership in your group of peers means more to you than you would have ever imagined when you first joined.

Here, then, is some preliminary information about the largest groups of massage therapists in the country. Call or write them for information yourself. Talk to them about the benefits of membership. Ask other therapists about their experiences with different organizations. You'll soon find a fit that's right for you.

American Massage Therapy Association

The oldest (and only not-for-profit, membership driven) nationwide association is the American Massage Therapy Association (AMTA). Founded in Chicago in 1943 with just 29 members, by 1980 it had a membership of 1,400, and in 2005 that number was over 46,000 with members in 27 countries (see Figure 10-1). This meteoric rise in recent years is a reflection of the phenomenal growth in popularity of the profession and its growing acceptance by the general public. Also, the thousands of new therapists who graduate from massage school each year are more aware than ever of the benefits they'll receive by joining an association.

Figure 10-1 | American Massage Therapy Association (AMTA) membership, 1943–2005.

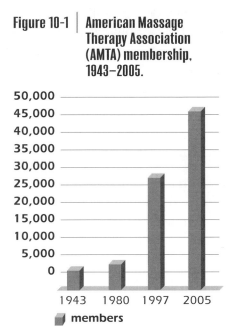

The AMTA is the group that the other associations compare themselves to and compete against. In general, the AMTA can be categorized as somewhat conservative. This doesn't mean that it isn't filled with innovative people, many of whom would be considered quite liberal by most standards. The AMTA takes on its collective shoulders the task of upholding the industry's respectability. For example, its members once confronted the publishers of *Playboy* magazine, who were planning on a pictorial of female massage therapists. The AMTA incited the profession as a whole to take action and petition the magazine's publishers to think again about their idea. The ensuing flood of calls and letters from therapists all over the country did the trick—*Playboy* sent a letter to the AMTA saying that it would not pursue the idea any further.

Two levels of membership are available in the AMTA: associate and professional. Professional membership is extended to those practitioners who have met at least one of the following criteria:

1. Graduation from a COMTA (Commission on Massage Therapy Accreditation) accredited training program

2. Licensure from a current AMTA accepted city, state, or province; accepted licenses include those from Alabama, Arkansas, Connecticut, Delaware, District of Columbia, Florida, Hawaii, Iowa, Louisiana, Maine,

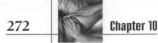

Maryland, Missouri, Nebraska, New Hampshire, New Mexico, New York, North Carolina, North Dakota, Ohio, Oregon, Rhode Island, South Carolina, Tennessee, Utah, Virginia, West Virginia, Washington, Wisconsin, Tucson, Arizona, and Ontario, Canada (local laws and ordinances may also apply, even in states with statewide licensure)

3. National Certification in Therapeutic Massage and Bodywork

4. Previous active AMTA membership status

Those not meeting these standards, such as graduates of nonapproved nor accredited COMTA schools and graduates of schools in foreign countries, could apply for associate membership. Associate annual dues are $169, including liability insurance, or $99 per year without insurance (in this case, members must prove they have liability coverage elsewhere). A maximum of three years of associate membership status is allowed before mandatory upgrading to professional status.

People still attending massage school can join as *associates* for $79 for three years. They can then upgrade to *professional membership* at anytime. Therapists who meet the standards can apply for professional membership. Dues in this case are $235 per year, plus any applicable chapter fees from the appropriate state chapter, which range from free to $30. In all, there are 50 state chapters plus Washington, D.C., and the Virgin Islands.

The association sponsors a yearly national convention with dozens of educational workshops. This convention is an excellent opportunity for networking and growth in your career, and you should certainly try to attend at least once. The cost may seem prohibitive at first ($300 for registration alone; travel, food, lodging, and entertainment can easily push the bill over $1,000), but remember your tax deductions (chapter 6) and consider the entire experience as an investment in your future. If you can't make it to one of the large national events, try making it to a regional one such as the AMTA New England Conference, where you'll still find plenty of value.

The AMTA has formed a Foundation that is dedicated to supporting the profession by promoting the development of scientific advances and community services. The Massage Therapy Foundation is separate from the AMTA itself, although they are closely linked. Funded by the AMTA plus individual and corporate donations, the foundation offers yearly grants given in three categories: research, community outreach, and scholarship. While

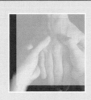

YOUR FIRST CONFERENCE

Heading out for your first convention or conference, especially if it's in another state or someplace you've never been before, can be a nerve-racking experience. You're likely to feel fine about going until just a day or two beforehand when you begin to think of all the strangers you're going to meet and the new experiences you're going to have. Then it's easy to get a case of the jitters.

When you first arrive at one of the megaevents sponsored by the AMTA and you look around at the hundreds of people all talking and laughing together, you may get the feeling that they all know each other already and you're somewhat of an outsider—and for the most part you'd be right. Many of the same people go to the shows year after year, and they've built up relationships and insider groups that may seem impenetrable at first glance.

You've got to remember, though, when you're standing frozen with shyness in the lobby of some strange hotel, that *they* need *you,* the new blood, to continue the growth of their business. Their livelihood depends on you, and they want to get to know you as much as you want to get to know them. Remember, too, that it's more comfortable for them to talk among the people they already know, just like it's more comfortable for you. The only difference is, all the people you know are back home!

Here are a few tips to help you feel more at home when you attend your first conference:

1. Go with a friend. Even if you don't know anyone who's going, call your local chapter and see if somebody else from your area will be attending.

2. If you want to save money on your trip, suggest sharing a hotel room with another attendee.

3. Call the AMTA office and ask for a list of other people attending alone who are looking for rides or roommates.

4. Mingle at luncheons, dinner banquets, and parties, introducing yourself to as many people as you can. People expect to be approached at conferences. There is no need to be shy.

5. Sign up for workshops that are hands-on so that you'll be paired up with a partner and have a chance to get to know someone in one of the ways you like best—through touch.

6. Spend a lot of time talking to vendors at the booths in the exhibit hall. They all want to meet you because you may be a potential customer or business partner. Stroll slowly through the aisles, spending time getting

(continues)

> to know each person and his or her products. Later, when you see them in the hallways or at functions, you'll have a basis for conversation.
>
> **7.** Have fun. Definitely partake of the social agenda created for each of these events. If people have seen you doing the limbo the night before, they'll be more likely to strike up a conversation the next day.
>
> **8.** If you notice any other people there alone, see if you can offer them a little company.

scholarship and research in massage have obvious benefits for the advancement of the profession, the more philanthropic efforts of the outreach program also help all massage practitioners by sharing the positive effects of massage with a wide range of individuals. For example, when a program funded by the Massage Therapy Foundation sends therapists into a hospital to massage elderly patients, nurses and doctors encounter massage as an adjunct to their care, perhaps for the first time. This awareness can help create employment openings for therapists in the hospital setting.

The AMTA has a detailed code of ethics that each member agrees to follow. To give you an idea of what will be expected of you as a massage professional, whether or not you join the AMTA, I'm reprinting that code here (see the sidebar, "The AMTA Code of Ethics").

The AMTA actively tries to raise public perception of massage therapy through proper use of the media and political channels. The group lobbies lawmakers and opinion molders on the profession's behalf. The AMTA has enough clout so that people in Washington listen, and even the people at *Playboy* have gotten the message.

National Massage Therapy Awareness Week, sponsored annually by the AMTA during the last full week of October, is designed to increase public awareness of the benefits of therapeutic massage and its value in health care and wellness. AMTA chapters and members hold public events to familiarize various segments of the population with massage therapy and its benefits—such as for relief of pain and stress and in recovery from injury and certain illnesses.

As a member of the group, your name will be placed in a directory. People who call the AMTA curious about massage are directed to therapists in their area, and you may receive more business this way. Chapters of the AMTA exist in all 50 states; the U.S. Virgin Islands; and Washington, D.C. You will receive a copy of this directory, which is an excellent tool for networking. Of course, you'll be

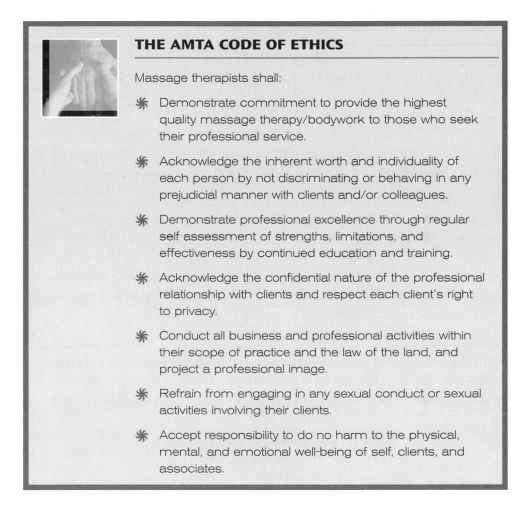

THE AMTA CODE OF ETHICS

Massage therapists shall:

✺ Demonstrate commitment to provide the highest quality massage therapy/bodywork to those who seek their professional service.

✺ Acknowledge the inherent worth and individuality of each person by not discriminating or behaving in any prejudicial manner with clients and/or colleagues.

✺ Demonstrate professional excellence through regular self-assessment of strengths, limitations, and effectiveness by continued education and training.

✺ Acknowledge the confidential nature of the professional relationship with clients and respect each client's right to privacy.

✺ Conduct all business and professional activities within their scope of practice and the law of the land, and project a professional image.

✺ Refrain from engaging in any sexual conduct or sexual activities involving their clients.

✺ Accept responsibility to do no harm to the physical, mental, and emotional well-being of self, clients, and associates.

eligible to purchase group health, disability, and life insurance. AMTA members also receive the quarterly magazine *Massage Therapy Journal* and a newsletter, *Hands On.* If you are interested in becoming a member or attending one of the conventions, contact:

> American Massage Therapy Association
> 500 Davis Street, Suite 900
> Evanston, IL 60201-4695
> Phone (877) 905-2700
> Fax (847) 864-1178
> http://www.amtamassage.org

(Note: The web address is *not* amta.com, which is for AMerican Travel Abroad.)

Associated Bodywork & Massage Professionals

Headquartered in Colorado, the Associated Bodywork & Massage Professionals (ABMP) group was founded in 1987; and, as of October 1997, it had quickly grown to over 20,000 members in the United States, plus a limited number of foreign countries. Membership in 2005 is over 50,000 (see Figure 10-2). The ABMP is dedicated to the support of practitioners in many types of touch therapies, some of which may not receive as much recognition in other organizations.

The ABMP's motto is "Expect More," which could be in reference to the AMTA. Members want therapists to feel more like a dynamic part of the association rather than a witness to its operations, and to that end they attract therapists to join by using such catchphrases as: Why settle for an association that stands behind you when you can have a partner who stands beside you? They are creating the image of a hip, responsive association that is not slowed down by politics or tradition.

In keeping with this all-embracing attitude, the ABMP is affiliated with over 25 specialty and local allied associations, which provides members with many networking opportunities. It offers five different levels of membership, including student; practitioner; professional; aesthetician; and the highest

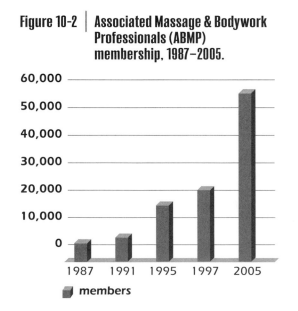

Figure 10-2 | Associated Massage & Bodywork Professionals (ABMP) membership, 1987–2005.

level, certified, ranging in price from $49 for students to $199 for practitioners to $229 for aestheticians and certified members. Supporting memberships are also available for allied professionals for $60 per year. Discounts are available for multiyear memberships.

The aesthetician membership category was the most recent, added in 1996 in response to the phenomenal growth of the spa industry and the growing number of therapists working in the spa setting. With over 12,000 spas and each one employing several massage and body treatment practitioners, a great number of qualified practitioners are needed in this area; many of them are receiving dual training as both massage therapists and aestheticians.

Just as with the AMTA, members receive liability insurance, plus the option to buy group health, life, and disability insurance. The quarterly magazine *Massage & Bodywork* and a newsletter, *Different Strokes,* are also included. Unlike the AMTA, there are no local chapters and no national meetings.

The ABMP has an extensive code of ethics, just like the AMTA does. In addition, it offers several extra benefits for members, including referral services for both job seekers and massage seekers; a practice management guide called *The Successful Business Handbook;* the *Massage & Bodywork Yellow Pages,* featuring many products and services, some at a discount; and *Thinking About Career Options,* a booklet that answers many questions for those considering massage as a career. The *Touch Training Directory,* found on http://www.massagetherapy.com, an associated Web site, offers one of the most complete listings of massage schools available.

The ABMP has a school accreditation program through its International Massage & Somatic Therapies Accreditation Council (IMSTAC). However, they also recognize the accreditation offered by other entities, including the COMTA.

Contact information for the ABMP follows:

> Associated Bodywork & Massage Professionals
> 1271 Sugarbush Drive
> Evergreen, CO 80439
> Phone (800) 458-2267
> E-mail: expectmore@abmp.com
> http://www.abmp.com

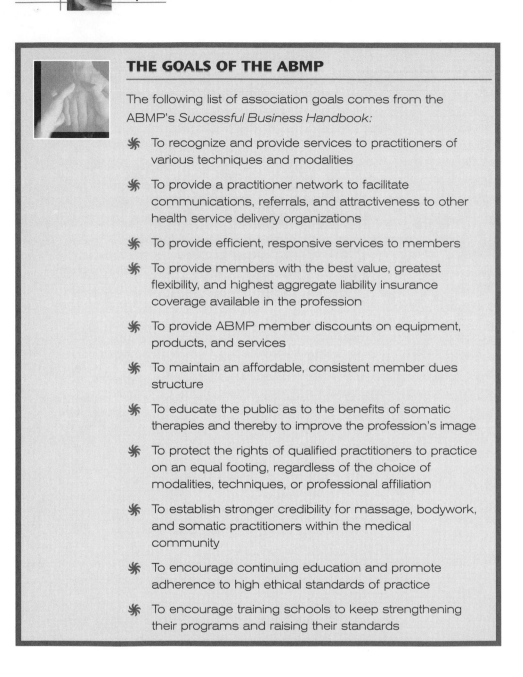

THE GOALS OF THE ABMP

The following list of association goals comes from the ABMP's *Successful Business Handbook:*

- To recognize and provide services to practitioners of various techniques and modalities

- To provide a practitioner network to facilitate communications, referrals, and attractiveness to other health service delivery organizations

- To provide efficient, responsive services to members

- To provide members with the best value, greatest flexibility, and highest aggregate liability insurance coverage available in the profession

- To provide ABMP member discounts on equipment, products, and services

- To maintain an affordable, consistent member dues structure

- To educate the public as to the benefits of somatic therapies and thereby to improve the profession's image

- To protect the rights of qualified practitioners to practice on an equal footing, regardless of the choice of modalities, techniques, or professional affiliation

- To establish stronger credibility for massage, bodywork, and somatic practitioners within the medical community

- To encourage continuing education and promote adherence to high ethical standards of practice

- To encourage training schools to keep strengthening their programs and raising their standards

International Massage Association

Will Green, head of the International Massage Association (IMA), feels that neither of the other associations offers exactly what most therapists are looking for today, which, among other things, is the lowest price on insurance.

He started the association in April 1994, requiring only 100 hours in school or work as an apprentice as qualification for membership. Within three and a half years, the IMA had 17,000 members (see Figure 10-3).

Will Green sees the IMA as the meeting point for a large collective of business-oriented therapists who want straightforward value for their dollar. IMA dues are $149, including liability insurance coverage, which is provided by an A++ carrier. Will aims to attract the entrepreneurial spirit of practitioners by offering them practice-building tools such as a three-part video series, produced in the IMA's own video production studio. Existing members can earn one of those videos for free by recruiting two new members, and many people have earned all three videos. State chapters have started in Texas, Indiana, California, Georgia, Florida, Delaware, New Jersey, New York, Alabama, Alaska, Illinois, Colorado, and Connecticut.

The IMA was the first massage association to set up its own internet server, and it now has several Web sites. The main one, http://www.imagroup.com, has an electronic referral service of therapists by area code. Learnmassage.com is for the general public who want some basic education in order to massage family and friends. A series of videos is available for this program as well.

A division of the IMA, the International Massage & Movement Schools Association, accredits massage schools and offers insurance for schools, as well.

Figure 10-3 | **International Massage Association (IMA) membership, 1994–2005.**

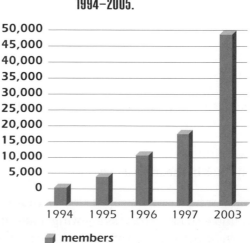

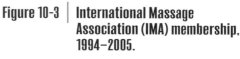
members

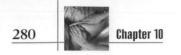

Contact information follows:

> International Massage Association, Inc.
> 25 South Fourth Street
> PO Box 421
> Warrenton, VA 20188
> (540) 351-0800
> http://www.imagroup.com

Smaller Associations

There are several smaller organizations dedicated to therapists who practice particular types of bodywork. Also, several states have their own associations. In fact, the oldest massage association in the country is the New York State Society of Medical Massage Therapists, which was founded in 1927. Refer to the appendix for a listing of several state and specialty associations.

Books

Another key way to stay connected to others in your profession is through books. Books are entry keys to a whole new understanding about massage, which has inspired a wealth of literature ranging from million-copy best sellers marketed to the general public like *The Book of Massage* to highly focused texts meant only for advanced practitioners of certain specialties. Because there are so many good texts available in the field, you may wonder which ones are right for you. Try these three quick tips when looking for your next massage read:

1. Check the book review columns in massage magazines.

2. Ask for recommendations from the clerks at massage book shops; they see what sells and what doesn't.

3. Call mail-order sources and ask for their top sellers in the category you're researching.

4. Visit the New Age and health sections of larger bookstores. They usually have a few good titles in the massage genre.

Many of the most popular books by therapists for therapists are listed in the appendix, and you'll find a section there suggesting a handful of books that are highly recommended for beginning therapists, as well as catalog resources where you can browse through hundreds of relevant titles.

Magazines

Three main magazines are published for people in the massage business. *Massage* magazine is an independent publication. *Massage Therapy Journal* is published by the AMTA, and *Massage & Bodywork Quarterly* is published by the ABMP. A subscription to just one of these will provide plenty of news and networking for the average therapist. If you read two or all three, you will be exposed on a continual basis to an avalanche of information that will keep you informed and updated about every aspect of your profession. Each magazine contains profiles of people who make a difference in the field; articles about various therapies and trends; columns about relevant treatment issues; massage-related travel pieces; legal and ethical issues; reviews of massage books, videos, and products; listings of schools; contact information for manufacturers, trainings, seminars, and conferences; plus much more. You should definitely make a promise to yourself to receive at least one of these publications. It will serve as a lifeline to your colleagues across the country and around the world.

Both of the association magazines come as part of membership, and all three can be ordered by regular subscription. See the appendix for details.

Newsletters

As mentioned throughout this book, there are many rich sources of knowledge shared from therapist to therapist through the medium of specialized newsletters. Many of them have highly targeted information for particular niche markets. You'll find a section listing them in the appendix.

BEYOND THE BASICS: ADVANCED TRAININGS

Because your time is limited and there are so many choices, you have to be discriminating when considering which career directions to follow. Which specialties will most help your clients? How will you know which modality is right for you? When is the right time to invest your money in advanced trainings, and when is it better to stick with what you already know?

When it comes time to choose which next step is right for you, you'll be using two distinct and sometimes opposing faculties: logic and intuition. Certain choices will make a lot of sense, and others will just plain *feel* right. Perhaps taking a course in neuromuscular therapy makes sense for advancing your career, but Thai massage tugs at your heart. Or taking three quick weekends of training in reflexology will add an immediate new source of income to your business, but you'd rather spend 10 times the money and time to study Trager, even though it will be more of a challenge to find new clients using that technique. Which way should you go?

Some therapists study extensively before making a choice. They interview graduates of various programs, read texts on the subjects that interest them, and pick a course based on how likely it is to advance their career. Other therapists act on their feeling about which direction to head in without really knowing how it will affect their business in the long run. An article they read may inspire them, or a chance encounter with another therapist may send them in a whole new direction.

In the following sections, we're going to look at some of the available avenues that you may choose to pursue as your career unfolds and you mature. Because the field is truly so diverse, with hundreds of massage, bodywork, and somatic techniques, the descriptions in this chapter are meant simply as an outline. They may give you a feeling for some of the major avenues you wish to travel down as you consider the steps that come next. Some of these directions actually lead out of the massage therapy field altogether; and perhaps you, like many therapists, will decide to continue your study in an allied modality such as acupuncture or nursing.

For simplification, I've categorized various therapeutic approaches under five main headings: "Mind/Body Practices," "Energy Work," "Deep Tissue/ Structural Therapies," "Movement-Oriented Bodywork," and "Techniques from the East." These categories are my invention and do not refer to any conventional classifications within the profession. Refer to the Advanced Trainings Chart in the appendix for information about specific courses and workshops.

Mind/Body Practices

Today, terms like "mind-body medicine" no longer strike fear into the hearts of the medical establishment. Institutions as venerable as Harvard Medical

School sponsor conferences entitled "Spirituality and Healing," and the acceptance of the mind/body/spirit unity is becoming fashionable and acceptable. But where does one go to *experience* that unity?

Many massage and bodywork practitioners focus their work on helping people have a "somatic," or body-based, realization of the mind/body/spirit connection. Their work has developed through generations of therapists, and the experiences their clients have can sometimes be called *spiritual* or *enlightening.* Although almost every form of massage is an aid to mind/body integration, these therapies in particular are extremely focused on that unity. People are often transformed through the experience of receiving this type of work.

If you are someone who likes to delve into the wholeness of other people and help them connect to their deeper resources, you may eventually want to explore some of these paths. The work can be emotionally demanding, somewhat like a minister's or counselor's, but the rewards can be profound.

The following are just a few of the mind/body practices with trainings that you can attend. For contact information and other details, consult the Advanced Training Chart.

✳ Jin Shin Do

✳ The Rosen Method

✳ Rubenfeld Synergy

✳ SHEN Physio-Emotional Release Therapy

✳ Somatosynthesis

✳ Vivation

Energy Work

A funny thing can happen when you spend all day every day working on human bodies through therapeutic massage. The reality of flesh and bones can sometimes fade away, and you begin to notice that everybody has a certain "energy" radiating from, or within, them. This can be felt in the form of heat or pulsations right in your hands, and it is more than the simple humming and flow of the blood. We are electromagnetic beings, and many types of massage have been developed to specifically work with the subtle

AN EXPERIMENT: FEELING THE FORCE

Without any special training or background, you can tune in and feel for yourself the energy emanating from another person. The first requirement for attunement is concentration, plus quietness. Begin your experience by following the instructions for meditation in chapter 7, but this time have a partner to act as your subject.

With your partner lying faceup on your massage table or on the floor, sit comfortably next to her. After several minutes of meditation, when your mind and body are relatively calm and relaxed, slowly raise your hands up, rub them together vigorously for 10 seconds, and then hold them just a few inches apart, palms facing together, feeling the stimulation and heat you've created. Experiment by increasing and decreasing the distance between your palms slowly, staying attuned to the subtle variations in heat.

When you're ready, shift your palms facedown and place them over your partner but not directly on her skin. Start six or eight inches away. Allow your hands to be still for a moment, then begin raising and lowering them slowly, feeling for the same sensations of heat you felt from your own palms. Close your eyes if this helps you concentrate. Try searching for the boundary of your partner's emanations, or "aura," where the sensation of heat stops, and run your palms along this area. You may begin to feel some strong sensations that will guide your hands in one direction or another. Let them move without trying to stop them. Your hands may naturally flow to particularly hot regions that contain some tension or injury in your partner's body. Or you may find your palms circling over certain areas that turn out to be "chakras," or concentrated energy centers.

The important thing during this exercise is to *just feel.* Although it's fine to pass some positive energy along to your partner, don't attempt to do specific healing if you haven't been trained in any particular energy modalities. Simply raise and lower your hands, and move them intuitively along the invisible pathways sensed by your palms. Don't worry if you don't feel anything on your first try. In fact, this kind of energetic awareness may sneak up on you when you are *not* trying, perhaps when you're giving a massage and find yourself extremely focused.

When you withdraw your hands from your partner, an appropriate way to finish is by putting your palms together once again, softly this time, in prayer position over your heart, acknowledging the interchange of positive energy.

currents of this energy in our bodies. Often the practitioner doesn't even need to physically touch the client to bring about the desired effects or exchanges because the energy fields of two people intersect beyond the barrier of the skin.

The following are just a few types of advanced therapy that pay close attention to the subtle energetic processes in the body:

- ❋ Reiki
- ❋ Polarity
- ❋ Craniosacral Therapy
- ❋ Therapeutic Touch
- ❋ Healing Touch

Deep Tissue/Structural Therapies

When most people look at a human body, they see various planes and curves intersecting to form a surface, underneath which lies a mystery. The therapist, on the other hand, sees into the structure. This process of looking beneath the surface can deepen for you if you decide to pursue one of the techniques in deep tissue therapies, which focus on the connective tissues within us. What is usually found through this type of work, of course, will be the same emotions and armoring that are uncovered through other forms of therapy. Sometimes, though, with deep tissue work, the powerful effects on the body's holding patterns can be very dramatic, even for observers.

Some of the more well-known deep tissue therapies include:

- ❋ Aston-Patterning
- ❋ Hellerwork
- ❋ Neuromuscular Therapy
- ❋ Postural Integration
- ❋ Rolfing®
- ❋ Trigger Point Therapy

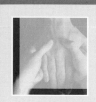

FINGERS THROUGH FLESH
A DEEP TISSUE EXPERIENCE

I once had a vivid experience that brought home the power of deep tissue therapies. At a yoga ashram in Pennsylvania, around 20 of us were gathered in a room to watch a demonstration of some neuromuscular techniques. The therapist was an instructor of the month-long residential bodywork training program we were taking part in. He told us to circle the massage table while he began working on a woman's neck and shoulder muscles. She had been complaining of chronic pain in her upper back for years, and her right shoulder was visibly higher than her left.

At first we were all in a "normal" state of consciousness, calmly watching our teacher perform the moves he had taught us earlier. But then something extraordinary happened. While we watched in fascination, the woman sighed loudly and long as the teacher's fingers seemed to melt a full inch deeper into her upper shoulder. Adjusting the direction of his pressure subtly, he was able to go even deeper a few seconds later, and we all started to breathe in unison with the woman on the table.

After two or three minutes of synchronized breathing and concentration, the woman sighed again, and we could see the tips of his fingers push even deeper, almost disappearing. A couple people in the room became light-headed. It seemed impossible for someone to push so deeply into the musculature. What normally appeared as solid substance was now dissolving right in front of our eyes, as if flesh were made of the softest dough. The woman seemed to be in an altered state, her face suffused with an expression beyond pleasure or pain.

This went on for 20 minutes or more, and when at last the woman sat up again, we were all amazed to see that her right shoulder had dropped completely back into alignment with the left one.

Movement-Oriented Bodywork

Swedish massage contains movement, particularly during joint mobilizations and stretches; and all touch techniques include movement to one degree or another. However, several forms of therapy incorporate movement more dramatically than others. Some of them include exercise routines in which the client moves his or her own body. Others teach movements that are aided by the therapist. The movements can include rocking, lifting, dropping, twisting, and cradling, among others.

What all of the movement-oriented therapies have in common is that they teach us how limiting our normal range of motion actually is. We move within boxes that we unconsciously keep closed. These techniques help open the box. Although everyone can benefit from learning how to move more freely, these techniques are especially recommended for people who use their bodies as an instrument, as in sports and the arts. In fact, a large number of people who become practitioners of these modalities came from exactly those backgrounds. Some of the techniques were invented by performers, such as the Alexander Technique.

Some of the most popular movement-oriented therapies include:

✳ The Alexander Technique

✳ Feldenkrais Method

✳ Pilates

✳ Trager

Techniques from the East

Many therapists feel a calling to study techniques from Asia, particularly Japan, China, and Thailand, and certain massage schools are dedicated exclusively to the teaching of these modalities. Shiatsu, in particular, is so popular that the state of New York requires therapists to study it to be licensed. All of the Eastern techniques are built on a profound knowledge of human anatomy, especially the energetic system, through which flows our life force energy, variously known as *chi, ha, prana,* and many other names.

Massage is taken seriously in the East. In China, for example, massage therapists study for three years and master several healing techniques before they can work in hospitals and clinics. In Thailand, massage is practiced by highly skilled therapists inside the temples, where it is considered a sacred art. Many great teachers have come to the United States from all over Asia to share the wisdom of their traditions. Also, many U.S. therapists take advantage of special massage-study-abroad trips sponsored by several different organizations and individuals. Groups often travel to China and Thailand in particular for this purpose. See "Massage Study Abroad" in the appendix.

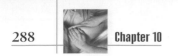

Some of the most popular Eastern techniques that are also taught in the West include:

- ✳ Acupressure/Acupuncture
- ✳ Ayurveda
- ✳ Chi Nei Tsang
- ✳ Hoshino
- ✳ Jin Shin Jyutsu
- ✳ Shiatsu
- ✳ Thai Massage

SPECIALIZED MASSAGE PURSUITS

Following are a few examples of what therapists can do with a little ingenuity and the desire to give. The types of massage mentioned here range from the compassionate touch of humanitarian massage to the nurturing touch of pregnancy massage to reaching out beyond humankind in animal massage to the fun, and yet deeply therapeutic, massage technique done in warm pools known as Watsu®. Also, in the medical field, nurse massage therapists have developed a network of their own, and new massage technology is offering therapists opportunities unheard of just a few years ago.

Humanitarian Massage

The massage profession is filled with people who are, at their very core, great humanitarians. That is the primary reason many people entered the field. In spite of the fact that the massage business will continue to explode in the near future, attracting its share of opportunists, even the most materialistic of therapists must occasionally hear a small voice inside saying "It is better to give than to receive."

Some of the most successful therapists feel obliged to give back in big ways. They finance their own trips to countries where people are struggling with poverty, war, and despair, literally reaching out their hands to do what they can. In many issues of the massage journals, articles have featured therapists on missions to El Salvador, Hungary, Bosnia, and other locations.

Many people have found that they can do something right here at home, as well, and they have founded organizations to bring therapeutic touch to those people who would otherwise not be able to afford it. One such organization is the Touch Foundation, founded by Shane Watson, owner of the Bodywork Emporium massage stores in California. Billed as the "Massage Peace Corps," this group of volunteers has set their sights on helping handicapped, elderly, and destitute people through the power of touch.

To find out more, contact:

> The Touch Foundation
> c/o Terry Solomon, Executive Director
> Phone (714) 754-9530

The American Massage Therapy Association (AMTA) also has a branch dedicated to helping worthy causes through massage. The Massage Therapy Foundation (see the listing in the "Professional Associations" section) gives Outreach Grants to bring massage to those who can't otherwise afford it or have never experienced it. Call (847) 889-5019 for more information.

Associated Bodywork & Massage Professionals (ABMP) have also instituted a charitable community outreach program, known as International Massage Week. For one week each year, usually in July, ABMP members donate their time toward humanitarian causes in a public outreach effort that helps spread the word about the benefits of massage at the same time. Call (800) 458-2267 to find out more.

Pregnancy Massage

I once had the honor of massaging one of my clients during her pregnancy, right up to her due date. In fact, she requested that I accompany her and her family into the hospital birthing suite to offer massage during her labor. I read books on prenatal massage, talked to friends who had gone through the experience, and prepared myself for the occasion. But when the big day finally arrived and I showed up at her bedside, I had barely placed one hand gingerly on her left foot before she yelled out, "Get your hands off me!"

Perhaps I was the wrong sex. Some massage therapists (all of them female) have acted as modern *doulas,* or labor helpers. Throughout history, in many parts of the world, women have been assisted through labor with the supportive presence of another woman, and many modern massage therapists have found that their nurturing skills have prepared them perfectly for that

PROFILE: Andrea Vladimir
from Massage to Acupuncture

Andrea Vladimir knew she wanted to diversify her massage career almost as soon as she became a therapist. Right after graduating from New York City's Swedish Institute, she looked in the *New York Times* want ads and found work in a clinic doing manual lymphatic drainage for lymphedema patients. "It was hard work," she recalls. "I saw seven or eight patients a day, twice a day, for 30-minute sessions. In addition to the massage, I changed their bandages and made sure they were moving enough. . . . These were people who'd received radical surgeries; they had extremely swollen limbs, and after several treatments many of them felt good about being seen in public again for the first time in months. Their swelling went down, and they really did recuperate much faster. So it was very satisfying work in that sense, but I was already in danger of developing repetitive stress syndrome, and I knew I had to take care of myself, as well.

"I was looking around for the right thing, both to increase my effectiveness as a therapist and to keep me interested in my work. Something about Oriental techniques always fascinated me, ever since I took a class with the shiatsu master Ohashi when I was still in high school. From an early age I liked the idea of medicine, but not the idea of painkillers. I liked helping people feel better, and I liked

Japanese tea ceremonies, even as a kid. All of these things led me eventually to the Pacific College of Oriental Medicine to study acupuncture."

Andrea had a feeling that acupuncture was a smart choice, but she didn't realize she'd soon be riding the crest of a large wave fueled by interest from the medical field, the media, and the public in general. When she began her acupuncture classes, there were fewer than a hundred students in the school. Just a few years later, that number was close to 400. Enrolling in one of the growing number of acupuncture schools across the country is considered a smart career move, one that many massage therapists are considering.

"Timing has been critical," says Andrea. "I started at massage school in the late '80s when it was still somewhat of a novelty. Then I enrolled in the acupuncture program at the perfect time, too, just as it was beginning to gain more acceptance. And now that I'm graduating, suddenly insurance companies are extremely interested in what I do. It's a great time to be branching into allied fields.

"The massage schools seem to be recognizing this trend. . . . Now the Swedish Institute, for example, has begun teaching classes in Chinese medicine. Many massage therapists are heading in this direction. Doing acupuncture gives you a broader base

(continues)

Andrea Vladimir (continued)

and adds to your viability as a therapist, especially in medical settings. Ten years ago you couldn't get a doctor to look you in the eye when you suggested working as a massage therapist in his office. Now when you tell them you're a therapist, they say, 'Are you available?'"

When asked what she recommends for other massage therapists who are looking to expand their careers, she has some practical advice. "The more skills you have under your belt, the more valuable you are," she states. "I've pursued training in sports massage as well as lymphatic drainage and acupuncture. Becoming an esthetician would be a smart investment, too. There's a lot of competition out there, and the more you have to offer, the better chances you'll have for success."

Andrea took a little time off when she had her first child, but now she is planning on using her new skills and getting to work in a clinical or spa setting. "The beauty industry is less stressful," she muses, "but I feel myself heading back to the preventive field. There are a couple new possibilities presenting themselves already, one with a plastic surgeon on the Upper East Side who wants to expand his practice into a day spa. The other is an internist who wants to make his practice more holistic. A lot of doctors today know that having a massage therapist on staff lets their patients know they're cared for.

"These two possibilities are just the beginning. Once I get going, there will be no stopping me. The same is true for all massage therapists who continue to follow their dreams, to expand and grow. I consider myself a professional student, and I want to study my whole life long in this field. It's not because I want another degree (although having those extra letters after your name is fun!) but because as you learn, your perception of yourself changes because you know so much more and can help that many more people. That's what really builds a reputation. My mother told me to become very good at just one thing, become the best you could be, and then when you branch out and do other things, you'll have that foundation to build upon. So you don't really leave massage when you study other modalities. You're just expanding upon the same theme, and you can still be the best.

"I used to think that being 'just a massage therapist' wasn't enough. Now I see that it's plenty. It's a career that allows you to help other people while continually improving yourself too. The more highly qualified you become, the better you'll feel, and the better you'll be able to make others feel!"

To reach the Pacific College of Oriental Medicine, call (800) 729-3468 or visit http://www.pacificcollege.edu. Campuses are located in New York, California, and Chicago.

role. Several books have been written on the subject (see the appendix), and weekend workshops are available, as well.

An entire mini-industry has sprung up around pregnancy massage. In addition to workshops, videos, and books, table manufacturers have developed special models for expectant mothers (you guessed it—they come with big holes in the center for the belly). As a natural adjunct to pregnancy massage, there is infant massage, traditionally practiced in countries like India and now quite popular in the United States. Studies from the Touch Research Institute show that touch is the single largest contributing factor to the healthy development of premature infants.

Before you jump in and start massaging your pregnant friends, you should familiarize yourself with the contraindications and with certain points that, when stimulated during pregnancy, are said to help induce labor.

One therapist who offers seminars for expecting mothers is Kate Jordan. She titles her program *Bodywork for the Childbearing Year,* and she focuses 75 percent on the hands-on aspect of the techniques. She has in-depth maneuvers for many different conditions and for different times before, during, and after pregnancy. Her students learn techniques from varying modalities (such as Myofascial Release and the Alexander Technique) adapted to the challenges of this specialty. She also covers postpartum therapy, cesarean recovery, postsurgical scar massage, and the marketing of this type of work. Kate has been on the board of directors of the National Certification Board for Therapeutic Massage and Bodywork, and she brings a high level of professionalism to this work.

To learn more, contact:

> Kate Jordan Seminars
> 8950 Villa La Jolla Drive, #A217
> La Jolla, CA 92037
> Phone (888) 287-6860
> E-mail: pregnancymassage@aol.com

Animal Massage Therapy

One of the most appreciative clients I ever worked on was the rescue dog used to search for buried survivors or bodies in the aftermath of Hurricane Andrew. The dog had thick black fur, and he was wearing a Day-Glo™ orange

PROFILE: Elaine Stillerman, LMT
MotherMassage®

Elaine Stillerman is one of the best-known practitioners of pregnancy massage in the United States. Her book and workshops called MotherMassage® are extremely popular. You may wonder how she raised herself to this exalted level. Like most people in the field, she got her start doing massage on a daily basis, then moved into new realms through a slow organic process, one step naturally leading to the next. Here, in her own words, is how the path unfolded for her.

"In 1980, when I had been out of massage school only two years, a client of mine became pregnant," says Elaine. "It was the first time I had ever worked on a pregnant woman and frankly I wasn't sure what to do. My massage school, like the other dozen or so schools in business at the time, never taught us about prenatal anatomy or massage techniques. So it was up to me to educate myself about what was safe and what wasn't.

"I initially turned to my first bodywork modality—shiatsu—and referred to (translated) Chinese texts that were very direct in their pregnancy, labor, and postpartum protocols. I read many interesting sociological and anthropological books that showed that massage accompanied childbirth throughout nearly the entire tribal world. Finally, I researched medical, nursing, and midwifery texts to learn about the physiological changes of pregnancy, labor, and postpartum. From these various sources, I pieced together the tapestry of what became MotherMassage® based upon anatomy and physiology and various massage techniques.

"My client told other pregnant friends about my massages and suddenly other massage therapists, who were uncomfortable treating their pregnant clients, started sending their expectant clients to this 'rogue massage therapist' who was not afraid of working with an especially deserving population. That's how MotherMassage® started.

"I recorded my findings and eventually turned these notes and massage routines into the book *MotherMassage: A Handbook for Relieving the Discomforts of Pregnancy* (Dell, 1992), written for the expectant couple. Urged to share my technique with other practitioners, I started teaching MotherMassage®: Massage During Pregnancy in 1990. In 2001, this workshop became a professionally certified course offering CEUs to participants. I have taught this class at dozens of prestigious massage schools, spas, and resorts.

"Prenatal massage is enjoying tremendous growth and interest. My classes are filled and the interest keeps

(continues)

intensifying. Pregnant women are aware of the numerous beneficial effects of prenatal massage and are booking appointments throughout their pregnancies and postpartum recovery periods. The medical community, prompted by new and innovative research, much of which originated with the Touch Research Institute out of the University of Miami Medical School, is also cognizant of the relief from common pregnancy-related discomforts that massage offers their patients.

"The popularity of prenatal massage extends from coast to coast and internationally as more massage schools present fundamental classes and/or continuing education programs. MotherMassage® is offered to massage professionals, advanced massage students, childbirth educators, nurse midwives, doulas, and other perinatal health professionals.

"The women who enjoy MotherMassage® during their childbearing years receive individualized care based upon what they need at the time of the appointment. In other words, since pregnancy is such a dynamic time of change, their needs vary from week to week as their pregnancies advance. The MotherMassage® practitioner also provides a safe, nurturing, nonjudgmental environment where clients are educated about decisions

they may have to make about their prenatal care.

"The workshop is three days long, eight hours each day, and provides 24 CEUs. Students must pass a take-home exam and massage two different pregnant women in order to receive professional certification. The course is approved by ALACE, CAPPA, DONA, FL Board of Massage, ICEA, Lamaze international, and the NCBTMB (Category A). MotherMassage® now provides a National Registry so expectant women all over the country can find certified bodyworkers who can provide them with the appropriate work for their special needs.

"The work itself is unique to each person who studies it. Practitioners come from a variety of backgrounds and have studied many different techniques. As long as the bodywork respects the anatomy and physiology of pregnancy and postpartum and incorporates the precautions and contraindications of prenatal massage, MotherMassage® is different with each person but is always safe and appropriate.

"In addition to MotherMassage®, I have written *The Encyclopedia of Bodywork* (Facts on File), the prenatal trilogy in *Massage Magazine* (2000–01), the "Womankind" column in *Massage Today,* and am now writing *Prenatal Massage: A Textbook of Pregnancy, Labor, and Postpartum Bodywork* (Mosby).

(continues)

Elaine Stillerman, LMT (continued)

"One of the most exciting aspects of doing prenatal massage is the profound impact the work has on these women. They come in with all sorts of aches and pains, questions and concerns, fears and phobias, and they leave feeling more confident, comfortable in their bodies, and looking forward to welcoming their babies. The bodywork also has a tremendous, far-reaching effect on the in utero environment. Whatever mom feels, the fetus feels through biochemical secretions. A stressed mother has a stressed child. Through the restorative MotherMassage® technique, a relaxed, stress-reduced mother has a baby who sleeps better, has a better disposition, and can deal with her own stress factors better.

"Our work reaches out to the next generation and is one of the most rewarding experiences a massage practitioner can have."

To find our more, contact:

Elaine Stillerman, LMT
Phone: (212) 533-3188
E-mail: Estillerman@cs.com
http://www.MotherMassage.net

vest that made him miserably hot in the Miami summer. He lay down panting amid all the emergency vehicles and commotion, submitting to my untrained ministrations with deep doggy groans of appreciation.

My massage on the rescue dog was simply an altered version of a normal massage for humans, and I was making it up as I went along. Over the years, there have been many people who wanted a protocol they could follow to treat animals. Those people who wish to work with animals usually follow the route of first becoming certified to massage humans, then branching out to treat nonhumans.

Most domesticated animals, as anyone who's ever scratched behind a dog's ears will know, love massage. They accept touch naturally, absorbing the pleasure and reacting positively to our attempts to soothe them. When they are experiencing an injury or trauma, though, they may need some special techniques that neither our love for them nor our human-based massage training has prepared us to offer. To address this problem, a handful of people have created trainings in animal massage techniques, most notably Linda Tellington-Jones, who offers workshops on the subject (see the Advanced Training Chart, appendix B, for contact information).

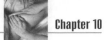

The majority of people interested in treating animals have focused their work on horses, for a number of reasons. First, horses are used for racing, jumping, hunting, showing, and heavy work, and they *need* massage more than most animals. Second, horses are accustomed to having humans tend to their needs, and they often *like* the extra attention of massage. Last, many people who own horses can *afford* to pay for massage for their animals.

Basic equine massage techniques were developed by Jack Meagher and then expanded on by other practitioners. Now several training systems are offered in horse massage. For example, Mary Schreiber, a certified massage therapist, started Equissage in 1989 and has graduated over 8,000 students who came from every state and 15 foreign countries.

Although there is no official licensing for equine massage therapists, horse owners generally prefer specially trained practitioners, and most of the people working on horses have graduated from one of the recognized equine programs. What's the most important trait of a good horse therapist? Sure, a good working knowledge of physiology is useful, and many years of experience with sports massage on humans is helpful, but good common horse sense is perhaps the most crucial prerequisite for any would-be equine therapist. As one practicing equine therapist stated, "The primary requisite for this work is loving horses."

If indeed you are a horse lover and are interested in this work, you'll be pleased to know that job opportunities are on the rise in this field. Therapists who take the courses and pass their examinations are finding work at ranches, farms, and race tracks all over the country. Some have even been lucky enough to work on horses that compete in the Olympics (see the story about Olympic massage in chapter 5).

Consult the Advanced Training Chart in appendix B for contact information.

Water Shiatsu (Watsu)

You may have thought, quite reasonably, that when you started your career in massage, you would be doing all of your work on dry land, in comfortable rooms, wearing clothes. While that is true in most cases, a growing number of therapists are slipping on their bathing suits and heading to the nearest warm-water pool to practice a modern technique based on an ancient healing system. Watsu, or water shiatsu, was conceived and developed by Harold Dull, a beat poet turned body therapist. After studying with Japanese Zen priests and shiatsu masters, Dull took the knowledge he had gained on land and translated it for use in a watery medium, finding that the added warmth and buoyancy helped loosen joints and support the spine. Freeing the spine is the cornerstone of a Watsu session.

Harbin Hot Springs, a clothing-optional resort in the hills just north of Napa Valley, was the ideal environment in which to refine and begin teaching his techniques. In addition to a thriving massage business, including a school, Harbin has a large pool filled with naturally warm spring waters. I visited this retreat and enrolled in a two-day introductory Watsu course to find out what the technique is like.

First observing Watsu as an outsider can be a slightly surreal experience. The main warm pool at Harbin is often filled with nearly 50 people at a time, all of them naked. Many of them are either students or practitioners of the technique, and they softly jostle for position with each other while floating their partners during Watsu treatments. When a class is in session, the pool can look like a training center for beginning water-ballet dancers. The practitioners cradle their partners, floating them on the surface, while engaging in a complex and graceful series of bends, rolls, and stretches, all in slow motion.

Watsu is not actually shiatsu under the water. Instead of focusing on the stimulation of specific points, practitioners glide their clients through the water, supporting them and gently coaxing the joints and muscles to relax and release, a result that is easier to achieve in water than on land.

While the atmosphere at Harbin is clothing-optional, Watsu is not always performed au naturel. In fact, many physical therapists and aquatics specialists use the technique to treat people with a wide range of disabilities, and everyone wears bathing suits. Some people have criticized Watsu because of the close physical contact that is required between practitioner and client in the water, but experience has shown that trust and nurturing can grow through this type of intimate yet nonsexual contact. Close bonds are formed quickly with Watsu, even more quickly than normally between therapist and recipient. I found that everyone involved at Harbin was professional, nonjudgmental, and nonthreatening, including the staff and all other participants. Even though no clothes were worn there, boundaries were respected.

Harold Dull has written a book on the subject, *Watsu: Freeing the Body in the Water* (Harbin Hot Springs Publishing, 2000), and he has traveled the world sharing the technique with people in many cultures. Dull visited Las Vegas for the annual Aquatic Therapies Symposium, and while there he found that many of the teachers were presenting techniques based on his work. "Watsu's popularity is mushrooming right now," Dull states. "Italy and Germany are the two countries outside the United States where it's doing best, and I just came back from Japan where it's going well, too. The Japanese are using it as a cool-down in the more strenuous aquatic exercise arena."

Dull says that many people around the country are teaching the technique, and recently a new program has been instituted to bring Watsu to more people in the general public than ever before. "We're trying to take Watsu in a horizontal direction as well as a vertical one," Dull says. "We've created modules in several areas across the country where people can come experience the technique for a couple days and then decide if it's something they want to pursue on the professional practitioner level or perhaps just for their own enjoyment and benefit. So far we have modules in Ventura, Houston, Vancouver, Chicago, Boston, and Philadelphia. People who learn at these centers can also use the facilities to offer sessions to clients."

When asked how Watsu can help massage practitioners in their careers, Dull points out that it is an ideal way to break the cycle of repetitive stress injuries that plague some therapists. "It's a way for some people to prolong careers that otherwise would be over. Besides teaching therapists new healthy ways to flow during their work, the water massage also takes the weight off of their limbs and joints. Therapists suffering from carpal tunnel syndrome, for example, have found that practicing the technique does not aggravate their condition, and often they can even improve while continuing to work."

Dull formed the Worldwide Aquatic Bodywork Association in 1993, and people from many countries have joined. Those wishing to practice professionally can become certified through a series of intensive programs. Some graduates have found work in the growing number of spas that offer Watsu to their guests. Others have used it in rehabilitative services through hospitals and physical therapy clinics, and some have built private clienteles.

For information about Watsu trainings and the Worldwide Aquatic Bodywork Association, or to order Harold Dull's books, contact the Massage School at Harbin Hot Springs, PO Box 570, Middletown, CA 95461; (707) 987-3801; e-mail: info@waba.edu; Web site: http://www.waba.edu.

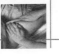

MOVING INTO OTHER PROFESSIONS

Massage and Nursing

For all of us who have ever spent any time in a hospital, we know that a simple soothing touch or sympathetic word from a compassionate nurse can turn a hellish experience into a more bearable one. A century ago, nurses had massage therapy included in their training. But then with the introduction of medical advances, everybody thought technology would take care of everything, so the element of human touch wouldn't be needed any more. That turned out not to be true, and now there is a renaissance happening as the two disciplines are utilized together once again. Many nurses have come to realize the power of their own touch, and they have embraced massage therapy as a part of their practice. On the other hand, some massage therapists have opted to join nurses on the front lines of health care, adding nursing degrees to their massage certificates. The professions have begun to overlap slightly, and everyone has benefited by the resulting symbiosis.

Perhaps the most well-known nurse to practice a form of massage is Dolores Krieger. She is a professor of nursing at New York University who implemented a five-step healing process called Therapeutic Touch. The technique, paradoxically, does not involve actual touch but rather the placing of the therapist's hands several inches away from the patient's body in sessions during which the "aura," or bioenergetic field, of the patient is assessed and affected. Ms. Krieger has taught her system to tens of thousands of health care professionals, particularly other nurses, who use it in hospitals. During the last 20 years, Therapeutic Touch has been offered in classes and workshops in more than 80 colleges and universities in the United States and about 70 foreign countries.

One way that massage has been integrated into the medical setting has been through volunteer programs in which students from local massage schools give treatments in area hospitals as part of their schooling. This, in turn, has exposed many nurses to the benefits of massage, and a good number of them have decided to explore a career in massage for themselves.

As more insurance companies and medical facilities embrace alternative therapies in general and massage in particular, this cross-pollination of the two fields will continue to flourish, to everyone's benefit. If you are interested in Therapeutic Touch, read Dolores Krieger's book, *Accepting Your Power to Heal: The Personal Practice of Therapeutic Touch*. If you would like to begin exploring a possible future in nursing, get a copy of *Healing Touch* newsletter at http://www.healingtouch.net. You can also learn more about the National Association of Nurse Massage Therapists by calling (800) 262-4017 or visiting http://www.nanmt.org.

If you haven't had an experience working in a hospital setting, you may want to volunteer at your local hospital before making a commitment to nursing school. If you want to work as a therapist in hospitals, see the information in chapter 3 for consultants who can help you.

New Medical Massage Technology

As science in general advances, so does the science of massage. Recently, new devices have been invented that far outperform the mechanical massagers of the past. Some of these have become advanced enough for use in medical settings, and physicians have begun to prescribe mechanized massage treatments as an additional way to address certain skin and subcutaneous tissue conditions.

For example, a French company called LPG sells a specialized massage machine primarily to plastic surgeons and dermatologists. The technology consists of dual motorized rollers in tandem with a true vacuum chamber that creates an effect similar to manual skin fold rolling, only much stronger. Massage therapists are familiar with the mechanics involved, and they are ideally suited to perform the maneuvers necessary for an effective treatment. The technique is known as *Endermologie*.

Hundreds of massage therapists who never thought about working in a medical setting were given the opportunity to do so when they were trained in the use of the device. The technique has been certified by the Florida State Department of Professional Regulation, Board of Massage, as a recognized massage modality, and therapists are given continuing education units when they take the training course. Physicians hire the trained therapists to work in their offices performing the procedure.

In today's technologically advancing marketplace, massage therapists are profiting in ways they never dreamed of just a short time ago. The company that makes this machine offers incentives to the therapists who they have trained in the technique. In a recent contest to determine who had achieved the most positive results for his or her patients, the grand-prize winner received a trip for two to Paris.

As the number of physicians who offer this procedure increases, so will the need for newly trained therapists, creating an entirely new job market. Therapists interested in this type of work can contact local physicians who offer Endermologie to inquire about the possibilities.

EXPANDING YOUR REACH

As the profession grows and more and more massage therapists spread the news about the benefits they can offer, we are in the process of creating an important new awareness about massage for people everywhere. This is being accomplished by therapists who engage in massage research to substantiate the benefits of massage; who write about massage for an ever-widening audience of practitioners and the general public; who teach workshops and seminars and massage school classes; who pass down their knowledge and dedication through the generations, making massage a family affair; who offer their expertise to other individuals and companies through consulting; and who finally make a name for themselves in the field, thus helping not only the people they touch directly but everyone who hears about them or their work.

Massage Research

Certain research-minded individuals have decided to aid massage therapists through the compilation of data supporting the use of massage throughout history. Richard Van Why of the Bodywork Research Institute has labored since 1988 on a encyclopedic work of 43 volumes with information about massage dating back to the year 1564 AD The Bodywork Research Institute also offers workshops in treating fibromyalgia.

For more information, contact:

> Richard VanWhy
> Phone (800) 400-0573

The Touch Research Institute, mentioned several times already, is worth mentioning again. As the first medical institute dedicated to the study of touch, it is an invaluable aid in our efforts to legitimize and popularize the positive benefits of massage. With a multidisciplinary staff of 40 scientists

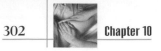
from the fields of medicine, biology, and psychology, the institute is in the midst of generating some important research. For example, studies have been undertaken to study the effects of massage in cases of newborns of cocaine-addicted mothers, infants of depressed mothers, infants with cancer, attention-deficit/hyperactivity disorder, adolescents with anorexia and depression, breast cancer, labor and childbirth, migraines, hypertension, eating disorders, spinal cord injuries, fibromyalgia, and chronic fatigue syndrome.

For more information, contact:

> The Touch Research Institute
> University of Miami School of Medicine
> Miami, FL
> Phone: (305) 243-6781
> http://www.miami.edu/touch-research/

Because massage is so often misunderstood in our society, it becomes necessary to substantiate our claims completely in as much detail as possible. Meticulous minds with academic strengths are needed in massage just like they are in other fields. If you are a research-oriented person, you may be able to help the profession of massage therapy more than you would have ever guessed, as the profile of Mirka Knaster in the next section explains.

Writing About Massage

Every field has its scribes, and massage therapy has been particularly blessed by the talents of many inspired, impassioned, talented writers. In fact, it seems that many of the people who have chosen massage are artists at heart, and they come to the profession with an artist's need to examine, reinvent, and share their experiences for the benefit and enjoyment of others.

If you have felt the slightest inclination to become a writer at any point in your life, massage may be the springboard upon which to initiate your efforts. If you've already done some writing, you can blend massage and writing to create an excellent synergy. Combined talents in these areas are in demand right now. We need massage crusaders, massage prophets, and massage storytellers. We need to spread the word, and writers are the ones who do that.

Traditionally, massage how-to books have done quite well by publishing standards, often becoming back-list favorites, which means they remain popular year after year. These are the books meant for a wide audience, the general public. They explain massage techniques along with their many benefits and usually include drawings or photographs for educational purposes. In some cases, the photographs themselves become the central selling tool of these books, and people buy them more for a certain aesthetic appeal than for their educational value. But people have a real desire to learn about massage, too, and some books do well with simple, helpful instructions. *The Massage Book* is one example, having sold over a million copies in 20 years. Beyond the how-to genre is a more in-depth class of massage books, many of them written specifically for practitioners and those interested in massage in a more serious way.

Of course, massage writing is not limited to books. In fact, probably the majority of words on the subject wind up in journals, magazines, and newsletters. One of the best ways to get started as a massage writer is by writing book reviews or penning a personal experience piece for one of the massage magazines. Simply by creating the intention to write such an article, you may inspire yourself to go out and have some particularly great experiences worthy to share with others. I began this way with a story for *Massage* magazine about training therapists at a new spa in Jamaica. That article, called "Massage in the Tropics," helped inaugurate my spa workshop career as well as my massage writing career. You'll find that publishing something automatically creates new credentials for you that may also help you in other aspects of your career.

When you approach magazines with story ideas, its best to follow certain traditional formats. Write to the editors of each magazine, enclosing a self-addressed stamped envelope (SASE), and request their writers' guidelines, which will tell you everything you need to know about sending material to them, such as the layout of your submission. This way, you'll stand a better chance of being accepted.

Magazine editors consistently state that the major reason they turn writers down is because they aren't familiar enough with the publication to write an appropriate article for its readers. Always read multiple issues of the magazines you want to write for. In this way, besides learning their style and tone, you'll also be updated on content. Sometimes the subject you were eager to write about for them was featured in a recent issue.

Some editors like to receive a "query letter," which describes your idea before you send an entire article. Others would rather see the whole thing. Find out

PROFILE: Mirka Knaster
Massage and Writing

What we learn in our bodies we can share with the world.

—*Mirka Knaster*

Mirka Knaster is widely known as the author of *Discovering the Body's Wisdom* (Bantam Books, 1996) and wonderful articles in *Massage Therapy Journal,* and as an instructor in the video, *Massage For Health,* hosted by Shari Belafonte. She travels extensively to speak and write about massage and "bodyways," the term she coined for all the Eastern and Western body therapies and movement arts. The following are her own words about the synthesis she has explored in the combined disciplines of massage, bodyways, and writing.

I've been blessed with insatiable curiosity. What excites me the most in life is learning, which makes me a born researcher. But that path hasn't always been easy. For example, I once was awarded a research grant from the Ford Foundation to conduct a project on women in Latin America. It took three years rather than the scheduled one year, and by the time I completed the reference book, I was so spent by the experience that I knew I needed to move on from academia. I sensed there was something one-sided, something unintegrated in my life. Even though I appeared to lead a natural or holistic lifestyle—I used herbs, exercised, grew vegetables,

backpacked, and camped—something was out of balance.

My work was strictly intellectual. I did not incorporate the body in a friendly way. In fact, I often denied my body's feelings and needs in order to get a lot done. I fulfilled my commitment and had my research published. But to explore other aspects of myself, I decided to leave my academic life at the University of California in Berkeley and at Stanford University, where I had earlier received my graduate degree. For a year, I lived in the more relaxing atmosphere of Santa Cruz and experimented with various body-mind practices. Then I traveled with my backpack and bicycle in the Northwest and visited friends in other areas.

Eventually I returned to the San Francisco Bay Area, but instead of going back to a university campus, I enrolled in massage school. That ended up being exactly what I needed—to connect to people with my hands, with my whole body. I have a desire to be of service. Although my academic work helped people on a certain level, it didn't feel direct and personal, the way massage did. Even so, I intuited from the beginning that actually doing massage was just a stepping stone, but I didn't know where it would lead me.

I moved to Napa Valley, established a private practice, and also led

(continues)

Mirka Knaster (continued)

workshops. In those days, I had to conduct my business "underground" because Napa was quite conservative. For example, to get a massage license, I would have had to go through the Napa police department, which meant wearing a photo ID and agreeing that they could come to my home at any time to check on me, I suppose to make sure I wasn't engaged in prostitution. Yikes! I kept wondering, "Why does massage have such a bad reputation? Why are we having this difficulty in America? Why, when I say the word 'massage,' do people raise their eyebrows at me, probably thinking of a 'red light district'?"

I realized that in order to help people see massage through different eyes, I had to play an educational role. I taught holistic health classes in the Continuing Education Department and set up a massage therapy program in the Health Occupations Department of Napa Valley College. I also spoke on local radio and to community groups— such as the Elks, Jaycees, Parents Without Partners, Ladies' Hadassah— about how massage has been a part of the history of Western medicine since ancient times and integral to cultures all over the world. By presenting these historical and cross-cultural aspects and demonstrating massage publicly, I thought that I would help remove the taint and stigma attached to massage because of massage parlors.

I was able to do this because I revisited my past. I remember thinking, "You can't keep a good researcher down." This is where my academic background was invaluable. I knew how to find the data I needed to present a different image of massage, one that would help transform public opinion. I spent endless hours poring through publications at the medical, anthropology, and public health libraries of Bay Area universities for reports on how massage has been used in other cultures. I read the earliest medical treatises by ancient Greek, Roman, and Arabic physicians because I wanted to find out how far back the practice went. I did the same for Asian systems of medicine. As I amassed this information, I began to piece together a broader, more positive picture of massage and also to understand where the problems had come from. Then, one day, my partner at the time said, "You're not going to be happy just doing library research; you're only going to be satisfied if you see for yourself." He was right, of course. So I had a garage sale, sold everything, rented out my house, and went to Asia in 1981, not knowing when I would return. I was gone for more than a year. I chose Asia because my library research revealed that it was the most likely area in the world where so many ancient practices were still alive and well. That turned out to be true. As I

(continues)

Mirka Knaster (continued)

traveled, everywhere I turned, I saw healing touch. I became a magnet for massage.

After that journey through Asia, I lived on the island of Maui and wrote a manuscript about my massage odyssey, but I couldn't get it published. There wasn't enough interest yet. As has often been the case in my life, I was ahead of the times. But I did get a letter from an editor at *East West Journal,* now called *Natural Health,* expressing interest in having me write for them. I turned parts of chapters from that manuscript into articles for the magazine. *Massage* magazine started in Hawaii around that time, too, and the publisher asked me to write a couple of columns, which I did for a few issues. Then I also began writing for *Massage Therapy Journal.* That's how sharing my information beyond my local community evolved. As far as I know, no one else was writing about massage and other cultures during that time. A producer in Los Angeles read my work in those publications and contacted me. He flew me to California to be a consultant, writer, and on-screen instructor in a massage video with Shari Belafonte.

For me, massage became a stepping stone back to writing, but from a whole different place, one that involves me spiritually, emotionally, intellectually, and physically. I learned how to write for the general public rather than for a critical dissertation committee sitting on my shoulder.

The work that I do and the life that I live are now in harmony. While writing *Discovering the Body's Wisdom,* for three-and-a-half years I lived in the woods in the Blue Ridge Mountains of western North Carolina. It was really important to nurture myself and my creativity with that quiet space in nature. I was able to watch the subtlest seasonal changes all year around. When I needed a break from my computer, I walked with my dogs among the trees, chancing upon wildflowers and mushrooms. I had a special spot in a tree over a stream where I'd stop to sit before heading back to my desk in the cabin.

I officially initiated my research in the field in 1978, and now, finally, my book has an audience. That means I've been working at it for over 20 years!

I no longer have a massage therapy practice. Instead, I apply the insights I've gained through my travels and my work with people in other ways. I incorporate my skills in cross-cultural research, writing, and communication into workshops, consulting, presentations at conferences, lifestyle Expos, health and retreat centers, and interviews on radio and television.

To promote *Discovering the Body's Wisdom,* I toured for a month in New Zealand. I'm interested in spreading the word about the importance of befriending the body and discovering

(continues)

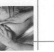
its wisdom, about joyfully and gratefully celebrating our embodiment. I want to inform health care professionals and consumers about the value of working with the body through massage and other bodyways. I have found that the best way to *use myself* is through all forms of *communication,* integrating the life of the mind and life in the body.

who wants what, and then give them what they want. Always print manuscripts in double-space and letters in single-space, and check for spelling and cleanliness. Make backup copies of your work. In query letters, be brief, but do tell the editor a little about yourself, especially anything that makes you especially qualified to have written what you wrote. Mention writing credits if you have them, and don't mention the lack of them if you don't.

In addition to massage magazines, you may try health magazines, as well. Also, local newspapers and magazines are often interested in stories from local authors. Even if they are in small publications, you can cut the stories out, copy them, and recirculate them as promotional material.

If you think you've got enough material for a book, or if you've already written a book and want to go about getting it published, you'll find many resources to help you. The how-to section for writers is located in the reference area of most bookstores. There you'll find such classics as *Writer's Market,* published by Writer's Digest Books, an annually updated guide to the people and places that buy what writers produce. Another useful source of information is Jeff Herman's book *Writer's Guide to Book Editors, Publishers, and Literary Agents* from Prima Publishing.

When seeking a publisher, you have the choice of either contacting a publishing house directly or trying to find an agent, who will then contact the publishers on your behalf. The best advice I can give is to be *extremely* professional and to constantly ask yourself how you can help the editors and agents you contact, not the other way around. How can you present your material in a more compelling, beautiful way? How can you make yourself and your book more high quality and marketable? How can you turn yourself into a more respectable authority? Tell people what you'll give them, not what you need them to give you.

Unless you have a connection with a publisher, seeking an agent first may be the best course. Michael Larsen, an agent in San Francisco, has written an insightful book called *Literary Agents: What They Do, How They Do It, and How to Find and Work with the Right One for You.* This is the book you need if you're serious about getting involved in the writer/agent relationship. If you are creating a book proposal to try to sell your project, Larsen's *How to Write a Book Proposal* is very helpful. It was the key that got me started as a book writer.

Even though it may sound more important and "real" to have your book published by an established house, many people are taking matters into their own hands and self-publishing their work. Creating your own book is no longer a second-class choice, and some of the most successful authors around are those who published their own material. With the growth of desktop publishing, accomplishing this is easier than ever. You don't have to wait until you've written a 500-page tome filled with thousands of references to print it. For one thing, it would be expensive, and readers today seem to prefer more easily digestible volumes. If you have a computer, you can start your very own book or booklet right now. There are people out there who can help you make it look good and get a shot at selling, too. If you're ready, call Para Publishing at (800) PARAPUB to order a copy of Dan Poynter's book, *The Self-Publishing Manual.* This book contains everything you need to know from how to organize and write your material to choosing printers and publicizing your work. Dan also offers workshops on the subject.

It's also a good idea to subscribe to one or more of the writers' magazines. *Writer's Digest* is a reasonably priced magazine filled with information about craft and contacts, while *Publisher's Weekly* is much more costly ($225 per year) and focuses on the business of book publishing and selling. All of these will help keep you informed about current news and outlets for your work.

Teaching Workshops and Seminars

With a conservative estimate of 25,000 newly graduated massage therapists entering the workplace each year, most of whom will seek out some form of continuing education to fulfill their licensing requirements as the years go by, a sizable market exists for teachers of workshops and seminars. Who leads these workshops? Is it exclusively the domain of mega-experienced old pros who live on an entirely different level than you do in the massage world? Will you have to wait many years before your chance comes to debut before a group of your peers, teach them something worthwhile, and receive the benefits (monetary and otherwise) for doing so? The answer to both of these questions is no.

After you've gained a reasonable amount of experience (only a year or two in some cases), you'll need just four ingredients to successfully create your own weekend workshop. Those ingredients are:

1. Extensive knowledge about one specific helpful technique or modality that others want to learn about

2. The ability to get across the essence and use of this technique to your students through written words, demonstrations, and lectures

3. The ambition and confidence to work with people in the creation and production of your workshop

4. A little knowledge about how the workshop scene works and whom to go to for help

If you are a beginning therapist, you may think that creating your own weekend workshop constitutes a romantic way to combine travel, fun, good work, and wide exposure in your field. At least partially, you'd be right. On the other hand, you'll need to do a lot of detailed planning and preparation to make a workshop happen in the first place. When it does happen, you'll almost always be surprised by the results. During my several years as a weekend workshop teacher, I've not only taught helpful treatments to hundreds of people in an atmosphere of support and trust but also have had many experiences I never planned on.

As a massage workshop instructor I:

- Literally got hit by a Mack logging truck on a highway in Maine

- Had to bail a student out of jail in a small town in central New Jersey

- Single-handedly moved all the furniture out of an office on the top floor of a Holiday Inn and carted 15 boxes of equipment in for the workshop (with a broken elevator)

- Got lost in traffic in Chicago and ended up at a Garth Brooks concert

- Had my left foot run over by a student's Ford Pinto

- Was locked out of the training room early in the morning with 20 impatient students eyeing me for almost an hour

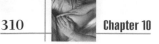
✳ Made several dear friends with some of the best folks you'll find anywhere in any profession

My favorite stop on the workshop circuit is Waldoboro, Maine, where the family who owns the massage school makes lobster dinners for me each time I stay in their home, which is always during fall foliage season.

You'll need to find a balance between pros and cons when you're considering a possible workshop lifestyle. Some people do extremely well at it and make a handsome living doing nothing but weekend gigs. Others, though, struggle for years before deciding to give up the idea. It takes a certain temperament, I think, to flourish in this niche; you have to like a constant change in scenery, enjoy being on stage, and care about teaching.

You'll face different types of students and different challenges with each class, yet there will be a certain sameness to your experiences as you present the same material to different groups.

If, knowing all this, you are inspired to get started, here are a few pointers. Put your proposed workshop into writing and present it to the appropriate board that administers massage in your state. Call or write them for the forms you'll need. The board will want to know your qualifications, the qualifications of any other teachers you propose to work with, the content of your course, the teaching methods, the hours, and any teaching aids you'll be using. Also, they'll want to verify that you will be keeping accurate records of your classes and students.

If you live in a state without massage licensing, you can send away to another state to be certified as a continuing education unit (CEU) provider. Florida and New York are good choices because many other states have reciprocity with them as regards CEU credits. Also, the National Certification Board for Therapeutic Massage and Bodywork (NCBTMB) offers certification for continuing education providers (see "Licensing" in Chapter 6).While it's true that you can teach a workshop without offering continuing education credits, being a CEU provider will give you a certain respectability, and it will draw a lot more students to your classes when they know that taking it will help them when it comes time to renew their license. (Two of the NCBTMB forms are shown in Figure 10-4 and Figure 10-5.)

Do a little arithmetic and you'll soon come to the conclusion that weekend workshops can be quite lucrative. Twenty students at $200 apiece makes $4,000, times 50 weekends a year (two off for holidays, because even people

Figure 10-4 | **NCBTMB CEU providership application form—Form A.**

Title of Course_____ Name of Organization/Individual_____

Name/Job/Title List name of instructor of above course. List current job title to correspond with each person.	Number of Continuing Education Hours the Participant will receive.	Course Description Give a brief description of the course being offered. Explain when course has been taught. *(Also, state whether course is offered in basic program, for organizations only.)*

Figure 10-5 | **NCBTMB providership form—Form B.**

Title of Course_____ Name of Organization/Individual_____

Learning Outcomes Each course must have clear and concise written statements of intended learning outcomes. Learning outcomes determine what it is the participants will know or be able to do as a result of a course. State the learning outcomes of the course below.	Teaching Method State the instructional methods as well as the instructional materials that will be used for this course.	Learning Environment The provider must provide an appropriate learning environment. Describe the learning environment that the provider uses when conducting the course.

making that much money have to rest sometime, right?) will have you making $200,000 a year—and you'll have Monday through Thursday off!

As you might have guessed, it doesn't work quite like that. While it is true that $4,000 is a reasonable amount to expect as proceeds from a weekend workshop (some of the more well-known seminars take in much more), all of that money won't go directly into your pocket. The massage school or other venue where the seminar takes place will take a percentage—and for those massage schools that do a bulk of the advertising and enrollment for their presenters, that percentage can be as high as 40 or 50 percent. If you produce your own workshops, you'll have to pay for space in a hotel, school, or conference center yourself; and you'll also be in charge of promotion and advertising, which can consume a good part of the proceeds. Keep in mind the expenses you'll encounter while on the road, as well—travel, food and lodging, entertainment, and the like. In addition, you may be splitting the pot with a cosponsor, such as the producer of the products you use in the seminar.

Even though the work is usually confined to the weekend, and sometimes Friday, too, workshops can be exhausting. Few therapists voluntarily choose to withstand the rigors of a dozen weekends in a row, much less a whole year's worth. However, you can work every other weekend, taking home half the total proceeds, and make a decent living from workshops alone. Some people do it, but most have learned to blend a more normal everyday lifestyle with occasional teaching trips throughout the year.

When you set forth on the workshop circuit, one thing is for sure: If your classes are not fun for you, they won't be fun for your students. You owe it to yourself and your students to upgrade your presentation skills and class content on a regular basis. As you may have guessed, weekend seminars are available to help you do just that.

Teaching in Massage Schools

Some therapists find that after massage school is over, they've received so much from the experience that they want to give something back. Others have discovered that massage school is the one place they felt most nurtured and comfortable in their adult lives. Still others came to massage from the teaching profession and found a natural niche in massage schools after their own graduation.

SELLING IS OK, EVEN FOR HEALERS

Some therapists have hit the road as weekend workshop warriors only to find that the extra work and time away from home weren't worth the added income unless they supplemented that income with commissions from the sale of products during the class. I was faced with this dilemma myself when I first started out.

The company I worked with, TouchAmerica, helped set up the workshops and supplied the products I used in class. Since they did the promotion, I received a smaller percentage, and we also split the proceeds with the school, which often didn't leave much for me on Sunday evening.

"That's OK," I was told. "You can make extra money by selling products in the class. You'll get 10 percent of the total."

My whole being reacted against the concept of selling products. Everyone was coming to learn, I assumed, not spend even more money. My partners at TouchAmerica were not happy with this attitude, and they encouraged me to change my concept of what selling was and regard it as a further service to my fellow therapists.

I couldn't do it. Weekend after weekend I fell short of the $1,000 goal for product sales. What's worse, it felt horrible having to stand in front of the class and give a sales pitch when my heart wasn't in it. There was nothing wrong with the products; I just didn't want to push anything on anybody. I had never been a salesman before.

A year went by in this manner, and everybody involved was questioning my ability to do the job, even me. Finally, at a workshop in Dallas one cold February on Friday night, the introductory evening, I confessed to the class. Instead of my normal, half-hearted, low-key sales pitch, I laid my heart on the line and told them how I really felt. "I'm not here to sell you anything," I told them. "And I don't want to waste any class time going over prices and dealing with products. All I want to do is teach. So if anybody wants to buy anything, you're going to have to let me know about it because I'm not going to mention it again." Then I proceeded with the course material.

That weekend I sold $9,000 worth of products.

Whatever the reasons, many therapists work as teachers at a massage school at some point during their careers. Usually the only requirement will be a massage certificate, often from the very school where you are applying for a job, and in many cases this makes becoming a massage instructor easier than becoming a teacher in other settings. Some people who get the chance to try it find out that they are natural-born teachers, and they do a great job. The experience can be quite rewarding, and it's a positive way to share with others what you've learned and assimilated into your own life. However, the massage school environment has its own challenges, and the job is not for everybody. The following are some of the pros and cons of working as a massage-school instructor.

On the Positive Side

1. Massage schools are run by some of the most wonderful people you'll find in any profession anywhere, and you're likely to form lifelong friendships with your bosses and coworkers.

2. You'll receive a certain amount of professional respect as an instructor, and the experience is good to have on your résumé.

3. Massage schools are usually run as somewhat "open" systems, the opposite of a closed corporate environment; if you're a person who blossoms outside of the typical work scene, massage schools may be for you.

4. Teaching in a massage school is a perfect opportunity to supplement your income within the field of massage without actually having to perform massage yourself. This is ideal for busy therapists who may be reaching their limit.

5. Some schools offer benefits like insurance and vacations.

6. The constant influx of new students with their own unique ways of doing things will help keep your own massage work open and alive instead of getting stuck in a routine.

7. As an instructor, you'll have many opportunities to help others grow in the profession and subsequently help their own clients. It's a way of multiplying your own positive influence as a therapist.

On the Negative Side

1. Massage schools, as a general rule, do not have vast endowments and are not cash-rich enough to pay large salaries to their teachers. Academia is not a field renowned for its high wage earners, and this applies equally to the massage academy. If you are not the owner or partner in the school, chances are your pay will be on the modest side, at least in the beginning (pay scales vary widely, but a rough median hourly wage is around $15).

2. You may be asked to teach some classes you aren't interested in.

THE WEEKEND WORKSHOP FORMAT
IS IT GOOD FOR US?

A large majority of the advanced training options you'll find for massage therapy are offered in the weekend-workshop format. This is a convenient way to be exposed to a good deal of information in a reasonably condensed period of time. Students can grow quickly in their understanding of a subject, and on Sunday evenings they eagerly return home with a lot of new information, inspired to integrate it into their practices.

The only problem with Sunday Evening Enthusiasm is Monday Morning Reality. Forced back into their regular routines right away, many therapists lose a lot of what they've learned. Here are a few hints to help with this dilemma:

1. Sign up for workshops that are taught as a series. By the time you feel the impact of your last training start to fade, you'll find yourself in a Part 2 classroom, ready to absorb more.

2. When you get home, use at least a little bit of your new knowledge *during the first week*. Even if you have to work late, practice the techniques. The sooner you do this, the better chance you'll have for retaining the knowledge.

3. On the weekend following your weekend workshop, break out the training manual and go over the entire thing again. One of the least utilized tools of most workshops is the manual, which the instructor has usually spent a great deal of time and care creating. Take advantage of it.

4. Try sharing what you've learned with someone else. The information you give may not be perfect, and it shouldn't be considered official, of course, but you may be able to supply a friend with some additional knowledge while at the same time solidifying it in your own mind. The best way to learn is to teach.

---

3. You'll be subjected to massage students on a continual basis. As you may have experienced in your own class, massage students can sometimes act as immaturely as grade-school children even though most of them are grown adults. Something about going back into a classroom and sitting at a desk seems to bring out the delinquent in certain people. They rebel against quizzes and complain about every detail of the learning process. Instead of being easier to deal with now that they've grown up, these students are harder to discipline.

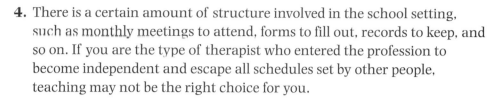
4. There is a certain amount of structure involved in the school setting, such as monthly meetings to attend, forms to fill out, records to keep, and so on. If you are the type of therapist who entered the profession to become independent and escape all schedules set by other people, teaching may not be the right choice for you.

If you are interested in teaching in a massage school, a good way to break in is by working there as a receptionist or at some other position first, especially if you are a new therapist. Some other positions available at most schools include workshop coordinator, retail-store manager, admissions officer, clinic coordinator, and office manager.

The best way to up your chances of being asked to work at a massage school is to concentrate on building your own reputation as a good therapist. Once you've done that, massage-school owners may come to you asking if you have enough free time to add your insights and acknowledged skills to their students' learning experience.

Massage As a Family Affair

When the people closest to you see how well you're doing with the massage business, you may become a role model for them, and you can end up with several generations of massage therapists in the family. Many massage-school owners have children who follow in their footsteps, and many therapists find that their children develop an interest in the career. Even the children of massage customers sometimes become curious when they see their parents relaxing in this unique way and enjoying the company of a stranger in the house who has them lie down on a table beneath a towel. It looks neat from a child's perspective, and they will often try to "help" mommy or daddy relax by adding their own unique maneuvers to the therapist's routine. Years later, when they're thinking about potential careers, the memory may help them decide on massage school.

On the other hand, the massage business has the potential to cause some friction between family members if everyone doesn't view the profession from the same perspective. For example, if a woman becomes a therapist but her husband doesn't understand her intentions, he may be threatened by her choice to "touch other naked men." This happens fairly frequently and has even caused relationships to break up. Some men, being unable to regard the touch of a female in a nonsexual light, can't believe it's possible for other men to do so. Women can feel similarly threatened if their boyfriend or husband practices massage. Of course, the same dynamics apply in same-sex relationships. If you have a family member or significant other who simply cannot fathom what therapeutic massage is all about, you may be in for some uncomfortable times ahead. Some people have forsaken their career for this reason alone. Others have forged ahead and eventually been able to explain the reality of the situation to their loved ones. Still others, it seems, can never get out of a cycle of recriminations and doubts.

Here are a couple of suggestions for helping a misguided mate see the light about your chosen profession:

1. Bring him or her to class at massage school. Listening to a long lecture about cell metabolism or muscle origins can go a long way in assuaging an overactive imagination.

2. Sign your partner up for a massage with a member of the sex he or she is attracted to, and make sure the therapist is an ethical practitioner. When your partner sees how professional this therapist is, he or she may realize that you work the same way.

If, like some therapists, you find yourself working side-by-side with family members, you'll face the same challenges encountered in any family business. However, you may find some consolation in knowing that, with this business in particular, some of the rough spots can be smoothed over when everyone involved focuses on their primary intentions, which are to relax, to heal, and to make whole. Doing this for each other, as well as the clients, can make this business more pleasurable than most.

Consulting

If you're willing to take the steps recommended in chapter 9 to create a professional image for yourself as a therapist, you can expand that process and create a professional image as an expert in your field, as well: You could become a consultant. What, you may be thinking, could a massage therapist possibly consult about? Would you be offering opinions to corporate executives about how they could relax their shoulders?

To conceive of yourself as a top-paid consultant, you first have to broaden your perceptions. If each of the people you massage individually benefits through the experience, it follows that almost everyone else would benefit, too.

PROFILE: Charlotte Applegate
a Family Massage Dynasty

When it comes to massage families, Charlotte Applegate has created her own dynasty in the Dallas area. She is the progenitor of three full generations of successful therapists, and the family continues to add new massage professionals to its ranks.

Over the years, Charlotte's love for massage and her commitment to the profession "rubbed off" on almost everyone in her family. Her son Jim and his wife both graduated from the family school, called the Institute of Natural Healing Sciences, which they now help manage. In addition, they own and operate a successful day spa in nearby Keller.

Charlotte's granddaughter Jennifer was fresh out of high school when she decided to take massage classes. She has now been a therapist for eight years, having worked in the family businesses in Texas and also branching out to find work in California at a large clinic and in a hotel. Back in Texas once again, she is going into partnership with Charlotte in yet another day spa.

Her grandson Rob also works at the school doing therapy. He has been a therapist for eight years. Her other grandson Michael has been a therapist for five years, and he works for a chiropractor. All of the grandchildren and her son Jim help with the teaching chores at the school.

As the latest addition to the massage ensemble, Charlotte's sister Rosemary attended massage school just last year and is now working at a day spa herself.

With so much daily interaction in hands-on situations, how does the family maintain a sense of peace and balance? "We have to be patient with each other," Charlotte states, "and we have to remember that nobody's perfect, especially when it comes to your family. Also, I think it helps when the younger people respect the older people with more experience. That can be a little difficult at times, especially when the older people have less experience, as was the case when my sister worked in Synergist, our store, before she went through her massage training. It all worked out fine, though, and we continue to work as a team."

Each member of Charlotte's family had his or her own reasons for attending the family school, making massage a part of his or her life, and contributing to the growth of the dynasty. Personal growth, career advancement, and family togetherness all played a part, not to mention some excellent discounts on their massage-school tuitions!

Now Charlotte is literally passing the torch of the business down through the generations. She is helping to finance

(continues)

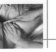

Charlotte Applegate (continued)

her granddaughter Jennifer in the day spa. After Jennifer pays her back, the business will be hers. She is watching her son and daughter-in-law, all of her grandchildren, and her sister prosper in an array of ventures—all made possible by massage. Recently, she sold the massage school to one of her instructors and is now building a spiritual retreat school with her new husband, a minister.

You can contact the Institute of Natural Healing Sciences at (817) 498-0716 or http://www.inhs.us.

You can't massage everyone, but you *can* help lead thousands of people to a discovery of massage and the benefits of body awareness.

The major requirement for work as a consultant is knowledge, and you needn't feel that the field is limited to those people with advanced degrees. As each year goes by, people become more aware of the role stress plays in their lives. Corporations lose thousands of hours of employee productivity and millions of dollars in profits to stress-related illnesses and absenteeism. If you could help an organization lower such losses by just 1 percent for one year through your example, advice, and enthusiasm, it would be well worth it for that organization to pay you many thousands of dollars. Speakers and consultants often make an extremely good living.

People want experts who can help them solve their problems, and since stress and stress-related dysfunctions are among the major problems all people and organizations face today, an expert massage therapist would be in high demand. How, then, do you become regarded as an expert? How do you position yourself as someone whom others should hire to help with their problems?

First, you have to believe passionately in what you do and what you stand for (for most massage therapists, this is not a problem). Then, you have to *create* something worthy of notice. Usually, your creation will be in the form of written material (books, booklets, training manuals) or other media (DVDs, audio programs, computer programs).

Once you've created some credentials, you have to get yourself noticed. The best way to do that is through magazines, newspapers, and news programs. Each time you appear anywhere and receive any kind of press, file it away in your press kit; when you have created a credible portfolio for yourself, you can present yourself as an expert. Of course, the beauty of consulting is that the very items that position you as an expert are the items you can sell to the people you consult with. You are recognized for your success, and that recognition brings you more success.

You'll most likely find your first job as a consultant through personal contacts. People need to trust you before they'll hire you and spend good money to hear your information. The first time somebody asks you if you're available for consultations, don't be surprised, *be ready!* Have an hourly or daily fee in mind, which should normally be at least twice as much as your massage fees. People expect to pay well for valuable information, and most beginning consultants undercharge for their services.

Great opportunities exist for therapists who are willing and able to position themselves as consultants. If you have a degree or expertise in another field—such as law, aesthetics, medicine, or business—you may already be thinking in terms of consulting work. Take the next step and put your massage skills together with your communication, motivation, and education skills.

Think for a moment about what the manager of a large corporation may be going through. Half of his staff is unmotivated and resentful. They call in sick a lot and complain behind his back. Most of the others are avidly climbing the same ladder the manager has climbed, and they threaten to take his position. This manager has been to dozens of corporate team-building seminars and brought in professional speakers to motivate his employees. Stress, he knows, is the number one reason why so many of the company's workers, including himself, are not performing at their best. Whom can he call?

The safest route for him to take is to contact the same sources that everyone else in his field uses. Speakers' bureaus and consultant organizations cater to people with exactly his needs. When he calls one of these agencies and asks for a consultant or speaker who specializes in teaching corporate employees how to reduce stress, he will most likely be put in touch with a professional who is extremely good at what he does and who may indeed help the company. But is that consultant truly an expert in the stress-reduction field? Does he know more than you, a massage therapist with years of experience at relieving stress one person at a time through your dedication, hard work, and enthusiasm?

As a therapist, you are probably more aware than 99 percent of all people about the mechanisms of stress and the positive effects of touch. Here is a partial list of some of the people who may benefit from your knowledge and consulting services, if you *position yourself* to fulfill their needs and offer them solutions to the particular problems they are facing:

❋ Physicians looking to incorporate alternative therapies into their practice, including massage

❋ Business people who are opening a spa or other health facility but who have no experience themselves with massage, spa therapies, training, and so on

❋ Corporations integrating a wellness program for their employees

❋ Organizations interested in stress-relief and quality-of-life improvements for their employees

❋ Attorneys who are trying cases involving massage issues and need massage therapists as expert witnesses (Read Dan Poynter's *Expert Witness Handbook* from Para Publishing, (800) PARAPUB.)

When it comes to consulting, *presentation* is important. You may have the knowledge that a company really needs, but if you don't present it in an acceptable form, nobody will be able to access it. Therefore, if you're beginning to think about the possibilities that consulting work may present for you, it will be worth it to go back over the material in chapter 9, "Creating a Professional Image." Build up your résumé, and get as many references as you can in the field you're trying to break into. Then invest in the resources listed in the sidebar, "Resources for Massage Speakers and Consultants," to help you hone your skills and meet the right people who can send you forward.

Making a Name for Yourself

The key to success—and what this book has been all about from start to finish—consists of a certain set of magic words that are spoken on a regular basis by people when you aren't around to hear them. They are the words that people use to describe what their experience was like on your massage table or reading the article you wrote about stress in the local paper or seeing you on television massaging relief workers after a disaster.

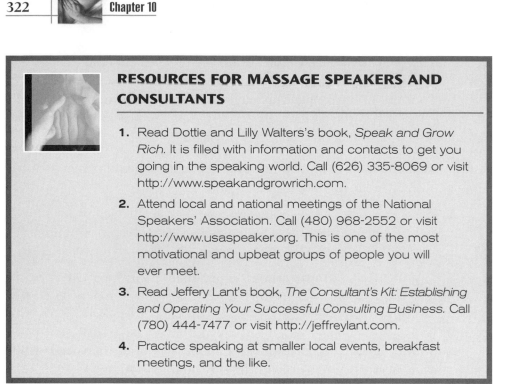

RESOURCES FOR MASSAGE SPEAKERS AND CONSULTANTS

1. Read Dottie and Lilly Walters's book, *Speak and Grow Rich.* It is filled with information and contacts to get you going in the speaking world. Call (626) 335-8069 or visit http://www.speakandgrowrich.com.

2. Attend local and national meetings of the National Speakers' Association. Call (480) 968-2552 or visit http://www.usaspeaker.org. This is one of the most motivational and upbeat groups of people you will ever meet.

3. Read Jeffery Lant's book, *The Consultant's Kit: Establishing and Operating Your Successful Consulting Business.* Call (780) 444-7477 or visit http://jeffreylant.com.

4. Practice speaking at smaller local events, breakfast meetings, and the like.

In the massage business, as in any business, the measure of your success will depend on the reputation you build and what people say of your work. Massage is very personal, at times ineffable, and no words are sufficient to describe exactly what effects your work has had on the people you touch; yet it's supremely easy for a client to make a simple, concrete judgment based on his or her experience. "Yes," they'll say, "you have *got* to have a session of massage therapy with Marianne. She's just . . . I can't find the words. She's *great.*"

On the other hand, they can shrug their shoulders and say, "Sure, it was nice."

In general, people won't voice too many negative opinions about you as a massage therapist because you'll be spending your time making them feel better to one degree or another, but the difference between "nice" and "great" can be the difference between an unending struggle and a satisfying career.

Although you spend your hours with one person at a time, your influence will float gradually outward and your work will become known. I hope for you that your clients become your fan club, your admirers, and your public relations team. If you make just a few people happy by offering the very best that you can give, your reputation will precede you and you will flourish and grow in this profession more spectacularly than you ever thought possible.

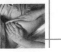

CONCLUSION

I welcome you to the end of this journey we've been on together. Now I'd like to welcome you to continue it. This is just the beginning.

Do you remember the words from chapter 1? Here they are again:

> The market for massage therapy in this country is *huge.* More people every day are discovering that massage is not a luxury but a necessity—and one that they can definitely afford. I can create a great lifestyle for myself doing massage therapy while at the same time helping the people I touch.

How do you feel about that statement now? Is it easier to believe? I hope so. There is a job out there for you, more than a job—a vocation, a lifestyle, and a meaningful way to contribute on an essential level to the lives of many.

For all of us here on the physical plane, there is nothing that is not touch. Every part of you touches on other parts within. On the fringes of our bodies, the thin separating membrane of our skin does more than form a barrier to exclude the world without; it invites the world in, as well. We were meant to connect. We were born to it. Massage therapists are the ones who have chosen to be the conscious embrace of our species, solidifying our bonds with each other and the planet through intentional compassionate touch. It is our mission, our blessing, our adventure.

I hope you keep growing in massage, as in all areas of your life, and that you fulfill your aspirations. The path ahead may still be somewhat unclear, but I urge you to proceed. Gradually, or perhaps all at once, the path will appear lit with candles, then lamplight, then a spotlight. You'll *know* where to go and whom to meet. When you do meet, there will be a spark of recognition in your eyes because you've been traveling similar paths all along.

I look forward to seeing you along the way.

To be continued*

I hope that our dialogue will not end when you finish reading this book. Send me an e-mail via my web site if you would like to stay in touch. www.royaltreatment.com

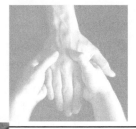

Appendix A
Resources

GENERAL RESOURCES

Scrip Massage and Spa Supply

Scrip carries just about anything that a massage therapist could hope to have in order to start and grow a thriving business. To make it easier for you, Scrip is offering 10 percent off your entire first order. Just call (800) 747-3488 and mention *Massage Therapy Career Guide*, source code (SC-1205). You can see Scrip's offerings on line at http://www.scripmassage.com.

Biofreeze

Biofreeze is the number one pain relieving product in the massage world. Discover what many therapists have already learned by visiting http://www.biofreeze.com or by calling (800) 246-3733.

Golden Ratio Woodworks

More than just a manufacturer or supplier, Golden Ratio has become synonymous with innovation in the massage industry. At its home base in Montana, Golden Ratio has developed a spa, guest house, factory, store, and product development plant. It is pretty cool. Visit http://www.goldenratiowood-works.com or call (800) 345-1129.

Downeast School of Massage

The Downeast School of Massage in Maine has a great massage therapy program and offers much good information on its Web site, including the DSM Store, which is dedicated to providing quality therapeutic supplies and alternative products for the enhancement of professional growth and personal holistic health. Visit http://www. downeastschoolofmassge.net or call (207) 832-5531.

Other Web Sites

The Web site for Steiner Trans-Ocean, the cruise ship spa employer is http://www. steinerleisure.com.

The Web site for the National Certification Board for Therapeutic Massage and Bodywork, http://www.ncbtmb.com, allows browsers to locate nationally certified therapists in their area as well as find out information about how to get certified. Call them at (800) 296-0664.

Lauriann Greene is a former musician turned therapist who specializes in helping therapists reduce work-related injuries. She developed the "Save Your Hands!" workshops for massage therapists and has taught hundreds of students and professionals across the United States and Canada. She later used her research and her work with injured massage therapists to write the book *Save Your Hands! Injury Prevention for Massage Therapists.* Lauriann wrote a regular column in *Massage* magazine called "Helping the Healers" and has published an important research study in *Massage & Bodywork Magazine* on the incidence and prevalence of work-related injury among bodyworkers and massage therapists. Contact Lauriann for more information via her Web site: http://www.saveyourhands.com.

The Touch Research Institute's site can be found at http://www. miami.edu/touch-research. Call (305) 243-6781.

Links and reference on reflexology can be found at http://www. reflexology-research.com. Call (505) 344-9392 for more information.

The Association of Labor Assistants & Childbirth Educators has a site at http://www.alace.org. Call (888) 222-5223.

The home page for the IRS is http://www.irs.ustreas.gov.

Information frequently changes, so you can search the site using keywords, such as "bartering."

The home page for BarterNet is http//barter.net.

BOOKS

Here is a list of six books that have proven valuable to many therapists over the years. This subjective selection does not reflect all tastes, but most therapists will find much of interest here:

1. Juhan, Deane. (2002). *Job's body: A handbook for bodyworkers.* Barrytown, NY: Station Hill Press.

2. Montagu, Ashley. (1971). *Touching: The human significance of the skin.* New York: Harper & Row.

3. Knaster, Mirka. (1996). *Discovering the body's sisdom.* New York: Bantam Books.

4. Tappan, Frances M. (2004). *Healing massage techniques: Holistic, classic, and emerging methods* (4th ed.). New York: Prentice Hall.

5. Thomas, Claire. (1995). *Bodywork: What type of massage to get—and how to make the most of it.* New York: William Morrow.

6. Kapit, Wyn, & Elson, Lawrence M. (2001). *The anatomy coloring book* (3rd ed.) New York: Benjamin Cummings.

These books and many of those that follow listed by category are available from http://www.amazon.com.

Spirituality/Healing

Krieger, Dolores. (1993). *Accepting your power to heal: The personal practice of therapeutic touch.* Santa Fe, NM: Bear & Company.

Thomas, Zach. (1994). *Healing touch: The church's forgotten language.* Louisville, KY: Westminster/John Knox Press.

Spas and Spa Therapy

Capellini, Steve. (1998). *The royal treatment: How you can take home the pleasures of the great luxury spas.* New York: Dell.

Miller, Erica. (1996). *Day spa operations.* Albany, NY: Milady Publishing.

Miller, Erica. (1996). *Day spa techniques.* Albany, NY: Milady Publishing.

Mother/Child

Sinclair, Marybetts. (1992). *Massage for healthier children.* Oakland, CA: Wingbow Press.

Stillerman, Elaine. (1992). *Mother massage: A handbook for relieving the discomforts of pregnancy.* New York: Bantam Doubleday Dell.

Waters, Bette. (2003). *Massage during pregnancy.* Deming, NM.

Self-Care for the Therapist

Butler, Sharon J. (1996). *Conquering carpal tunnel syndrome and other repetitive strain injuries.* Oakland, CA: New Harbinger.

Greene, Lauriann. (2000). *Save your hands: Injury prevention for massage therapists.* Seattle, WA: Gilded Age Press.

Sexual Abuse Issues

Ford, Clyde. (1999). *Compassionate touch.* Berkeley, CA: North Atlantic Books.

Herman, Judith L. (1997). *Trauma and recovery.* New York: Basic Books.

Katherine, Anne. (1993). *Boundaries: Where you end and I begin.* St. Louis: Fireside Parkside Books.

Business/Finances/Consulting

Battersby, Mark E. (1996). *SalonOvation's tax & financial primer.* Albany, NY: Milady Publishing.

Lant, Jeffery. (1991). *The consultants kit, establishing and operating your successful consulting business.* Cambridge, MA: JAB Publishing.

Laut, Phil. (1999). *Money is my friend.* New York: Ballantine Books.

Poynter, Dan. (2004). *The expert witness handbook.* Santa Barbara: Para Publishing.

Wilde, Stuart. (1995). *The trick to money is having some.* Carlsbad, CA: Hay House.

Walters, Dottie & Lillie. (1997). *Speak & grow rich.* New York: Prentice Hall.

Insurance/Medical Billing

Madison-Mahoney, Vivian. *Comprehensive guide to insurance billing for massage professionals.* Order at http://www.massageinsurancebilling.com.

Writing

Herman, Jeff. (2004). *Writer's guide to book editors, publishers, and literary agents.* New York Writer Inc.

Larsen, Michael. (1996). *Literary agents: What they do, how they do it, and how to find and work with the right one for you.* New York: John Wiley & Sons.

Poynter, Dan. (2003). *The self-publishing manual: How to write, print and sell your own book.* Santa Barbara: Para Publishing.

Writer's Market. (Published annually). Cincinnati, OH: Writer's Digest Books.

Medical Massage

Thompson, Diana L. (2002). *Hands heal, documentation for massage therapy, a guide to SOAP charting.* Lippencott, Williams and Williams.

Massage Training

Beck, Mark. (2006). *Theory and practice of therapeutic massage* (4th ed.). Clifton Park, NY: Thomson Delmar Learning.

Aromatherapy

Davis, Patricia. (2000). *Aromatherapy: An A to Z.* Essex, Great Britain: C. W. Daniel Co.

Lavabre, Marcel. (1997). *Aromatherapy workbook.* Rochester, VT: Healing Arts Press.

Rose, Jeanne. (1992). *The aromatherapy book.* Berkley, CA: North Atlantic Books.

Tisserand, Robert B. (1978). *The art of aromatherapy.* Rochester, VT: Healing Arts Press.

Worwood, Valerie Ann. (1991). *The complete book of essential oils and aromatherapy.* San Raphael, CA: New World Library.

Miscellaneous

Benjamin, Ben E. (1984). *Listen to your pain: The active person's guide to understanding, identifying, and treating pain and injury.* New York: Penguin Books.

Fernandez, Ernesto. (1998). *The healer's journey: Transforming your bodywork career*

through mentoring and supervision. Lutz, FL: Roldan-Bauta Press.

Scott, Mike. (2003). *Equine massage, muscle therapy.* Bolton, MA: Massageshill Muscles Therapy Productions.

BUSINESS TOOLS

Hemingway Publications
Phone (815) 877-5590
http://www.hemingwaypublications.com
Hemingway Productions offers a full line of
  brochures that you can use in your
  waiting room or as handouts for clients.
  Representative titles include *Your First
  Massage* and *Benefits of Therapeutic Massage.*
  Many other items are also available.

Information for People
Phone (800) 754-9790
http://www.info4people.com
Presentation videos, greeting cards, display
  cases, brochures, gift certificates, and post
  cards are all aimed at helping massage
  therapists increase their business.

WaterColors Printers
Phone (800) 804-2019
http://www.watercolorscards.com
WaterColors offers a full line of greeting
  cards, post cards, special occasion cards,
  and gift certificates with a massage theme.

Dr. Jeffery Lant
(780) 444-7477
http://www.worldprofit.com
Jeffery Lant publishes an extensive line of
  books and tapes to motivate people for
  success as consultants, speakers, writers,
  and more.

MAGAZINES

Massage magazine
Phone (800) 533-4263
http://www.massagemag.com
$26/year United States, $30/year
  Canada/Mexico, $47/year international

Massage Therapy Journal (quarterly
  publication of the AMTA)
Phone (877) 905-2700
http://www.amtamassage.org/journal/
  home.html
$25/year or $45/2 years United States,
  $70/year or $120/2 years international

Massage & Bodywork Quarterly (publication
  of the ABMP)
Phone (800) 458-2267
http://www.massageandbodywork.com
$26/year or $45/2 years United States

American Spa magazine
Phone (866) 344-1315
http://www.americanspamag.com
An excellent magazine for therapists
  thinking about going into the spa field.

ASSOCIATIONS

American Massage Therapy Association
  (AMTA)
Phone (877) 905-2700
http://www.amtamassage.org

Associated Bodywork & Massage
  Professionals (ABMP)
Phone (800) 458-2267
E-mail: expectmore@abmp.com
http://www.abmp.com

International Massage Association, Inc. (IMA)
Phone (540) 351-0800
http://www.imagroup.com
http://www.learnmassage.com

American Organization for Bodywork
    Therapies of Asia (AOBTA)
Phone (856) 782-1616
http://www.aobta.org
Members must graduate from a 500-hour
    program in one of the oriental bodywork
    traditions.

Florida State Massage Therapy Association
Phone (877) 376-8248
http://www.fsmta.org

New York State Society of Medical Massage
    Therapists
Phone (877) NYS-SMMT
http://www.nysmassage.org
Oldest massage association in country,
    founded in 1927.

SCHOOLS

The Touch Training Directory compiled by Associated Bodywork and Massage Professionals (ABMP) features hundreds of massage schools and bodywork training institutes. It can be viewed free of charge on line at http://www.massagetherapy.com/careers/training.php.

MASSAGE EQUIPMENT MANUFACTURERS

Comfort Craft
Phone (800) 858-2838
http://www.comfortcraft.com

Custom Craftworks
Phone (800) 627-2387
http://www.customcraftworks.com

Earthlite
Phone (800) 872-0560
http://www.earthlite.com

Golden Ratio Woodworks
Phone (800) 345-1129
http://www.goldenratiowoodworks.com

Living Earth Crafts
Phone (800) 358-8292
http://www.livingearthcrafts.com

Oakworks
Phone (800) 916-4613
http://www.oakworks.com

Pisces Productions
Phone (800) 822-5333
http://www.piscespro.com

Stronglite
Phone (800) 289-5487
http://www.stronglite.com

TouchAmerica
Phone (800) 678-6824
http://www.touchamerica.com

Ultra-Lite
Phone (800) 999-1971
http://www.ultralightcorp.com

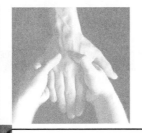

Appendix B
Advanced Trainings Chart

This chart provides information about specific courses, workshops, and advanced areas of study that are mentioned in this book. It is a quick reference guide and was created to provide you with an easy overview of some of the choices available.

If you are interested in . . .	Contact
Horses, and you feel an intuitive connection to them already, take the next step and become a horse massage therapist.	EquiTouch Systems http://www.equitouch.net (800) 483-0577
	Equissage http://www.equissage.com (800) 843-0224 Don Doran's Equine Sports Massage (352) 591-4735 http://www.equinesportsmassage.com
Providing massage services to people in public settings such as offices, airports, storefronts, and others, chair massage (or on-site massage, as it is sometimes called) may be the perfect addition to your practice.	TouchPro Chair Massage Workshops created by David Palmer (800) 999-5026 http://ww.touchpro.com
	Seated Massage Experience seminars Raymond Blaylock (888) 407-6287 http://www.mytouchresources.com

If you are interested in . . .	Contact
Plunging into the fast-growing spa world and you want to become an extremely knowledgeable therapist on the subject, contact Anne Bramham at the American Spa Therapy Education and Certification Council (ASTECC). She offers detailed instruction in all modalities, blending of treatments, business concerns, client specifics, creation of spa menus, and much more.	Anne Bramham ASTECC (888) 241-2095 http://www.asteccse.com
Learning how to care for newborns with specific massage techniques	International Loving Touch (503) 253-8482 www.lovingtouch.com
Becoming a trained professional labor assistant	Association of Labor Assistants & Childbirth Educators (888) 222-5223 http://www.alace.org E-mail: info@alace.org
How your touch can benefit women all through their pregnancies and into the delivery room	Elaine Stillerman Mother Massage (212) 533-3188 http://www.mothermassage.net
Becoming trained in the art of Japanese finger pressure massage, called Shiatsu, and other Asian modalities	American Organization for Bodywork Therapies of Asia (AOBTA) (856) 782-1616 http://www.aobta.org
Learning how to strengthen the internal organs and raise spiritual energy with the Taoist system originated by Mantak China	Healing Tao USA (888) 999-0555 http://www.healingtaousa.com
Helping relieve pain for people suffering from fibromyalgia	Richard VanWhy (306) 569-2077 http://www.fibrohugs.com
Helping older people with your massage services and your caring	Dietrich Miesler Daybreak Geriatric Massage Project http://www.daybreak-massage.com
Finding out more about how to help people in emergency situations with massage therapy	AMTA (877) 905-2700 http://www.amtamassage.org
Learning how bodywork done in the water can help free people in chronic pain, ease certain fears, and also feel incredible	Massage School at Harbin Hot Springs (707) 987-3801 E-mail: info@waba.edu http://www.waba.edu

If you are interested in . . .	Contact
Tapping into the pulsations of the craniosacral rhythm to help restore free-flowing energy and release from long-held pain and tension	Upledger Institute (800) 233-5880 http://www.upledger.com
Learning the ancient Chinese system that utilizes needles to stimulate points on the "meridians" or energy pathways of the body	http://www.healthwwweb.com/schools/oriental.htmp
How you can utilize elements of the ancient natural healing system from India	Ayurvedic Institute (505) 291-9698 http://www.ayurveda.com
Tuning the human instrument for ultimate performance (often, through not exclusively, for athletes and actors) through redefining an awareness of movement and habitual patterns	American Society for the Alexander Technique (AmSAT) (800) 473-0620 http://www.alexandertech.org
Improving the functionality of the human body through acute attention to the smallest details of movement, thus repatterning bad habits and creating greater awareness, lightness, and ease	Feldenkrais Educational Foundation of North America (866) 333-6248 http://www.feldenkrais.com
Using gentle rocking and other movements to create waves of pleasurable sensations and re-educate the body into a more effortless way of being	Trager International (250) 337-5556 United States Trager Association (440) 834-0308 www.trager.com
Understanding the body's relationship to gravity and how to repattern certain long-standing structural problems so that the body can move with more ease	Institute of Structural Integration (800) 530-8875 http://www.rolf.org Guild for Strutural Integration http://www.rolfguild.org
A softer form of Rolfing® that includes an integrated system of massage and lifestyle principles	Aston Enterprises (775) 831-8228 http://www.astonenterprises.com
Using connective tissue manipulation to rebalance the entire body	Hellerwork Structural Integration http://www.hellerwork.com
Developing skills in using a highly developed system of trigger point and deep-tissue therapy	St. John Neuromuscular Therapy (NMT) Seminars (888) 668-4325 http://www.stjohnseminars.com

If you are interested in . . .	Contact
Becoming proficient at releasing the hypersensitive points found in muscles	Bonnie Prudden Myotherapy (800) 221-4634 http://www.bonnieprudden.com
Balancing the human energy system through an understanding of the positive/negative currents flowing through us, to restore health and vibrancy	American Polarity Therapy Association (303) 545-2080 http://www.polaritytherapy.org
Developing an attunement to "universal life energy" and using it to help yourself and others	The Reiki Alliance (208) 783-3535 http://www.reikialliance.org
Passing healing energy to someone's bioenergetic field without the need to directly touch that person, with a system taught to thousands of health care professionals	Nurse Healers & Profesisonal Associates International (509) 693-3537 http://www.therapeutic-touch.org
Opening people up to their true selves through working with the emotions stored in muscles	The Rosen Method Center (510) 845-6606 http://www.rosenmethod.org
Combining intuitive awareness, gestalt therapy, movement-oriented bodywork, and gentle touch to release deep-seated "holding patterns" in people	The Rubenfeld Synergy Center (877) 776-2468 http://www.rubenfeldsynergy.com

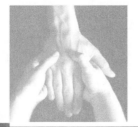

Index

ABMP. *See* Associated Bodywork & Massage Professionals (ABMP)
accreditation of massage schools, 44–46
acquaintances, as potential clients, 102–3
acupuncture, 290–91
ADAM Interactive Anatomy (CD), 196
advanced trainings, 281–88
    deep tissue/structural therapies, 285–86
    Eastern techniques, 287–88
    energy work, 283–85
    mind/body practices, 282–83
    movement-oriented bodywork, 286–87
advertising, 106, 258–59, 262
    See also marketing
AIDS and HIV, 66, 112–13
ALTAR factors, for choosing massage school, 44–46
American Massage Therapy Association (AMTA), 270–75
    code of ethics, 275
    liability insurance, 146, 274–75
    Massage Emergency Response Team, 118
    members, 12, 271
    See also Massage Therapy Foundation
anatomy CDs, 196
animal massage therapy, 292, 295–96
Applegate, Charlotte, 318–19
aromatherapy oils, 191
Associated Bodywork & Massage Professionals (ABMP), 276–78
    humanitarian massage, 289

liability insurance, 146, 277
members, 12
preprinted newsletters, 254
training institutions guide, 44
associations, professional, 268–80
athletes as clients, 108, 113–17
attire, 244, 247–48
attitude, positive, 34–35

baby boom generation, 13–14
back pain, 108
bartering, 102, 223–28
    See also fees; income
"becoming established" career stage, 29–31
Benjamin, Ben, 112
BestSpaJobs.com, 92
Bindi Body Oil, 192, 193
Biotone Dual Purpose Massage Creme, 192, 193
body mechanics, 230
Bodywork Emporium, 183, 289
Bodywork Research Institute, 301
BodyWorks (CD), 196
books
    on finances, 237
    resources, 280–81
    on speaking and consulting, 322
    on writing, 302–3, 307–8
Bottorf, Bob, 119–20
boundaries, establishing, 122–23, 124, 125
Brennan, Teresa, 170–71

brochures, 253, 254
budgets
    one-room massage office, 172–74
    two-room massage office, 174–75
    See also finances
Burke, Mike, 87
burnout, combating, 228–32
business cards, 253, 254, 258, 261
business contacts, as potential clients,
        102–3, 104
business management, 60, 133
business plans, 264–65
business stationery, 252, 253

cancer, 108, 121
candles, 177–78
career stages, 26–34
    becoming established, 29–31
    long-term success, 33–34
    mid-career crisis, 31–32
    neophyte, 26–29
Cayce, Edgar, 190, 193
Central Florida School of Massage
        Therapy, 246–47
certification
    continuing education providers,
        310, 311
    and licensing, 143
    national, 143–44
    and payment for massage, 101
    sports massage, 116–17
    See also licensing
chair massage, 68–70
chairs, massage, 186, 188, 189
Chesky, Eric, 96
chiropractic adjustments, 131
chiropractors, 67, 170–71
chronic fatigue syndrome, 121
Clean Again oil remover, 195
client information forms, 212
client records, 211–15
clients, 99–125
    and advertising, 106
    choosing, 230–31
    co-opting of, 97
    consultations and evaluations,
        107–8
    establishing boundaries, 122–23,
        124, 125
    feedback from, 96

getting referrals and introductions,
        105–6
    honoring requests and objections
        of, 132
    less-than-desirable, 27–28
    listening to, 123–24
    marketing to, 264
    potential, 100–105
    referring to other therapists, 229
    special cases, 107–22
    who become friends, 124–25
clinics, massage rooms in, 169, 171
club spas, 88–89
co-op advertising and marketing, 262
codependence, 130
commandments for beginning therapists,
        131–34
Commission on Massage Therapy
        Accreditation (COMTA), 44
competencies, 60–61
complementary and alternative medicine,
        15–17
*Comprehensive Guide to Insurance Billing for
        Massage Professionals* (Madison-
        Mahoney), 148–49
computers, 195–97, 209
    See also Internet; Web sites
COMTA (Commission on Massage Therapy
        Accreditation), 44
concierges, hotel, 74–75
conferences, 273–74
consulting, 317, 319–21, 322
continuing education
    benefiting from, 315
    in chair massage, 69
    to combat burnout, 232
    encouraging, 96
    importance of, 133
    and marketing, 261
    opportunities for, 17
    provider certification, 310, 311
    requirements for, 144–45
    on vacation, 233
    See also massage schools
conventions, 273–74
corporate headquarters, 70–71
cover letters, 248, 249
Cowan, Julia, 170–71
cruise ship spas, 86–87
crusader (personality type), 129

daily planners, 208–9
day spas, 85–86, 166–69, 210–11
Daybreak Geriatric Massage Project, 121
December (Winston), 179
deductions, tax, 151–55
deep tissue/structural therapies, 285–86
dental spas, 89
destination spas, 83–84
diagnoses, 132
disabilities, clients with, 109, 147
disaster victims and relief workers, 34,
        117–18, 119–20, 292, 295
discounts, 258, 263, 264
Discovering the Body's Wisdom (Knaster),
        304, 306
disfigurements, clients with, 109
distractions, 178–79
doctors' offices, 15–17, 68
draping techniques, 125
dream day scenario, 239–42
Dull, Harold, 296–98
dying people, as clients, 121–22

earning trap, 51–52
East West College, 55–58
Eastern techniques, 287–88
Edgar Cayce Aura Glow oil, 190, 193
educational goals, 48–50
elderly clients, 118, 120–21
Ellis, Susie, 89
emergencies, client, 125
emotionally needy clients, 109–10
employee status, 63–64
Endermologie, 300–301
energy work, 283–85
equipment
    linens, 189–90
    massage chairs, 186, 188, 189
    massage tables, 181–82, 185–86,
        187–88
    oil removers, 195
    oils and lotions, 190–93
    retailing, 183–85
Esalen Institute, 11, 160
establishment licenses, 64–65, 145–46
exercise, 229

family members
    helping them understand massage
    therapy, 316–17

as massage therapists, 316, 318–19
as potential clients, 101–2
Fanuzzi, John, 187–88
feedback, client, 96
fees
    and income, 222–23, 224
    increasing, 33
    and saving for vacation, 235
    setting, 215–20
    for terminated sessions, 36
    See also bartering; free massages;
    income
fellow victim (personality type), 130
female clients, and sexual issues,
        37–38
Fernandez, Ernesto J., 59–61
fibromyalgia, 121
finances, 233, 235–39
    See also budgets
floor plans
    massage room in salon environment,
        167–68
    one-room massage office, 173
    two-room massage office, 176
Florida
    insurance billing and reimbursement,
        148
    licensing and regulation, 141
Florida State Massage Therapy
        Association, 246, 261
flyers, 253, 254
forms
    client information forms, 212
    client record forms, 213, 214
    continuing education providership
    forms, 311
    SOAP forms, 214–15
free massages
    for advertising space, 258–59
    for family and friends, 101
    as marketing, 259
    and philanthropist personality type,
        129–30
    for referrals, 102, 104, 106
    volunteer massage work, 257
    See also fees
friends
    clients who become, 124–25
    and massage school choice, 50
    as potential clients, 101–2

gift certificates, 263–64
Glotsbach, Brian, 115–16, 117
God, massage as communication with,
    24–25
Golden Ratio Woodworks, Inc., 187–88
Green, Will, 278–79
groups, marketing to, 264

hand pain, 232
Harbin Hot Springs, 297
headache, 108
Healer's Journey, The (Fernandez), 59,
    60–61
Healing Touch (Thomas), 24
health, safeguarding, 133
Heart Aroused, The (Whyte), 50
heart conditions, 108
Hewton, Camille, 227
Hill, Napoleon, 237, 257
HIV/AIDS, 66, 112–13
hobbies, 231–32
home studios, 71–72, 159–61
horse massage, 296
*Hospital Based Massage Network
    Newsletter,* 66
hospital/hospice work, 65–66
hotel calls, 74–75
hotel/resort spas, 84–85
house calls, 73–74, 97
How to Write a Book Proposal (Larsen), 308
humanitarian massage, 288–89
Hurricane Andrew, 34, 117, 292, 295

identity crisis, 28
illnesses, 108, 121
IMA (International Massage Association),
    146, 278–80
IMSTAC. *See* International Massage &
    Somatic Therapies Accreditation
    Council (IMSTAC)
income
    in chiropractor's offices, 67
    goals, 257
    income expectation chart, 220–21
    in long-term success stage, 33
    as neophyte, 27, 28
    in spas, 82–83
    variations in, 221–23, 224
    while becoming established, 30
    See also bartering; fees

independent contractors, 63–64
infant massage, 292
Institute of Natural Healing Sciences,
    318–19
insurance
    billing and reimbursement, 147–50
    coverage of massage, 67
    liability, 146, 269, 274–75, 277
    offered by professional associations,
        269, 274–75, 277, 279
intention, 36, 37–38
International Massage & Somatic
    Therapies Accreditation Council
    (IMSTAC), 44, 277
    See also Associated Bodywork &
    Massage Professionals (ABMP)
International Massage Association (IMA),
    146, 278–80
International Massage Week, 289
International Spa Association (ISPA), 79
Internet, 196, 197, 255, 262
    See also Web sites
introductions, getting, 105–6
Island Software, 197
ISPA (International Spa Association), 79

Jesus, healing touch of, 23
Job's Body (Juhan), 135, 239–40
Jordan, Kate, 292
Juhan, Deane, 135, 239–40

"kidding around," sexual, 36–37
Knaster, Mirka, 304–7
know-it-all (personality type), 130–31
Krieger, Dolores, 299–300

Larsen, Michael, 308
late policy, 205
laundry, 235
Laut, Phil, 237
law, 120, 132
    See also certification; licensing; taxes;
    zoning
    learning trap, 51–52
    letterhead, 252, 253
    liability insurance, 146, 269,
        274–75, 277
    licensing
    and continuing education, 96
    establishment licenses, 64–65, 145–46

and massage schools, 45, 47
and payment for massage, 101
private practice in your home, 72
requirements, 134–35, 141–43
of salons, 64–65
state boards, 135–41
See also certification
lighting, 177–78
linens, 189–90, 235
listening to clients, 123–24
literary agents, 307, 308
logos, 248, 251–53
long-term success career stage, 33–34
lotions and oils, 190–93
LPG (company), 300–301

Madison-Mahoney, Vivian, 148–50
magazines, 281, 303, 307, 308
male therapists
    challenges for, 38–40
    sexual issues, 37–38, 39
managers of massage therapists, 94–97
Manipulate Your Future (Madison-
    Mahoney), 148
marketing, 259–64
    See also advertising; self-promotion
Martin, Noel, 183–85
Massage & Bodywork Quarterly, 44, 277,
    281
Massage Adventures, 251, 252
"Massage and Bodywork with Survivors of
    Abuse" (Benjamin), 112
Massage Book, The, 303
massage chairs, 186, 188, 189
Massage Company, 183–85
massage dollars, 263–64
Massage Emergency Response Team
    (MERT), 118
Massage Magazine, 44, 281
massage networks, 75
massage rooms
    in clinics, 169, 171
    in salons or day spas, 166–69
massage schools, 41–61
    accreditation, 44–46
    administration, 46
    business savvy, 57
    character and personality, 56–57
    facilities, 52
    faculty, 52–53

learning trap *versus* earning trap, 51–52
and licensing, 45, 47
location, 46, 50
mentors, 58–61
mission, 57–58
private, 47
quality of education and interaction, 56
reputation, 46
researching, 41–47, 55–58
setting educational goals, 48–50
size, 55–58
standards, 53–55
teaching in, 312–16
as transformational experience, 48
tuition, 46
See also continuing education
massage tables, 181–82, 185–86,
    187–88
massage therapists
    bonding with other, 133–34
    personality types, 129–31
    physical limits of, 31, 32
    talking about other, 132–33
    traits, 20–21
massage therapy
    demand for, 13–14
    development of, 10–12
    growth rate, 12–13
    number of adults receiving, 9–10, 13
    opportunities in, 17–18
    psychology of, 21–22
    versus psychotherapy, 123–24
    receiving, 134, 230
    trading, 227
    Web sites, 255
    See also touch
Massage Therapy Foundation, 272,
    274, 289
    See also American Massage Therapy
    Association (AMTA)
Massage Therapy Journal, 43–44, 112,
    275, 281
Mathenia, Kara, 90
McGillicuddy, Michael, 245–47
medical/dental spas, 68, 89
medical massage technology, 300–301
meditation, 163–65
Meisler, Dietrich, 121
memories, somatic, 22
mentors, 58–61

MERT (Massage Emergency Response Team), 118
mid-career crisis career stage, 31–32
mind/body practices, 282–83
Moll, Edie, 56–58
Money is my Friend (Laut), 237
monthly planners, 206–7
MotherMassage, 293–95
movement-oriented bodywork, 286–87
moving into other professions, 290–91, 299–301
muscle aches and pains, 32, 108
muscular dystrophy, 121
music, 178–80, 232

National Center for Complementary and Alternative Medicine, 66
National Certification Board for Therapeutic Massage and Bodywork (NCBTMB), 56, 143–44, 310, 311
National Certification Exam, 12–13, 45, 144
National Massage Therapy Awareness Week, 274
National Speakers' Association, 322
nature, reconnecting with, 229, 231, 234, 235
NCBTMB (National Certification Board for Therapeutic Massage and Bodywork), 56, 143–44, 310, 311
neophyte career stage, 26–29
nervous disorders, 108
networking, 104–5, 261, 264
New Age movement, 160
newsletters, 254, 281
Newton, Don, 56
nightmare day scenario, 202–4
nudity, 122–23, 125
nursing, 299–300
nutritional advice, 132

obese clients, 110–11
off-menu service items, 263
offices, massage, 72–73, 161, 162, 169, 171–77
oil holsters, 193
oil removers, 195
oils and lotions, 190–93
Oklahoma City bombing, 34, 118, 119–20

Olympic Games, 113, 114, 115–16
on-site massage, 68–70
open house, 263

Pacific College of Oriental Medicine, 290, 291
pain, 32, 99–100, 108, 232
Palmer, David, 68–69
Paper Direct, 253
Paralympics, 113
personal injury cases, 149
philanthropist (personality type), 129–30
photographs, 253–54
Playboy, 271
Porr, Ellen, 234–35
positive attitude, 34–35
postsurgery clients, 108
Poynter, Dan, 308, 321
pregnancy massage, 108, 289, 292, 293–95
press kits, 254, 256, 262, 319–20
private house calls, 73–74, 97
private practice
    incorporating spa services, 89–91
    in separate studio, 72–73
    in your home, 71–72
products, selling, 183–85, 313
professional associations, 268–80
professional image, creating, 243–65
    advertising, 258–59
    business plans, 264–65
    image enhancers, 244–56
    marketing, 259–64
    promotion with heart, 256, 258
promotion. *See* self-promotion
prostitution, 135, 142
psychiatric disorders, 108
psychotherapy, 123–24

radio shows, appearing on, 104
Rasmusson, Doug, 191
records, client, 211–15
Red Cross, 34, 117, 118
referrals, 102, 104, 105–6, 107, 229
religion, 11, 23–24
    See also spirituality
research, 65–66, 301–2
    See also Touch Research Institute
resort/hotel spas, 84–85

resources, 268–81
    books, 280–81
    magazines, 281
    newsletters, 281
    professional associations, 268–80
résumés, 248, 250
retailing, 183–85
retirement funds, 238–39

safety concerns, 147
Safety Harbor Spa, 76–77
salons, 64–65, 166–69
Sasso, Valerie, 210–11
saving money, 235, 236, 238–39
scheduling. *See* time management
seasonal promotions, 263
self-promotion
    as competency, 60
    as consultant, 319–20
    with heart, 256, 258
    in long-term success stage, 33
    with potential clients, 103–5
self-publishing, 308
selling massage products, 182–85, 313
seniority system, 95–96
serotonin, 66, 112
session notes, 213, 214
sexual abuse survivors, 111–12
sexual issues, 35–38, 39, 75
sheets, 189–90, 235
shyness, 104–5
skin conditions, 108
SOAP forms, 214–15
Social Security, 239
Solien-Wolfe, Lynda, 260–62
sores, 108
spa industry, 76–92
    beyond pampering, 79–81
    changes in, 76–77
    club spas, 88–89
    cruise ship spas, 86–87
    day spas, 85–86
    destination spas, 83–84
    employers, 83–91
    growth of, 77, 79
    medical/dental spas, 68, 89
    opportunities in, 91–92
    private practice incorporating spa
        services, 89–91
    profit sharing, 82–83

resort/hotel spas, 84–85
    Web sites, 87, 92
space, creating the perfect, 157–95
    christening with meditation, 163–65
    equipment, 181–82, 185–90,
        192–93, 195
    general guidelines, 157–58
    lighting, 177–78
    location, 158–62
    music, 178–80
    one-room massage office, 172–74
    setting up, 163, 165–77
    temperature, 194
    two-room massage office, 174–77
spine pain, 108
spirituality, 23–26, 24–25, 50
    See also religion
sports massage, 108, 113–17
state boards of massage therapy, 135–41
Stillerman, Elaine, 293–95
stress management, 108, 320–21
studios, massage, 72–73, 161, 162, 169,
    171–77
success guidelines, 257
supervisors of massage therapists, 94–97

tables, massage, 181–82, 185–86,
    187–88
talk radio shows, appearing on, 104
taxes, 150–55, 225–26
teaching
    in long-term success stage, 33
    as marketing, 263
    in massage schools, 312–16
    workshops and seminars, 308–12
temperature, 194
10 commandments for beginning
    therapists, 131–34
terminally ill clients, 121–22
test massages, 92–94
Therapeutic Touch, 299–300
Thermophore heating element, 189, 194
Think and Grow Rich (Hill), 237, 257
third-party billing, 147–50
Thomas, Zach, 23–24, 26
time management, 204–11
    and burnout, 230
    computerizing, 209
    daily planners, 208–9
    in day spas, 210–11

keys to, 205–6
monthly planners, 206–7
weekly planners, 207–8
See also computers
tipping, 75, 82
tiredness, 108
touch
power of, 127–28
psychology of, 21–22
spirituality of, 23–26
taboos against, 11, 22
See also massage
Touch Foundation, 289
Touch Research Institute
cost-effectiveness of touch
therapies, 148
elderly people study, 118, 120
HIV study, 112
infant massage studies, 292
research, 65–66, 301–2
Touch Training Directory, The, 44, 277
TouchAmerica, 313
towels, 190, 235
trading massages, 227
training. *See* advanced trainings;
continuing education; massage
schools
Trick to Money Is Having Some, The
(Wilde), 237

Ulrich, Dan, 141–42
undercapitalization, 163
University of Miami Medical School Touch
Research Institute. *See* Touch
Research Institute
Upledger Institute, 260

vacations, 30, 231, 232–33, 234–35
Van Why, Richard, 301
Vermont, licensing not required in, 101,
134–35
Vladimir, Andrea, 290–91
volunteering, 34, 257, 261
See also free massages

Washington State insurance billing and
reimbursement, 149
water, drinking, 229
water shiatsu (Watsu), 296–98
Web sites, 87, 92, 255
See also Internet
weekly planners, 207–8
Whole Life Expo, 183, 187
Whyte, David, 50
Wilde, Stuart, 237
Windjammer Barefoot Cruises, 87
Winston, George, 179
word of mouth, 258
work hours, 125
See also time management
workers' compensation, 148, 149
workspace, 63–97
chiropractors, 67
corporate headquarters, 70–71
doctors' offices, 68
hospital/hospice work, 65–66
hotel calls, 74–75
independent contractor *versus*
employee status, 63–64
massage networks, 75
on-site massage, 68–70
private house calls, 73–74, 97
private practice in separate studio,
72–73
private practice in your home, 71–72
salons, 64–65
spa industry, 76–92
test massages, 92–94
tips for managers, 94–97
Worldwide Aquatic Bodywork
Association, 298
wounds, 108
wrist pain, 232
writing, 103–4, 259, 302–8

zoning regulations, 71–72, 145